Bristol-Myers Squibb/Zimmer Orthopaedic Symposium

Biological, Material, and Mechanical Considerations of Joint Replacement

Bristol-Myers Squibb/Zimmer Orthopaedic Symposium Series

Biological, Material, and Mechanical Considerations of Joint Replacement

Editor

Bernard F. Morrey, M.D.
Professor and Chairman
Department of Orthopaedics
Mayo Clinic
Rochester, Minnesota

Raven Press ● New York

Raven Press, Ltd., 1185 Avenue of the Americas, New York, New York 10036

Made in the United States of America

Library of Congress Cataloging-in-Publication Data
Biological, material, and mechanical considerations of joint replacement /
   editor, Bernard F. Morrey.
       p.   cm. — (Bristol-Myers Squibb/Zimmer Orthopaedic Symposium
series)
   Includes bibliographical references and index.
   ISBN 0-7817-0008-6
   1. Artificial joints—Congresses.   I. Morrey, Bernard F., 1943–
   II. Title.   III. Series.
   [DNLM: 1. Joint Prosthesis—congresses.   WE 312 B615 1993]
   RD686.B56   1993
   617.5′8059—dc20
   DNLM/DLC
   for Library of Congress   93-20466
                                                                   CIP

9   8   7   6   5   4   3   2   1

Contents

*Figures 2B–E, 3C, 4A–D appear in color following p. 138.

New Approaches: Clinical and Basic Research

Closing Summaries and Future Directions

Contributing Authors

T. Albrektsson, M.D., Ph.D. *Department of Handicap Research, University of Gothenburg, Brunnsgatan 2, S-413 12 Gothenburg, Sweden*

James M. Anderson, M.D., Ph.D. *Institute of Pathology, Case Western Reserve University School of Medicine, 10900 Euclid Avenue, Cleveland, Ohio 44106-4907*

Donald L. Bartel, Ph.D. *Department of Mechanical and Aerospace Engineering, Cornell University, 219 Upson Hall, Ithaca, New York 14853*

Jonathan Black, Ph.D. *Department of Bioengineering, Clemson University, 301 Rhodes Engineering Research Center, Clemson, South Carolina 29634-0905*

Gordon Blunn, Ph.D. *Department of Biomedical Engineering, University College London, Royal National Orthopaedic Hospital, Brockley Hill, Stanmore, Middlesex HA 74LP, United Kingdom*

J. D. Bobyn, Ph.D. *Jo Miller Orthopaedic Research Laboratory, Montreal General Hospital, McGill University, 1650 Cedar Avenue, Room LS1, 409 Livingston Hall, Montreal, Quebec, Canada H3G 1A4*

Mark E. Bolander, M.D. *Department of Orthopaedics, Mayo Clinic, 200 First Street Southwest, Rochester, Minnesota 55905*

Barbara D. Boyan, Ph.D. *Department of Orthopaedics, University of Texas Health Science Center at San Antonio, 7703 Floyd Curl Drive, San Antonio, Texas 78284-7774*

Charles Bragdon, B.S. *Orthopaedic Biomechanics Laboratory, Massachusetts General Hospital, 15 Parkman Street, Boston, Massachusetts 02114*

Bryan Brooks, B.S. *Department of Orthopaedics, University of Texas Health Science Center at San Antonio, 7703 Floyd Curl Drive, San Antonio, Texas 78284-7774*

Stanley A. Brown, Ph.D. *Department of Biomedical Engineering, Case Western Reserve University, Cleveland, Ohio 44106-7207*

Gottfried H. Buchhorn, M.D. *Orthopaedic Department, University Hospital of Goettingen, Robert Koch Strasse 40, D-3400 Goettingen, Germany*

L. V. Carlsson, M.D., Ph.D. *Departments of Handicap Research and Orthopaedic Surgery, University of Gothenburg, Brunnsgatan 2, S-413 12 Gothenburg, Sweden*

Jungi Chiba, M.D. *Institute of Rheumatology, Tokyo Women's Medical College, KS BLD, 9-12 Wakamatsu-cho, Shinjuku-ku, Tokyo 162, Japan*

Pascal Christel, M.D., Ph.D. *Department of Orthopaedic Surgery, Lariboisière Saint-Louis Medical School, University Paris 7, 10 Avenue de Verdun, F-75010 Paris, France*

John P. Collier, D.E. *Dartmouth Biomedical Engineering Center, Dartmouth College, Hanover, New Hampshire 03755*

Richard Coutts, M.D. *7920 Frost Street, #200, San Diego, California 92123*

Roy D. Crowninshield, Ph.D. *Zimmer, Inc., P.O. Box 708, Warsaw, Indiana 46581-0708*

J. E. Davies, Ph.D. *Centre for Biomaterials, University of Toronto, 124 Edward Street, Toronto, Ontario, Canada M5S 1A1*

A. R. Dujovne, Ing., M.Sc. *Jo Miller Orthopaedic Research Laboratory, Montreal General Hospital, McGill University, 1650 Cedar Avenue, Room LS1, 409 Livingston Hall, Montreal, Quebec, Canada H3G 1A4*

C. Anderson Engh, Jr., M.D. *Anderson Orthopaedic Research Institute, 2445 Army Navy Drive, Arlington, Virginia 22206*

Charles A. Engh, M.D. *Anderson Orthopaedic Research Institute, 2445 Army Navy Drive, Arlington, Virginia 22206*

Jorge O. Galante, M.D., D.Sc. *Department of Orthopedic Surgery, Rush-Presbyterian-St. Luke's Medical Center, 1653 West Congress Parkway, Chicago, Illinois 60612*

Steven R. Goldring, M.D. *Department of Medicine, Harvard Medical School, Medical Services (Arthritis Unit), Massachusetts General Hospital, Boston, Massachusetts 02114 and Department of Medicine, New England Deaconess Hospital, Boston, Massachusetts 02215*

Stephen L. Gordon, Ph.D. *Musculoskeletal Diseases Branch, National Institute of Arthritis and Musculoskeletal and Skin Diseases, National Institutes of Health, Westwood Boulevard, Room 407, Bethesda, Maryland 20814*

Jeffrey Hambleton, D.D.S. *Wilford Hall Medical Center (USAF), Lackland Air Force Base, Lackland, Texas 78236*

Amy Hanson, B.S. *Orthopaedic Biomechanics Laboratory, Massachusetts General Hospital, 15 Parkman Street, Boston, Massachusetts 02114*

William H. Harris, M.D. *Hip and Implant Unit, Massachusetts General Hospital, 15 Parkman Street, Boston, Massachusetts 02114 and Department of Orthopaedics, Harvard Medical School, Boston, Massachusetts 02114*

Arne Hensten-Pettersen, Ph.D. *NIOM, Scandinavian Institute of Dental Materials, Kirkeveien 71B, N-1344 Haslum, Norway*

Donald W. Howie, Ph.D., M.B.B.S., F.R.A.C.S. *Department of Orthopaedic Surgery and Trauma, University of Adelaide, Department of Orthopaedic Surgery and Trauma, Royal Adelaide Hospital, North Terrace, Adelaide 5000, South Australia*

Michael H. Huo, M.D.   *Joint Replacement Center, Waterbury Hospital, 1201 West Main Street, Waterbury, Connecticut 06708*

Joshua J. Jacobs, M.D.   *Department of Orthopedic Surgery, Rush-Presbyterian-St. Luke's Medical Center, 1653 West Congress Parkway, Chicago, Illinois 60612*

M. Jacobsson, M.D., Ph.D.   *Department of Handicap Research, University of Gothenburg, Brunnsgatan 2, S-413 12 Gothenburg, Sweden*

Murali Jasty, M.D.   *Orthopaedic Biomechanics Laboratory, Massachusetts General Hospital, 15 Parkman Street, Boston, Massachusetts 02114*

Kathleen Kidd   *Dartmouth Biomedical Engineering Center, Dartmouth College, Hanover, New Hampshire 03755*

Kang Jung Kim, M.D.   *Institute of Rheumatology, Tokyo Women's Medical College, KS BLD, 9-12 Wakamatsu-cho, Shinjuku-ku, Tokyo 162, Japan*

Stefan Kreuzer, M.S.   *Department of Orthopaedics, University of Texas Health Science Center at San Antonio, 7703 Floyd Curl Drive, San Antonio, Texas 78284-7774*

J. J. Krygier, C.E.T.   *Jo Miller Orthopaedic Research Laboratory, Montreal General Hospital, McGill University, 1650 Cedar Avenue, Room LS1, 409 Livingston Hall, Montreal, Quebec, Canada H3G 1A4*

Louis M. Kwong, M.D.   *Harbor-UCLA Medical Center, 1000 West Carson Street, Torrance, California 90509*

J. M. Lee, Ph.D.   *Centre for Biomaterials, University of Toronto, 124 Edward Street, Toronto, Ontario, Canada M5S 1A1*

Kyla Lee, Ph.D.   *Orthopaedic Biomechanics Laboratory, Massachusetts General Hospital, 15 Parkman Street, Boston, Massachusetts 02114*

Jack E. Lemons, Ph.D.   *Laboratory Research, Division of Orthopaedic Surgery, Departments of Surgery and Biomaterials, University of Alabama at Birmingham, 509 Medical Education Building, 1813 Sixth Avenue South, UAB Station, Birmingham, Alabama 35294-3295*

Monica Luna   *Department of Orthopaedics, University of Texas Health Science Center at San Antonio, 7703 Floyd Curl Drive, San Antonio, Texas 78284-7774*

Grace E. Macalino, M.P.H.   *Anderson Orthopaedic Research Institute, 2445 Army Navy Drive, Arlington, Virginia 22206*

W. Macdonald, M. Phil., C.P.Eng.   *Department of Handicap Research, University of Gothenburg, Brunnsgatan 2, S-413-12 Gothenburg, Sweden and King's College Hospital, Markhill, Camberwell, London SE5 9RS, United Kingdom*

Archie J. Malcolm, F.R.C.Path., M.D.   *University Department of Pathology, Royal Victoria Infirmary, Queen Victoria Road, Newcastle-upon-Tyne NE1 4LP, United Kingdom*

William J. Maloney, M.D.   *Palo Alto Medical Clinic, 300 Home Avenue, Palo Alto, California 94301-2794*

Donald E. Marlowe, M.S.E. *Center for Devices and Radiological Health, U.S. Food and Drug Administration, 12200 Wilkins Avenue, Rockville, Maryland 20852*

Michael B. Mayor, M.D. *Dartmouth Biomedical Engineering Center, Dartmouth College, Hanover, New Hampshire 03755*

Thomas F. McGovern, M.S. *Anderson Orthopaedic Research Institute, 2445 Army Navy Drive, Arlington, Virginia 22206*

Mark N. Melkerson, M.S. *Orthopedic Branch, Division of General and Restorative Devices, Office of Device Evaluation, Center for Devices and Radiological Health, U.S. Food and Drug Administration, HFZ-410, 1390 Piccard Drive, Rockville, Maryland 20850*

Katharine Merritt, Ph.D. *Department of Biomedical Engineering, Case Western Reserve University, Cleveland, Ohio 44106-7207*

Nirmal K. Mishra, Ph.D. *Orthopedic Branch, Division of General and Restorative Devices, Office of Device Evaluation, Center for Devices and Radiological Health, U.S. Food and Drug Administration, HFZ-410, 1390 Piccard Drive, Rockville, Maryland 20850*

Bernard F. Morrey, M.D. *Department of Orthopaedics, Mayo Clinic, 200 First Street Southwest, Rochester, Minnesota 55905*

David H. Mueller, M.S. *Medtronic, Inc., 7000 Central Avenue Northeast, Minneapolis, Minnesota 55432*

Jack E. Parr, Ph.D. *Zimmer, Inc., P.O. Box 708, Warsaw, Indiana 46581-0708*

R. M. Pilliar, Ph.D. *Centre for Biomaterials, University of Toronto, 124 Edward Street, Toronto, Ontario, Canada M5S 1A1*

Clare M. Rimnac, Ph.D. *Department of Biomechanics, The Hospital for Special Surgery, 535 East 70th Street, New York, New York 10021*

Michael G. Rock, M.D. *Department of Orthopaedics, Mayo Clinic, 200 First Street Southwest, Rochester, Minnesota 55905*

Harry E. Rubash, M.D. *Department of Orthopaedic Surgery, University of Pittsburgh, 3601 Fifth Avenue, Pittsburgh, Pennsylvania 15213*

Eduardo A. Salvati, M.D. *Hip and Knee Service, The Hospital for Special Surgery, 535 East 70th Street, New York, New York 10021 and Cornell University Medical College, New York, New York 10021*

Thomas P. Schmalzried, M.D. *Harbor-UCLA Medical Center, 1000 West Carson Street, Torrance, California 90509 and Joint Replacement Institute, 2400 South Flower Street, Los Angeles, California 90007*

Zvi Schwartz, D.M.D., Ph.D. *Department of Orthopaedics, University of Texas Health Science Center at San Antonio, 7703 Floyd Curl Drive, San Antonio, Texas 78284-7774 and Hebrew University Hadassah Faculty of Dental Medicine, P.O. Box 1172, Jerusalem 91-010, Israel*

Jona Sela, D.D.S. *Department of Orthopaedics, University of Texas Health Science Center at San Antonio, 7703 Floyd Curl Drive, San Antonio, Texas 78284-7774 and Hebrew University Hadassah Faculty of Dental Medicine, P.O. Box 1172, Jerusalem 91-010, Israel*

Manfred Semlitsch, Ph.D. *Sulzer Medical Technology, Ltd., CH-8401 Winterthur, Switzerland*

Dale R. Sumner, Ph.D. *Department of Orthopedic Surgery, Rush-Presbyterian-St. Luke's Medical Center, 1653 West Congress Parkway, Chicago, Illinois 60612*

Helene P. Suprenant *Dartmouth Biomedical Engineering Center, Dartmouth College, Hanover, New Hampshire 03755*

Russell T. Turner, Ph.D. *Department of Orthopaedics, Mayo Clinic, 200 First Street Southwest, Rochester, Minnesota 55905*

Robert M. Urban *Department of Orthopedic Surgery, Rush-Presbyterian-St. Luke's Medical Center, 1653 West Congress Parkway, Chicago, Illinois 60612*

Peter S. Walker, Ph.D. *Department of Biomedical Engineering, University College London, Royal National Orthopaedic Hospital, Brockley Hill, Stanmore, Middlesex HA 74LP, United Kingdom*

Jeng-Tzung Wang, M.D. *Department of Medicine, Harvard Medical School, Medical Services (Arthritis Unit), Massachusetts General Hospital, Boston, Massachusetts 02114 and Harvard School of Dental Medicine, Boston, Massachusetts 02215*

John E. Wennberg, M.D. *Center for the Evaluative Clinical Sciences, Dartmouth Medical School, Hanover, New Hampshire 03755*

Leo A. Whiteside, M.D. *Department of Orthopaedic Surgery, DePaul Biomechanical Research Laboratory, DePaul Community Health Center, Missouri Bone and Joint Center, 3165 McKelvey Road, Suite 240, Bridgeton, Missouri 63044*

Hans-Georg Willert, M.D. *Orthopaedic Department, University Hospital of Goettingen, Robert Koch Strasse 40, D-3400 Goettingen, Germany*

Ian R. Williams, B.A. *Dartmouth Biomedical Engineering Center, Dartmouth College, Hanover, New Hampshire 03755*

Halina Witkiewicz, Ph.D. *Department of Orthopaedics, Mayo Clinic, 200 First Street Southwest, Rochester, Minnesota 55905*

Timothy M. Wright, Ph.D. *Department of Biomechanics, The Hospital for Special Surgery, 535 East 70th Street, New York, New York 10021*

Martin A. Yahiro, M.D. *Orthopedic Branch, Division of General and Restorative Devices, Office of Device Evaluation, Center for Devices and Radiological Health, U.S. Food and Drug Administration, HFZ-410, 1390 Piccard Drive, Rockville, Maryland 20850*

D. L. Young, B.Eng. *Jo Miller Orthopaedic Research Laboratory, Montreal General Hospital, McGill University, 1650 Cedar Avenue, Room LS1, 409 Livingston Hall, Montreal, Quebec, Canada H3G 1A4*

Foreword

The generally high rate of orthopaedic implant success is the result of the cross-fertilization of skills and knowledge between surgeons and researchers and device manufacturers. This applies to the surgical process, as well as to the design and application of these devices.

During the seventh annual Bristol-Myers Squibb/Zimmer Orthopaedic Research Symposium, clinical, scientific, and regulatory experts devoted attention to biological materials, mechanical responses, and product design of orthopaedic implants.

The symposium, "Biological, Material, and Mechanical Considerations of Joint Replacement: Current Concepts and Future Directions," was chaired by Bernard F. Morrey, M.D., of the Mayo Clinic in cooperation with the American Academy of Orthopaedic Surgeons' Council on Research and Scientific Affairs, the American Society for Biomaterials, and the American Orthopaedic Society.

Annual symposia are a part of our support for orthopaedic research. Since 1983, Bristol-Myers Squibb and its Zimmer subsidiary have contributed more than $3.75 million in orthopaedic research through the Orthopaedic Research and Education Foundation. Since 1988, we have presented the annual Bristol-Myers Squibb/Zimmer Award for Distinguished Achievement in Orthopaedic Research, a peer-judged prize of $50,000 given to a researcher who has made outstanding contributions to the field of orthopaedic research.

We hope these proceedings will lead to a greater understanding of the importance of a multidisciplinary approach to the development of improved orthopaedic implants.

RICHARD L. GELB
CHAIRMAN AND CHIEF EXECUTIVE OFFICER
BRISTOL-MYERS SQUIBB COMPANY

Editor's Foreword

Today's science of biomaterials is in large measure reflected by the history of orthopaedic total joint replacement. As a result of the evolution of biomaterials, there are more accepted international standards for orthopaedic biomaterials and product designs than for any other medical implants.

Very early attempts at replacing or resurfacing joints were fraught with material or design problems. Sir John Charnley, the father of modern total joint replacement, experienced biomaterial wear phenomena in his early patients in the 1960s, which were unpredicted by extensive preclinical testing. Although these early difficulties were rapidly overcome, biocompatibility still remains of interest for modern-day devices that will become long-term implants in the human body.

The symposium, chaired by Bernard F. Morrey, M.D., Chairman and Professor of the Department of Orthopaedics at the Mayo Clinic, dealt with this very timely subject of total joint implant biocompatibility. Dr. Morrey and his associates created an excellent forum of world experts to examine the topic of biomaterials from a multidisciplinary approach focusing particularly on biomaterials research, orthopaedic surgery, and medical device legislation. This free and open discussion of key issues led to recommendations from each field of expertise on the future application of biomaterials and designs for use in orthopaedic total joint replacement.

ROBERT L. FUSON, M.D.
SERIES EDITOR

Preface

Despite the incredible impact that joint replacement arthroplasty has had on patients suffering from arthritic conditions and on the orthopedic profession, significant issues and questions remain. As a matter of fact, few of the innovations and changes from the original Charnley design have been shown to have any real value. This has given rise to the well-recognized dictum that change and progress are not synonymous.

Numerous reports have emerged that have critically analyzed joint replacement arthroplasty from three perspectives: clinical outcome, basic research from the material scientist and biomechanician, and in recent years, investigative research of the biologist.

The specific goal and focus of the symposium documented in this volume are first to integrate the disciplines of clinical investigation, material and biomechanical insights, and biological techniques to address the pressing questions regarding joint replacement arthroplasty. With the integration of these three disciplines, three specific goals or questions are addressed: (i) What is the standard and accepted knowledge base of these three areas of expertise at this moment in time? (ii) How can the information and insights of the three disciplines be integrated and interpreted? (iii) Based on a recognition of the depth of information and its integration and interpretation, what can be told about future directions from a clinical practice and basic investigative perspective?

In addition to these scientific questions, regulatory aspects of joint replacement are assuming increased significance and exploration.

The specific format of the symposium and this volume consists of several chapters defining the clinical, material, biomechanical, and biological perspectives of the various components of joint replacement arthroplasty. A discussion of experts involved in these areas then summarizes the topic at the conclusion of each section.

In this context, the book is organized according to the following: (i) keynote addresses introduce each of the three areas of investigation; (ii) the cement interface, ultrahigh molecular weight polyethylene, metal debris, and the interface of uncemented devices are discussed; (iii) the current concerns with respect to the articulation and wear debris are then discussed; (iv) a thorough discussion on adverse and toxic effects of the implants or their component part follows; (v) manufacturing, funding, and regulatory issues are then addressed; (vi) brief closing remarks concisely summarize the essence of the symposium and the material presented in this volume.

The discrete intent of this volume is to provide a benchmark to both the orthopedic surgeon and the scientist of the status of joint replacement at this time. It is hoped this can serve as a reference document for these disciplines and provide a direction for fruitful investigations in the future.

BERNARD F. MORREY, M.D.

Acknowledgments

I would specifically like to express my most sincere appreciation to the Bristol-Myers Squibb/Zimmer Company for its most generous grant that allowed the development and execution of this symposium.

This symposium topic and program were endorsed by the American Academy of Orthopaedic Surgeons' Council on Research and Scientific Affairs, the American Orthopaedic Society, and the American Society for Biomaterials.

Bristol-Myers Squibb/Zimmer Orthopaedic Symposium

Biological, Material, and Mechanical Considerations of Joint Replacement

Biological, Material, and Mechanical
Considerations of Joint Replacement,
edited by B. F. Morrey.
Raven Press, Ltd., New York © 1993.

1

Keynote Address: Clinical Considerations

William H. Harris

Hip and Implant Unit, Massachusetts General Hospital, Department of Orthopaedics,
Harvard Medical School, Boston, Massachusetts 02114

It has been said that success has a thousand fathers. Failure is an orphan. Among the many remarkable things about total joint replacement is the fact that in total joint replacement almost the opposite of that statement is true. For most patients, over long periods of time, the uniformity and quality of success are so high and so common that success is the norm, the expected, the routine. The failures are dissected, analyzed, and reported. In general, it is the concerted effort to understand and eliminate the failures that has driven the field for the past 30+ years.

It is particularly enlightening to consider the changing sequence and changing understanding of what has been perceived as the number one mechanism of failure of total joint replacement during this period of time. I will use total hip replacement as my source of examples, simply because the clarity of the illustration is so vivid in the development of total hip replacements.

IMPLANT FAILURE: A HISTORICAL PERSPECTIVE

Lysis

Beginning with the polytetrafluorethylene experience, which started in 1959, the number one problem in total joint replacement of that day was, interestingly enough, bone lysis secondary to granuloma formation. Those terms were not used. The role of the macrophage was only vaguely perceived. Cytokines were unknown. Nevertheless, the first, dominant problem of total joint replacement was lysis secondary to granuloma formation caused by particulate debris.

With the serendipitous introduction of ultrahigh molecular weight polyethylene 30 years ago, the problem of lysis disappeared, or, at least, it went into hiding.

Sepsis

The next number one problem was that of sepsis. Because of a series of environmental circumstances and the decision against the use of prophylactic antibiotics, Charnley's initial rate of sepsis was 8.9% (3). The first series of total hip replacements done in this country carried a 13% sepsis rate (24). By a combination of both ordinary and extraordinary means, the problem of sepsis has been vanquished, or nearly so. Contemporary sepsis rates are well under 1% (13,14,19). The extraordinary means involved Charnley's efforts in creating a new field in operating-room environmental control including laminar flow, body exhaust systems, plus the added feature of the use of prophylactic antibiotics.

Loosening

The third issue to emerge as the dominant problem was that of loosening. In total hip replacement, this meant loosening on the acetabular side and loosening on the femoral side. And it was, indeed, loosening coupled with the reemergence of lysis that led to the decade of the eighties being termed the decade of "cement versus cementless." The erroneous concept of that day was that cement caused the lysis.

It was, of course, a gross misunderstanding to call the lytic process "cement disease," but the concept of that time was that eliminating the cement would eliminate the lysis. This idea was coupled with the belief that bony ingrowth would provide a better, and biologic, form of fixation.

Another of the important misconceptions of the early years of total hip replacement was the belief that loosening represented a single or common process. Conversely, one of the most important observations among the recent explosion in basic research in total hip replacement has been our demonstration that the initiating mechanism of failure of fixation of cemented *femoral* components (15) is exactly the opposite mechanism of that for cemented *acetabular* components (18).

Based primarily on radiographic findings and observations made at revision surgery, the common belief existed that failure of fixation of cemented femoral components was identical in nature to that of cemented acetabular components and originated at the cement-bone interface. This widely held concept is completely false.

Basic information about the originating event in failure of fixation cannot be discerned from radiographs. They are too coarse and too late in the process. Nor can it come from surgically retrieved specimens. They are too coarse, too late in the process, and too many other secondary events have taken place. Nor can it be derived from the study of simulated total hip replacements done in cadaver bones, since they are incapable of a loading history or biologic responses. The only way to gather this crucial information is from the analysis of autopsy-retrieved, successful implants after years of *in vivo* service in which the mechanism of loosening has *begun* but has not reached completion.

From such studies we were able to establish a number of key observations (15,18).

Debonding: Mechanism of Femoral Loosening

On the femoral side, the proximate event that leads to loosening of cemented femoral components (assuming that any sort of reasonable cementing technique had been used) is, in fact, *debonding*. Failure begins as a separation between the cement and metal. The cement-bone interface remains absolutely pristine, or nearly so. What happens is that the metal debonds from the cement and, to a lesser extent, cracks originate from pores or voids within the cement. Debonding has certain universal characteristics. It initiates at only two places, unless there is a defect in the cement mantle. Those two locations are (i) proximally, primarily from the very high strains that exist secondary to the torsional forces associated with stair climbing and rising from a chair, and (ii) near the tip where very high stresses exist secondary to the loading forces that occur both in stair climbing and in single-leg stance during gait (10). Debonding progresses distally from the proximal area and proximally from the distal area. When the debonding has become complete, the femoral component is loose.

Debonding causes the single most common x-ray manifestation of loosening of a femoral component, namely the radiolucency between the cement and metal in the proximal-lateral area of the anteroposterior (AP) film or the proximal anterior portion of the lateral film. Proximal debonding with persistent distal fixation leads to the circumstances that created stem fractures in the time when cast chrome cobalt stems were used.

With debonding, the strains in the adjacent cement rise rapidly (9), which accelerates the progression of the debonding process and the fragmentation of the cement. Eventually, failure takes place at the cement-bone interface, but only late in the process and distinctly secondary to debonding.

In short, in cemented femoral components, the initiating event is proximal and distal debonding, with some help from cracks in the cement that arise from pores. Notably, the cement-bone interface remains intact. Strain changes secondary to the debonding accelerate the debonding process, accelerate fragmentation of the cement, and ultimately lead to loosening, failure of the cement-bone interface, particulate methacrylate, a grossly loose component, and lysis.

A much smaller subset of patients may have fragmentation of the cement and lysis adjacent to a defect in the cement layer or a very thin layer of methylmethacrylate while the component remains grossly well fixed. This subset we have termed *lysis without looseness* (11).

Mechanism of Acetabular Loosening: Bone Resorption

The situation on the acetabular side is exactly the opposite of that on the femoral side. The mechanism of loosening of cemented acetabular components is that of the ingress of polyethylene debris at the periphery of the cement-bone interface circumferentially around the acetabular component (18). This is followed by macrophage invasion, bone resorption, and progression of the process as a cutting wedge moving relentlessly toward the dome of the acetabular component. When this process reaches the dome, the entirety of the interface is destroyed and the acetabular component is loose.

Cemented acetabular components do not become loose secondary to mechanical issues such as increased or decreased stress, trabecular or cement fractures, or altered loading conditions. Neither do they become loose secondary to monomer or heat toxicity or other forms of biologic response, nor does disuse osteoporosis play an important role. The proximate cause of acetabular loosening is biologic, not mechanical. The proximal cause of femoral loosening is mechanical, not biologic.

It is also important conceptually to appreciate that the *remote* cause of acetabular loosening is also mechanical. It is the generation of the particulate polyethylene debris. Thus, in the broad sense, one can say that both femoral and acetabular components fail ultimately because of a mechanical process, but the proximate cause on the femoral side remains mechanical, and the proximate cause on the acetabular side is biologic.

Now, return to the issue of tracking the history of total hip replacement from the point of view of the remarkable changes that have occurred in what has been viewed as "the number one problem" at different phases of the history of total hip replacement. After sepsis was brought under control, the "next" number one problem was loosening.

Associated with loosening of cemented femoral components emerged the destructive bone process, which has been termed lysis. It was, indeed, the issues of loosening (and primarily femoral loosening) plus the associated lysis that led to the revolution in the mid-seventies, which ultimately became known during the eighties as cement versus cementless.

IMPORTANT NEW ADVANCES

Three new observations become very important in terms of the definition of the "next number one problem" or "the current number one problem." These are observations concerning (i) the mechanisms of loosening of *cementless* acetabular components, (ii) data on improved fixation of femoral components, and (iii) the first true understanding of the generic nature of the lysis process.

Cementless Acetabular Loosening

First, why do *cementless* acetabular components become loose? The fascinating thing is that the mechanism is exactly the same as for cemented acetabular components. Specifically, polyethylene debris works its way into the interface, macrophages follow, lysis of a slow and diffuse nature takes place, which produces the radiolucent zone, and ultimately the acetabular component comes loose. The nature of this process is absolutely the same as it is on cemented acetabular components. It is biologic. It is "particulate disease."

Cemented Femoral Durability

What has happened to femoral loosening? Have improved cementing techniques resulted in better fixation? The decade of the eighties established that in fact femoral loosening in cemented femoral components can be virtually eliminated. Instead of a 30% to 40% figure with first-generation femoral cementing (20,22), it is a 3% figure with second-generation femoral cementing at 11 years (16). The eighties also established that a fully porous-coated femoral component can lead to a very high incidence of femoral fixation, at least over the intermediate term (5 to 8 years). Thus, selected contemporary techniques for both cemented and cementless implants can lead to nearly uniform success in the fixation of femoral components.

Particulate Disease

What about a better understanding of the generic nature of lysis? It is now quite clear that the lytic process associated with total joint replacement is "particulate disease." It can be caused by fragmented cement, polyethylene particles, or metal particles. There is no such thing as cement disease; there is fragmented cement disease. There is no such thing as polyethylene disease; there is particulate polyethylene disease. There is no such thing as metal disease; there is particulate metal disease. The process involves ingestion of the particles by the macrophages, failure to dissolve the particles, and the elaboration of a complex series of enzymes (8) and cytokines (7), which, in an effort to consume the particles and repair the process, leads to bone resorption.

As an aside, one of the most exciting areas of this conference is the extraordinary advances in the understanding of the complex biology of this resorptive process. But without going into those details, the major observation that comes from the synthesis of these three observations is the concept that the single remaining number one problem in total joint replacement is lysis secondary to particulate disease.

Loosening, as noted above, used to be considered a single problem. It now is recognized as two entirely different problems. Femoral loosening is predominantly a mechanical problem, but acetabular loosening is a biologic problem. However, the biologic problem on the acetabular side, namely, particulate debris and the macrophage response, is identical in nature with the other major problem, namely, lysis. In other words, socket loosening and bone lysis are the same problem. They represent different degrees and different rates, but the mechanism is identical. It is biologic and identical in nature. Thus, with femoral fixation assured at very high levels on the femoral side by selected cemented or cementless techniques, the two remaining problems, namely, socket loosening and bone lysis, have become one; the single remaining problem is particulate disease. It is, therefore, fascinating that we have come full cycle. In 1960–1962, the number one problem in total hip replacement was lysis from particle disease.

It then became sepsis.

It then became loosening.

We then learned that femoral loosening and socket loosening were different.

We then learned that femoral loosening can be solved and that socket loosening is caused by particulate debris.

We now know that the current number one problem in total joint replacement is particulate disease, which leads to both lysis and socket loosening. We have come full circle. The number one problem is lysis. One must now extend that position further, based on the very disturbing fact that lysis of the femur, in association with cementless femoral components, regardless of type, design, or metallurgy, is prohibitive in its incidence, time of onset, rising numbers, and extent.

The second qualifier concerning the current number one problem, namely, lysis secondary to particulate disease, is the fact that it is occurring earlier and with greater damage to the acetabulum in many of the contemporary cementless systems than we have previously experienced.

Thus, the number one problem of total hip replacement in its infancy was particulate disease. Lysis secondary to particulate disease is back with us and dominates total joint arthroplasty today.

GENERATIONS OF HIP REPLACEMENT

Now I would like to look at where we stand today from an entirely different point of view. This is the concept of assessing both the history of total hip replacement and the confusing and conflicting data that confound rational understanding of the current scene, through the eyes of a new concept, namely, the concept of "generations of total hip replacement." Consider, if you would, five generations, three involving the use of cement and two involving cementless implants.

First-generation cementing involved the original techniques of the 1960s, which, for example, on the femoral side involved no cement plug, finger packing the cement, no pressurization, and the use of femoral stems that frequently had narrow medial borders and sharp corners and were made of cast material.

Second-generation femoral cementing consisted of the introduction of a medullary plug, the use of a cement gun, the early efforts at pressurization of the cement, and the improvement of the femoral stem by having a broad medial border without sharp corners, the use of a superalloy, and generally the presence of a collar.

Third-generation femoral cementing involves all of those features of second-generation plus the routine use of pressurization, porosity reduction to reduce the pores in the cement, precoating the implant, a rough surface on the implant, and centralization of the implant to assure a minimum thickness and complete cement mantle.

First-generation cementless femoral components include a wide variety of designs, ranging from Mittelmeier to AML "fully coated, one size fits all," AML proximally coated, APR, PCA, HGP, and others.

Second-generation cementless femoral components involve AML "fully coated, multiple sizes," Multilock, Anatomic, PCA E series, Omniflex, and others.

THE CEMENTED GENERATION

What do we learn from such a grouping? Look first at the cemented series. The first thing we learn is that second-generation femoral cementing makes an enormous difference. Loosening rates of femoral components at 10 years varied from 30% to 40% in first-generation techniques (20,22). In second-generation femoral cementing, our femoral loosening rate decreased to 3% at 11 years in primary total hip replacements in the older age group (16). The Mayo Clinic and the Brigham and Women's Hospital found identical improvement. The femoral loosening rate is only 2% in patients under the age of 50 (average age 41 years) at 12 years (1) and only 20% at 12 years in revision surgery (6). Does it make a difference how the cement is used? Absolutely.

Does this division of the experience into generations help to clarify the confusing and conflicting data? Absolutely. First-generation femoral cementing data are outmoded, cannot be used for comparison with contemporary experience, and represent the past. Second-generation femoral cementing sets the worldwide standard. Basically up to 11 years, the femoral loosening problem has been solved with second-generation femoral cementing.

Why then go to third generation?

The answer is simple. Virtually none of our patients has longevity expectations that stop at 11 years. The figures for longevity in North America are the following: At age 65, 60% of the patients will live 20 years, 40% will live 25 years, and 20% will live 30 years. To be content with 11-year data is folly.

If, then we are to extend the durability of cemented femoral components, we must attack the basic mechanism by which they come loose. That, of course, is debonding and the initiation of cracks through pores in the cement. Thus, it is obligatory, if we are to meet the expectations and needs of our patients, to use third-generation femoral cementing when we use cement on the femoral side.

LESSONS FROM CEMENTED IMPLANTS

What do we learn from looking at the femoral cementless experience when considered in terms of generations?

We have clearly learned the lesson that 2-year data on cementless implants are not definitive. Every cementless system looks excellent at 2 years. Five-year data are minimum to make differentiations between success and failure in a cementless series. That very important statement means that we have useful data only on first-generation cementless femoral components. No useful data exist on second-generation cementless systems except the AML fully coated, multiple sizes.

What have we learned so far? First-generation femoral cementless components have a higher incidence of loosening, subsidence, thigh pain, disuse osteoporosis, heterotopic ossification, and revision compared with second-generation cemented femoral components.

Even more important is the single dominating observation concerning cementless femoral components that femoral lysis begins earlier, increases in incidence rapidly, and is far more extensive at 5 to 7 years in all cementless femoral components than in second-generation cemented femoral components.

The incidence of lysis in all cementless femoral components at 5 to 7 years is high and climbing. The incidence of lysis in the femur for the AML prosthesis has been reported as 19% and 56% (2,17), for the PCA as 26% (5), for the HGP as now 31% (12), for the APR prosthesis as 16% (4) and so forth. Both the incidence and the extent are severe. With AML prostheses, the greater trochanter has spontaneously pulled off in several cases and the lesser trochanter has done so similarly.

So, if we look at the lesson of first-generation cementless femoral components, it is quite clear that first-generation femoral cementless components are not comparable to second-generation cemented femoral components.

The decade of the eighties was described as cement versus cementless. More appropriately, it was, in relation to femoral components, the decade of first-generation cementless femoral components competing with second-generation cemented femoral components.

That battle is over. Second-generation femoral cementing won. Second-generation femoral cementing won in terms of thigh pain, subsidence, disuse osteoporosis, heterotopic ossification, and reoperations. But even more important, and dominating the entire scene, second-generation femoral cementing won overwhelmingly in terms of bone lysis. At a comparable time period, the incidence of femoral lysis in second-generation femoral cementing is 2%, all focal and all associated with well-fixed femoral components (16). In terms of the major first-generation femoral cementless components, the figures are those just presented above. And they are climbing.

That battle of the eighties in terms of cement versus cementless is over for the femoral side. The new form of that contest will be shaped as the competition between third-generation femoral cementing and second-generation cementless femoral components. It will be 5 years before that issue can be resolved.

THE YOUNG PATIENT

Let us look at two other subsets of the general aspects of femoral components for total hip replacements. What about total hip replacements in the young? This was an area in which cementless was widely advocated for the femoral reconstruction.

Long-term data covering an average 8- to 12-year follow-up (1) show that cement when used well is excellent for the femoral component in the young. Our figures at 12 years show 98% solidly fixed and 100% in place.

REVISION ARTHROPLASTY

What about revisions? Second-generation femoral cementing here makes an enormous difference. At 12 years, 80% of the femoral components are solidly fixed and 90% are still in place (6). This also is a remarkable advance over first-generation cementing for aseptic loose cemented femoral components. In short, second-generation femoral cementing dominates the field.

Now let us look at the current status of the situation on the acetabulum. In terms of cemented acetabular components, no changes in technique have made a significant difference in the incidence of radiographic evidence of acetabular loosening. All figures show that in the neighborhood of 40% or 50% of the acetabular components are loose by radiographic criteria at 10 years or so (16,20,22), but only a small number, generally in the neighborhood of 5% to 10%, have been revised.

Beyond 10 years, revision rates, loosening rates, and lysis increase. The question is whether or not this is a glass half full or a glass half empty. Are we to emphasize that 50% are loose, or that 5% to 10% have been revised? My belief is that, particularly in view of the real need for longevity at the 20- to 30-year level of total joint reconstructions, we should view it as half empty. We must do better than 50% loose at 10 years.

Can cementless sockets do this? No one knows. No one has 10-year data. However, we do know that threaded rings have an extremely poor record and that many of the other first-generation cementless acetabular components, which are not threaded-ring types, at 5 to 7 years are loose, show migration of the femoral head in the polyethylene, and/or have extensive lysis in the innominate bone.

What are some representative figures? With the AML cup, the incidence of lysis in the innominate bone (2) has been reported at 14% at 5 to 7 years. With the PCA acetabular component, Stulberg et al. (21) have reported a very high incidence of innominate lysis including the arresting figure that among those cases 7 years *in situ*, 47% have pelvic lysis.

We must ask two questions: What are the causes of these adverse findings and do all systems show the same results?

The major categories of potential causes of these adverse results are the following: poor design features, three-body wear, and unidentified changes in the polyethylene itself.

Clearly in the first-generation cementless acetabular components of many designs, there were many gross design errors. A number of companies created acetabular components with large holes at the back of the shield, which both left the polyethylene unsupported and left it exposed to tissue. Some manufacturers, in order to accommodate surgeons using a 32-mm head, were willing to reduce the polyethylene thickness down as thin as 2.5 mm. Many designs did not provide good support for the polyethylene. Others did not provide good fixation for the polyethylene. Many had a cylindrical section, which, if the socket were placed in a high degree of abduction, meant that load bearing was against a thin layer of polyethylene.

In addition, all of the modular designs of acetabular components created the possibility of increased particulate debris arising from multiple sites, a factor absent from solid polyethylene acetabular components.

Three-body wear may well be increased from the use of modular systems. Particulate metal debris can come from the Morse cone or from the cementless implants themselves, which could migrate into the joint and accelerate polyethylene wear.

Finally, we are, to a large extent, ignorant of the techniques and, more important, changes in techniques of the manufacturers and processors of ultrahigh molecular weight polyethylene. Who knows the effect on wear characteristics of deciding to fuse the polyethylene flakes at 500 psi versus 1,000 psi? All of these issues are critical.

The second question is: are all cementless acetabular systems the same? No, some of the cementless acetabular systems have excellent records up to 5 to 7 years.

The next issue is the role of press-fit acetabular components. We have carried out a comparative study of two groups of patients. One group was done with a socket using an exact fit and screws, the other using press fit and no screws. The average follow-up on the first group was 5 years. The average follow-up on the second group was 6 years. None of these cases showed discernible polyethylene wear. None showed lysis in the acetabulum. No cup was loose, had migrated, or had been revised for loosening in either series. Even more important was the critical observation that the press-fit group had a statistically significant reduction in radiolucent zones. This information, when coupled with our experimental studies showing that press fit increases the stability peripherally and our dog studies show that press fit increases the bone growth peripherally, creates a strong scientific base for the concept that press fitting has a high probability for reducing the ingress of polyethylene, reducing the radiolucent zones, and reducing the loosening of this type of acetabular component. It is our belief, without direct data, that this type of acetabular component press fit will provide better long-term results than the use of cement. However, it will be 3 more years before we will be able to establish that statement.

We can, however, establish already, although at a shorter time interval, that a hemispherical cementless socket fixed with screws is vastly better than cementing for revision of the acetabular component. All of the studies using cement have shown in the neighborhood of 25% to 40% of the acetabular components loose at 3.5 years following cemented revision of a loose, nonseptic acetabular component. A hemispherical cementless socket fixed with screws in comparable patient populations shows a 2% loosening rate (23). Thus, at least in the short term, it is clear that this type of cementless acetabular component is much better than the use of cement for acetabular revisions. Longer term data will be needed to establish that these excellent results continue.

I pointed out previously that 5-year data are needed to have reliable information on cementless components. The data noted above on cementless acetabular revisions are at an average of 3.5 years, not 5. However, here is an instance in which data on follow-up durations shorter than 5 years are valuable. They are valuable because the cemented acetabular data at the same time duration are so poor. Data at 3.5 years are valuable if they show that socket loosening has been reduced from the 30% to 40% figure at 3.5 years using cement to 2% at 3.5 years using a hemispherical cementless socket with fiber mesh fixed with screws.

THE PRESENT

Where is total hip replacement at this time? As of November 1, 1992, almost exactly 30 years since the beginning of the modern era of total hip replacement surgery and 33 years since the first total hip replacement, on the femoral side, the data overwhelmingly support the use of contemporary cementing for primary operations in the older age group, for the young, for revisions, independent of diagnosis, independent of sex, and independent of age. For acetabular revisions, the data are very strong establishing the superiority of the hemispherical cementless socket fixed with screws in the short term. Long-term data will be necessary.

For primaries the optimal choice for acetabular reconstructions remains unproven. My own bias favors a solid-backed, press-fit hemispherical cementless socket with thick polyethylene that is well fixed.

Tomorrow's issues will be assessing on the femoral side to see if third-generation femoral cementing or second-generation cementless femoral components are better.

The issue of accelerated polyethylene wear must be urgently addressed, evaluating design features, three-body wear, and the polyethylene itself. I foresee a major increase in investigation of polyethylene and wear, and a strong movement to establish new manufacturing techniques to permit the successful reintroduction of metal on metal articulations.

The explosive contemporary biology of the lytic reaction will be extremely important and may very well provide us with modes of diminishing, inhibiting, or abolishing this adverse biologic response while, simultaneously, every effort is made to eliminate the generation of particulate debris.

I foresee also exciting advances in the local control of osteogenesis, which could play a dramatic role in enhancing the fixation of cementless components.

Finally, I see vigorous efforts at attempting to establish composite femoral stems in an effort to address the one other remaining issue, which I have not spoken of at all, the long-term changes associated with stress shielding and its related disuse osteoporosis.

The past 30 years have been enormously exciting. The current scene is enormously capable and effective in the dramatic resolution of most of the problems of severe arthritis of the major joints. Tomorrow, because of the efforts of dedicated investigators and conferences such as this, it will be even better.

REFERENCES

1. Barrack RL, Mulroy RD Jr, Harris WH. Improved cementing techniques and femoral component loosening in young patients with hip arthroplasty: a 12 year radiographic review. *J Bone Joint Surg [Br]* 1992;74:385–389.
2. Beauchesne RP, Kukita Y, Knezevich S, Suthers K. Roentgenographic evaluation of the AML porous coated acetabular component: a six year minimum follow-up study. Presented at the 59th Annual Meeting of the American Academy of Orthopaedic Surgeons in Washington, DC, February 25, 1992, paper no. 416.
3. Charnley J, Eftekhar N. Postoperative infection in total prosthetic replacement arthroplasty of the hip-joint. With special reference to the bacterial content of the air of the operating room. *Br J Surg* 1969;56:641–649.
4. Cox CV, Dorr LD. Five-year results of proximal bone ingrowth fixation total hip replacement. Presented at the 59th Annual Meeting of the American Academy of Orthopaedic Surgeons, Washington, DC, February 25, 1992, paper no. 415.
5. Crutcher JP, Borden LS, Hedley AK, Hungerford DS. Minimum five year follow-up of unce-

mented total hip arthroplasty for primary osteoarthritis. Presented at the 58th Annual Meeting of the American Academy of Orthopaedic Surgeons, Anaheim, CA, March 9, 1991, paper no. 198.

6. Estok DM, Harris WH. Long-term results of cemented femoral revision surgery using second generation techniques: average 11.7 year follow-up. *Clin Orthop (in press)*.

7. Goldring MB, Goldring SR. Skeletal tissue response to cytokines. *Clin Orthop* 1990;258:245–278.

8. Goldring SR, Schiller AL, Roelke M, Rourke CM, O'Neill DA, Harris WH. The synovial-like membrane of the bone-cement interface in loose total hip replacements and its proposed role in bone lysis. *J Bone Joint Surg [Am]* 1983;65:575–583.

9. Harrigan TP, Harris WH. A three-dimensional non-linear finite element study of the effect of cement-prosthesis debonding in cemented femoral total hip components. *J Biomechanics* 1991;24:1047–1058.

10. Harrigan TP, Kareh J, O'Connor DO, Burke DW, Harris WH. A finite element study of the initiation of failure of fixation of cemented total hip components. *J Orthop Res* 1992;10:34–44.

11. Jasty M, Floyd III WE, Schiller AL, Goldring SR, Harris WH. Localized osteolysis in stable, non-septic total hip replacement. *J Bone Joint Surg [Am]* 1986;68:912–919.

12. Jasty M, Haire T, Tanzer M. Femoral osteolysis: a generic problem with cementless and cemented components. Presented at the 58th Annual Meeting of the American Academy of Orthopaedic Surgeons, Anaheim, CA, March 9, 1991, paper no. 222.

13. Lidwell OM, Lowbury EJL, Whyte W, Blowers R, Stanley SJ, Lowe D. Effect of ultraclean air in operating rooms on deep sepsis in the joint after total hip or knee replacement. A randomized study. *BMJ* 1982;285:10–14.

14. Lidwell OM, Lowbury EJL, Whyte W, Blowers R, Stanley SJ, Lowe D. Infection and sepsis after operations for total hip or knee-joint replacement: influence of ultraclean air, prophylactic antibiotics and other factors. *J Hyg* 1984;93:505–529.

15. Maloney WJ, Jasty M, Burke DW, et al. Biomechanical and histologic investigation of cemented total hip arthroplasties. A study of autopsy-retrieved femurs after *in vivo* cycling. *Clin Orthop* 1989;249:129–140.

16. Mulroy Jr RD, Harris WH. The effect of improved cementing techniques on component loosening in total hip replacement. *J Bone Joint Surg [Br]* 1990;72:757–760.

17. Oh J-H, Kim Y-H, Kim VEM. Endosteal osteolysis in cementless porous coated femoral components. Presented at the 59th Annual Meeting of the American Academy of Orthopaedic Surgeons in Washington, DC, February 25, 1992, paper no. 407.

18. Schmalzried TP, Kwong LM, Jasty M, et al. The mechanism of loosening of cemented acetabular components in total hip arthroplasty. *Clin Orthop* 1992;274:60–78.

19. Schutzer SF, Harris WH. Deep-wound infection after total hip replacement under contemporary aseptic conditions. *J Bone Joint Surg [Am]* 1988;70:724–727.

20. Stauffer RN. Ten-year follow-up study of total hip replacement. With particular reference to roentgenographic loosening of the components. *J Bone Joint Surg [Am]* 1982;64:983–990.

21. Stulberg BN, Buly RL, Howard PL, Stulberg SD, Wixson RL. Porous coated anatomic acetabular failure: incidence and modes of failure in uncemented total hip arthroplasty. Presented at the 59th Annual Meeting of the American Academy of Orthopaedic Surgeons, Washington, DC, Feb. 24, 1992, paper no. 282.

22. Sutherland CJ, Wilde AH, Borden LS, Marks KE. A ten-year follow-up of one hundred consecutive Muller curved-stem total hip-replacement arthroplasties. *J Bone Joint Surg [Am]* 1982; 64:970–982.

23. Tanzer M, Drucker D, Jasty M, McDonald M, Harris WH. Revision of the acetabular component with an uncemented Harris-Galante porous-coated prosthesis. *J Bone Joint Surg [Am]* 1992; 74:987–994.

24. Wilson Jr PD, Amstutz HC, Czerniecki A, Salvati EA, Mendes DG. Total hip replacement with fixation by acrylic cement. A preliminary study to 100 consecutive McKee-Farrar prosthetic replacements. *J Bone Joint Surg [Am]* 1972;54:207–236.

Biological, Material, and Mechanical Considerations of Joint Replacement, edited by B. F. Morrey. Raven Press, Ltd., New York © 1993.

2

Keynote Address: Biomaterials for Total Joint Replacements

Jack E. Lemons

Laboratory Research, Division of Orthopaedic Surgery, Departments of Surgery and Biomaterials, University of Alabama at Birmingham, Birmingham, Alabama 35294-3295

Metals and alloys, polymers, ceramics, carbons, and combinations and composites of these classes of materials are all utilized as biomaterials for the construction of total joint replacement (TJR) devices. Analysis of the transfer of elements and force across the devices and through the tissues (interfacial studies) provides one method for establishing relative biocompatibility profiles and identifying opportunities for improvements of existing or for inventing new device systems. Two current research and development goals within the biomaterials discipline include (i) anisotropic composites with stable attachments to viable tissues and (ii) minimization of biodegradation and wear debris.

Overall evaluations of biomaterial chemical and the associated biochemical reactions to elemental compositions show cell and tissue tolerances for most elements released from devices at biodegradation debris concentrations to be below 100 parts per million (ppm). Confounding influences of particulates and/or local strain (motion) complicate these types of correlations, and TJR interactions have been shown to depend also on debris form (e.g., ions, mers, compounds), tissue and host type, alterations of the local and systemic environment, and time. The relative importance of some of these factors has been realized only within the past few years.

Mechanical properties, when compared to similar test values from compact bone, show ratios of tensile strength from 2 to $11\times$ for alloys and inert ceramics and 0.05 to $1\times$ for polymers; elastic moduli from 7 to $11\times$ for alloys, 1 to $20\times$ for ceramics, and 0.0003 to $0.5\times$ for polymers; and ductilities from 8 to $55\times$ for alloys, 0 to $1\times$ for ceramics, and 2 to $900\times$ for polymers. These biomechanical properties provide a wide range of opportunities and thereby dominate the initial criteria for device-based design, biomaterial, and application selections.

The introduction of composites that provide three-dimensional mechanical and chemical anisotropies (biomechanics more like tissues with stable bonding to bone and soft tissues) and a complete reevaluation of bearing interfaces and designs for TJR articulation should result in significantly altered devices before the year 2000. Improvements will require continued coordination and collaboration among the orthopaedic surgery, biomechanics, and biomaterials disciplines.

BACKGROUND

Biocompatibility profiles of the synthetic materials (biomaterials) utilized for TJR devices in orthopaedic surgery have been characterized in terms of the elements and forces transferred during function. This theme will be emphasized throughout the following discussions. Characteristics associated with elemental compositions of synthetic materials can be further described in terms of the element-dependent chemical (material) properties and the affiliated biochemical (biological) responses. An analogous association can be made for the material-based mechanical properties and the related biomechanical interactions. To validate theoretical and experimental aspects of these biomaterial and biomechanical concepts, requests have been made for detailed publication of biomaterial bulk and surface characteristics of devices, including relevant physical, mechanical, chemical, electrical, and biological properties. These requests have been made, in part, to maximize basic science information during research and development phases and to provide opportunities to describe mechanisms of interactions. Restated, for research and development, biomaterial surface and bulk properties should be known prior to experimental surgical implantations and subsequent *in vivo* applications (24).

Interfacial reactions along the synthetic biomaterial and tissue contact zones have been used to describe both anticipated and unanticipated interactions (22). Critically, laboratory environmental testing conditions can provide only basic simulations for subsequent clinical applications. However, if fundamental property data are available for the implant at the time of placement *in vivo,* relative changes in structure and properties over time can result in mechanism-based insights regarding limitations of functionality and longevity and, thereby, through reiterative processes, can suggest opportunities to improve existing systems and to develop new prosthetic devices for patient treatment modalities (17).

ROLES OF SCIENCE, TECHNOLOGY, AND APPLICATIONS

Orthopaedic surgery, biomechanics, biomaterials, and other directly supporting disciplines, more recently, molecular biology, have evolved significantly over the past three decades. This has been demonstrated by the ever-increasing numbers of TJR types, designs, surgical procedures, and rehabilitation regimes. Importantly, the basic sciences have provided information to enhance technology transfer. For example, existing knowledge of biomaterial surface chemistries and the related characteristics of force transfer (static and dynamic) have resulted in new surfaces for device bonding-to-bone and relatively normal kinematics for TJR (4,15). However, several hundred different designs of TJR devices exist within hospital inventories, and this general trend has been one of ongoing expansion. Clearly, a single optimal system for each joint or patient condition has not yet been made available to the profession.

Criteria for device selection have evolved from both the physical and biological disciplines and again present the issue of interactions along device biomaterial-to-tissue interfaces and the additional concept that biocompatibility can be defined as minimal harm to the device and the host. That is, the biomaterial and the device should satisfy the intended functional results; however, since the device and the host are both changing over time, optimizations of implant longevities require a balance of orthopaedic, biomechanical, and biomaterial considerations (8). Clinical experience following prospective analysis protocols most often provides validation for the basic scientific theories and technological applications; therefore, controlled clinical studies represent one important step in the development of new or improved TJRs.

As the keynote to the topic of biomaterials, this chapter will summarize the biomaterials used for the construction of TJR, compare biomaterial and biological properties, give examples of element- and force-based interfacial reactions, and review some critical issues related to biocompatibility.

TJR DEVICE BIOMATERIAL AND BIOMECHANICAL CHARACTERISTICS

Musculoskeletal joint replacements include a wide range of designs and biomaterials (15,17). To provide some specific examples, schematic representations of hip (THR), knee (TKR), and finger (MP) devices are shown in Fig. 1. These schematics are intended to be general, with emphasis on the recent expansion to modular multicomponent and multimaterial designs.

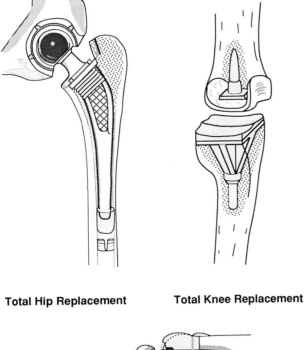

Total Hip Replacement   **Total Knee Replacement**

Finger (MP) Joint Replacement

FIG. 1. Schematic drawings of hip, knee, and finger joint replacements showing multiple concepts of modular designs (ball-socket or plateau; porosity for ingrowth; fin, rod, and collar stabilizers; centralizers, restrictors, and spacers; and various attachment methods) and materials (metals, polymers, and ceramics).

The biomaterials for TJR devices include metals and alloys, ceramics, polymers, and combinations and composites of these classes of materials (1). These biomaterials contact one another and/or tissues and tissue fluids to provide attachment, articulation, and motion. Normal function requires force transfer among and across all of the device parts and the associated tissues, and, because function is cyclic at variable rates, the dynamics of motion and force transfer become key issues. Since three-dimensional geometric features and normal joint kinematics introduce multi-directionally oriented forces, one result is the dissipation of compression-, tension-, and shear-type mechanical stresses. Also, because biomaterials and tissues respond quite differently to each type and magnitude of biomechanical stress, device designs must be optimized to decrease adverse force transfer conditions. This requires a combination of material and mechanical criteria within each TJR construct. Another aspect is that biomaterials do not "heal" when damaged, and, therefore, properties such as fatigue, creep strengths, and contact motion-based wear must be fully optimized to increase *in vivo* stabilities.

RELATIVE BIOMATERIAL AND TISSUE PROPERTIES

Chemical and Biochemical Considerations

Elements contained within the biomaterials used for device construction include the primary substances that make up 99 (or more) wt % of the compositions. Minor additions (intentional) or residual impurities (bulk and surface) seldom exceed 1 wt % (1). In all cases, the elements have tissue interaction profiles that can be assessed in terms of their potentials for biological host toxicity, hypersensitivity, and carcinogenicity (7). These characteristics, which are quantity related, are also known to depend on form (ions, mers, compounds, particulates), tissue and host types, and time. For TJR, the biomechanical environment (e.g., local strain) can introduce synergistic conditions that directly influence biocompatibility reactions.

As an example of relative toxicity considerations, the toxicities of some metallic elements (ions in solution as corrosion products) that were evaluated in tissue culture experiments (10,11) are shown in Fig. 2. The relationship presented demonstrates a comparison for fibroblast responses to concentrations, shown as reciprocal, of metallic elements (ppm ions in solution) added to culture systems. Significant differences existed among the elements, with chromium (+6 valance state) and vanadium showing cellular changes at concentrations below one ppm. Other ionic concentrations did not introduce measurable cellular reactions until magnitudes exceeded 12 ppm or more. Clearly, these types of experiments have limited applicability to the complex TJR conditions because of the *in vitro* tissue culture environment. However, the relative trends in cultures have been judged to be valid and associated *in vivo* experiments have shown correlations with these data (11).

Interestingly, elements like nickel, in which *in vivo* hypersensitivity reactions are known (7), show mild relative toxicity reactions (similar to cobalt and aluminum) within these types of cell culture test systems. Another observation made from these studies was that metallic elements in combination showed more adverse conditions at lower concentrations in comparison to the same elements when tested alone. Subsequent experiments using laboratory animal models and human clinical trials have further defined local and systemic pathways for elements from implant biomaterials

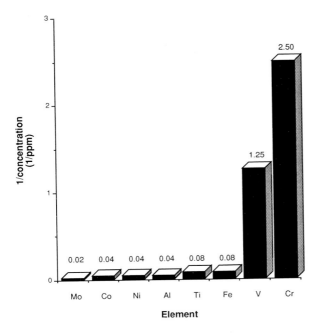

FIG. 2. Graphic relationship showing the relative elemental concentrations of metallic elements added to fibroblast tissue cultures that introduced significant changes in cell morphology and number. Critical concentrations were 50 ppm for molybdenum (Mo), 25 ppm for cobalt (Co), nickel (Ni), and aluminum (Al), 12.5 ppm for titanium (Ti) and iron (Fe), 0.75 ppm for vanadium (V), and 0.38 ppm for chromium (Cr).

(6,8). When present as a biodegradation product in a charged (ionic) form, local interactions with polar or oppositely charged species normal to the biological environment (e.g., chlorides, phosphates, biomolecules) would form reaction products that have been shown to strongly influence *in vivo* responses. For example, nickel has been shown to be transported systemically, whereas chromium reacted within the local environment (6).

Because of localized degradation and surface-specific phenomena (21), biodegradation products do not have a simple relationship to nominal biomaterial chemical analyses (bulk compositions), and elements of higher toxicity profiles can exist within bulk compositions without introducing adverse tissue reactions (e.g., antimony, lead, and vanadium). However, if particulates are generated, the relative surface areas per volume of original implant and the reaction rates can be greatly altered. This topic is further discussed below as similar issues related to electrochemical corrosion and wear are examined.

Mechanical and Biomechanical Considerations

Forces transferred across biomaterial-to-tissue interfaces depend on host, device, and biomaterial interrelationships. The overall type and shape of the device components and the functional force vectors dominate the macroscopic strain distributions across interfaces. Therefore, host and device-design factors must be evaluated as a first line of consideration. Interfacial stability also depends on the microscopic strain distributions where the biomaterial factors such as modulus of elasticity and surface attachment (e.g., porosity, bioactive coating) strongly influence the local strain distributions.

The basic material properties (e.g., tensile, fatigue, creep and fracture strengths, ductilities, hardnesses, and contact wear susceptibilities) also determine *in vivo* stabilities and, therefore, biocompatibility profiles. Comparisons of mechanical properties of several metallic, ceramic, and polymeric biomaterials (1) are presented as a ratio-to-compact bone in Figs. 3 to 5.

The ratio values for tensile strength demonstrate magnitudes that significantly exceed bone ($1.5-13 \times$) for most of the metallic and ceramic biomaterials. Polymers, in contrast, often have tensile strengths that are about the same or lower than compact bone ($0.05-1 \times$). Therefore, tensile and shear load-bearing conditions, in which higher magnitude values exist, require the selection of metallic or ceramic biomaterials. Moduli of elasticity ratios also show a wide range ($5-11 \times$ for alloys, $0.5-20 \times$ for ceramics, and $0.0003-0.5 \times$ for polymers). Once again, biomaterial selection must be coupled with design parameters such as size, shape, and loading to minimize the influences of relative differences in properties. Capabilities for ductility (plastic deformation) are the greatest for the polymers (except for polymethylmethacrylate [PMMA]) and the least for ceramics and carbons. Therefore, compressive loading considerations must be emphasized for the ceramic biomaterials or, if loaded in tension or shear, the local stresses must be within the biomaterial property limits (lower magnitudes). In contrast, if damping or stretching (elastic deformation) of higher magnitudes is required, polymers or composites are the best choice.

Contact wear properties are quite material and environment-condition dependent (3,12). The relative values given for the biomaterial surfaces in Fig. 5A–C are provided on a comparative basis within the specific biomaterial group (metals and alloys, ceramics, and polymers). Within the alloy grouping, titanium alloy is most susceptible, requiring selective surface treatment for wear resistance, whereas the cobalt alloys are least susceptible (24). Inert ceramics, such as aluminum and zirconium oxides, with high indentation hardnesses are most resistant to wear during two-body wear processes (14). Calcium phosphate ceramics are, in general, not resistant to wear and therefore are not intended for application where any contact wear would be present (4). Polymers have demonstrated higher wear rates for polytetrafluoroethylene and relatively lower rates for polyethylene, when considered as a bearing with smooth surfaced alloys and ceramics (3). In general, when overall wear magnitudes are compared under *in vivo* circumstances, inert ceramics demonstrate the lowest wear rates, whereas polymers exhibit the highest wear rates. This comparison is made for two-body wear conditions. If three-body wear is considered, all biomaterials, including inert ceramics, show relatively high rates for abrasive contact-mediated wear processes (12).

Environment-Dependent Biomaterial Stabilities

The characteristics demonstrated by the previous figures can be significantly altered by local environments (5,13). For example, if the supporting bone anatomy changes over time, regional compressive forces may be altered to become tensile or shear, and static contact may be converted to dynamic motion. Local damage to the region may occur because of biodegradation products, and such situations often result in alterations of pH, oxygen concentration, and motion (21). These alterations can introduce destructive mechanisms that otherwise would not have been anticipated. Since most biomaterials function at relatively high ratios of mechanical loading within a reactive and corrosive environment for millions of cycles, destructive

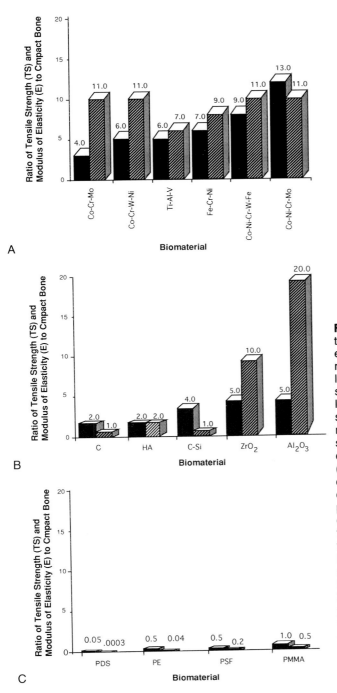

FIG. 3. A: Graphic comparison of tensile strength (■) and modulus of elasticity (▨) for cobalt- (Co), titanium- (Ti), and iron- (Fe) based alloys expressed as a ratio of the same property for compact bone. Alloys are presented in increasing tensile strength magnitudes from left to right. **B:** Graphic comparison of tensile strength (■) and modulus of elasticity (▨) for ceramic aluminum (Al_2O_3), zirconium oxide (ZrO_2), hydroxylapatite (HA: $Ca_{10}(PO_4)_6(OH)_2$), carbon (C), carbon-silicon (C-Si) expressed as a ratio of the same property for compact bone. The biomaterials are shown with increasing tensile strength from left to right. **C:** Graphic comparison of tensile strength (■) and modulus of elasticity (▨) for polymeric polydimethylsiloxane (PDS), polysulfone (PSF), polyethylene (PE), and polymethylmethacrylate (PMMA) expressed as a ratio of the same property for compact bone. The biomaterials are shown with increasing tensile strength from left to right.

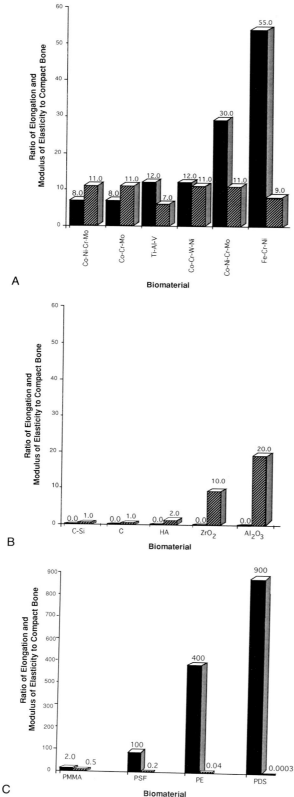

FIG. 4. A: Comparison of elongation (■) and modulus of elasticity (▨) for cobalt- (Co), titanium- (Ti), and iron- (Fe) based alloys expressed as a ratio of the same property for compact bone. Alloys are presented in increasing tensile strength magnitudes from left to right. **B:** Comparison of elongation (■) and modulus of elasticity (▨) for ceramic aluminum (Al_2O_3), zirconium oxide (ZrO_2), hydroxylapatite (HA: $Ca_{10}(PO_4)_6(OH)_2$), carbon (C), and carbon-silicon (C-Si) expressed as a ratio of the same property for compact bone. The ceramics are presented in increasing moduli of elasticity from left to right. **C:** Comparison of elongation (■) and modulus of elasticity (▨) for polymeric polymethylmethacrylate (PMMA), polysulfone (PSF), polyethylene (PE), and polydimethylsiloxane (PDS) expressed as a ratio of the same property for compact bone. The polymers are presented in increasing elongation magnitudes from left to right.

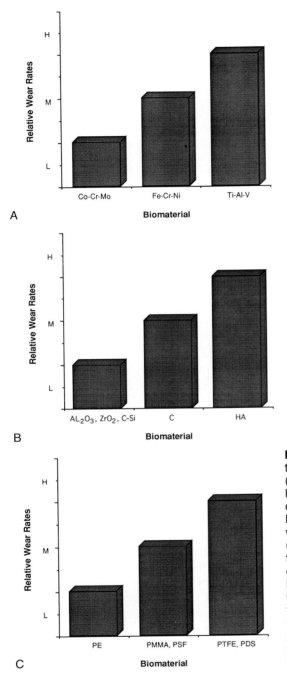

FIG. 5. A: Graphic comparison of relative two-body wear susceptibilities of cobalt- (Co), iron- (Fe), and titanium- (Ti) based alloys. Magnitudes are shown in ascending order from left to right. L, low; M, medium; H, high. **B:** Comparison of relative two-body wear susceptibilities of ceramic aluminum (Al_2O_3), zirconium oxide (ZrO_2), hydroxylapatite (HA: $Ca_{10}(PO_4)_6(OH)_2$), carbon (C), and carbon-silicon (C-Si). Magnitudes are shown in ascending order from left to right. **C:** Comparison of relative two-body wear susceptibilities of polyethylene (PE), polymethylmethacrylate (PMMA), polysulfone (PSF), polytetrafluoroethylene (PTFE), and polydimethylsiloxane (PDS). Magnitudes are shown in ascending order from left to right.

mechanisms can be anticipated over the long term. Many currently available TJR device longevities exceed two decades and opportunities to increase lifetimes by a factor of four may require new-generation biomaterials, designs, and treatment modalities.

CRITICAL ISSUES

Two critical issues normally discussed within orthopaedic surgery and other disciplines are (i) the attachment of devices to tissues and (ii) conditions of device-based articulation, wear, and wear debris.

Attachment to Bone and Soft Tissues

TJR devices at the outset (e.g., Charnley) utilized mechanical lutes (bone cements) such as autocuring PMMA for fixation (2,25). The PMMA biomaterial has limited strength and ductility, and its use for mechanical stability depends on bulk and comprehensive interpositional loading characteristics. The clinical advantages of an autocuring, space-filling material are numerous, and recent interests in modified or new bone cements are certainly justified (23). Since PMMA has an elastic modulus that is lower than that of bone and the TJR alloys, the interposition of the PMMA lute also provides a damping and redistribution of mechanical forces; therefore, the use of particulate- or fiber-reinforced composites as TJR lutes could have an important place in future developments.

Attachment through device surface porosities and tissue ingrowth continues to have a significant appeal (8). The porosity results in a localized decrease in modulus of elasticity or a regional change in stiffness, where multioriented forces can be distributed through complex geometrical features and in a renewable attachment capability (continual tissue ingrowth and regeneration).

Additions of bioactive surfaces such as calcium phosphate ceramics, glasses, and glass-ceramics also have significant theoretical advantages from the standpoint of interfacial bonding and force transfer (4). These types of biomaterials are much more similar to bone from both a chemical and mechanical standpoint. Also, the elements are natural to biological environments (e.g., $Ca \cdot PO_4$); they are insulators to heat and electricity; they can act as barriers to diffusion. Stable interfacial bonding to bone should result in active force transfer along all attachment sites and a minimization of biomaterial-to-bone tensile or shear force-based motions. This could be a significant advantage with respect to long-term function and maintenance of tissues regionally. Most expressed concerns associated with TJR over the past few years relate to the tensile and shear fatigue strengths of these types of biomaterials during long-term, *in vivo* functional load cycles. Once again, composites with lower moduli of elasticity and increased strengths could hold answers to coating-to-substrate interfacial improvements.

Articulation and Wear

One of the most pressing issues relates to TJR articulation and contact surface wear (20). Biomaterial surface articulation for existing TJR results in a mixture of secondary substances being generated that include particulates. Within limits, the host tissues appear to tolerate these types of biodegradation products. However, with modular designs, surface porosities for ingrowth, combinations of materials, third-body-mediated wear, increased functional conditions (younger and more active patients), and biodegradation debris, these factors have been shown to adversely influence both bone and soft-tissue regions. Some aspects are poorly understood, such as: (i) the introduction of active electrochemical potentials for alloys along articulating areas where passive oxides are removed and reformed during cyclic motions, (ii) minor articulating surface irregularities introduced by postsurgical bone or cement (PMMA) particulate debris, (iii) pH and synovial fluid alterations related to local environmental reactions, and (iv) normal and abnormal biochemical products introduced by systemic enzymatic processes. Overall, relatively good *in vivo* stabilities have been achieved for existing devices through the control of environmental reactions and biodegradation products of available biomaterials, combined with enhanced designs and clinical treatment regimens.

As the disciplines progress, the extension of data to better understand the interrelated phenomena should result in improved functions and associated longevities. One short-term objective is to provide incremental improvements (15–20%) within existing devices as the new systems evolve. Relatively small magnitude improvements can reduce the need for a revision within any given device's lifetime. However, since multiple revisions represent a major area of concern, primary TJR device lifetimes need to be significantly improved.

Roles of Biomaterial Characteristics

The introduction of TJR modifications, such as porosity for tissue ingrowth and attachment and modular designs for improved sizing, placement (and replacement), and function, may be indirectly associated with some recently identified adverse sequelae (e.g., multicomponent particulate debris and osteolysis). For example, when an alloy is annealed or sintered at an elevated temperature for the attachment of porous surfaces, microstructural features (e.g., internal grain size) may be altered in proportion to time and temperature exposures. Previous metallurgical studies (e.g., Hall-Petch relationship) (16,18) have shown significant changes in strength, hardness, and wear resistance as a direct function of grain (or microstructure) dimensions. (This is also true for the redistribution or solution of carbides.) The larger the grain size for some metals and alloys, the lower the strength and hardness and the higher the relative wear rate. Also, some modular designs introduce interfaces where micromotion and fretting zones may be increased. When combined (porous surfaces, annealed structures, and modular designs), conditions more adverse than anticipated may have been unintentionally introduced. Also, when processing, changes in local concentrations of elements (e.g., carbon and chromium for cobalt alloys, or oxygen and hydrogen for titanium alloys) could significantly influence surface and bulk properties (especially contact wear phenomena).

A confounding situation for TJR relates to recent studies that have shown variable material conditions associated with the polyethylene(s) used for TJR (9,22). Fabrication methods, residual contaminants, and irregular internal microstructures, combined with increased patient functional requirements, have enhanced wear and particulate generation for some devices. Since identified through device retrieval analyses, major improvements in these types of biomaterials have been introduced to the profession.

The comments above are intended to be critically constructive from a viewpoint of long-term involvement with device biomaterials. In each instance, the conditions described may, or may not, relate to potential improvements for any given device. In that regard, devices and biomaterials have, in general, been optimized by the manufacturers of TJR devices. However, combination of ideas, when considered from a thorough base of manufacturing experience, could result in improvements for existing systems.

SUMMARY

Biomaterial and biomechanical property requirements for TJR devices have been shown to push the limits of existing designs and applications. Thus, limitations associated with long-term function in younger and more active patient populations have resulted in concerns about existing *in vivo* longevities. In this regard, properties and functional interactions have been reviewed to assess some of the relative magnitudes and possible limits. In each situation encountered for device construction using existing metals and alloys, ceramics and carbons, polymers, and combinations and composites, phenomena can be described that have resulted in loss of tissue support, motion, pain, and in some device revisions. It appears that functional design-based efficiencies can be maintained, while adverse biomaterial-based sequelae are minimized for existing systems. However, to accomplish lifetime improvements of two-to-four times, a new generation of biomaterials, designs, and treatment modalities will probably be required. Within the biomaterials discipline, new generation, three-dimensional composites should become available where the chemical and mechanical properties are anisotropic and more like the tissue being replaced. An equally important consideration is the availability of basic mechanical data, from biomechanical evaluations of tissues and models of TJR, that also provide important basic and applied information (19). Current theories propose that anisotropic biomechanical properties should be similar to the tissues replaced, whereas chemical and biochemical bonding to tissues could help to optimize conditions of force transfer, tissues maintenance, and function. Surface treatments and combinations of highly wear-resistant materials for articulation could also result in acceptable (little or no) magnitudes of wear-based debris. These goals appear to be reasonable and are anticipated to be accomplished prior to the year 2000.

REFERENCES

1. *Annual book of ASTM standards: vol 13.01, medical implants*. Philadelphia: ASTM Publications, 1992.
2. Charnley J, Kamangar A, Longfield M. The optimum size of prosthetic heads in relation to the wear of plastic sockets in total replacement of the hip. *Med Biol Eng Comput* 1969;7:31–67.
3. Clarke IC, McKellop HA. Wear testing. In: von Recum A, ed. *Handbook of biomaterials evaluation*. New York: Macmillan, 1986:114–130.
4. Ducheyne P, Lemons JE, eds. *Bioceramics: material characteristics versus in vivo behavior.* [*Ann NY Acad Sci* 1988;523].
5. Griffin CD, Buchanan RA, Lemons JE. In vitro electrochemical corrosion study of coupled surgical implant materials. *J Biomed Mater Res* 1983;17:489–500.

6. Hensten-Pettersen A, Merritt K. *International workshop on biocompatibility and hypersensitivity to alloy systems*. Ann Arbor: University of Michigan Press, 1985:143–247.
7. Lang BR, Morris HF, Razoug ME, eds. *International workshop on biocompatibility and hypersensitivity to alloy systems*. Ann Arbor: University of Michigan Press, 1985.
8. Lemons JE. *Quantitative characterization and performance of porous implants for hard tissue applications*. STP 953. Philadelphia: ASTM Publications, 1988.
9. Li S, Nagy V, Wood B. Chemical degradation of polyethylene in hip and knee replacements. *Orthop Res Soc Trans* 1992;17:41.
10. Lucas LC. Biocompatibility investigations of surgical implant alloys. Ph.D. dissertation, University of Alabama at Birmingham, Birmingham, 1982.
11. Lucas LC, Bearden LJ, Lemons JE. Ultrastructural examination of in vitro and in vivo cells exposed to solutions of 316L stainless steel. In: *Corrosion and degradation of implant materials*. STP 859. Philadelphia: ASTM Publications, 1985:208–223.
12. McKellop H, Clarke I, Markolf K, Amstutz H. Friction and wear properties of polymer, metal and ceramic prosthetic joint materials evaluated on a multichannel screening device. *J Biomed Mater Res* 1981;15:619–653.
13. Meers DC. *Materials and orthopaedic surgery*. Baltimore: Williams and Wilkins, 1979.
14. *Metals handbook, failure and prevention,* vol 8. Metals Park, OH: American Society for Metals, 1975.
15. Morrey BF, ed. *Total joint arthroplasty*. New York: Churchill Livingstone, 1991.
16. Petch NJ. Petch theory and Hall-Petch relationships. In: *Mechanical properties of metals*. New York: John Wiley, 1967.
17. Petty W, ed. *Total joint replacement*. Philadelphia: WB Saunders, 1991.
18. Rhines FN, Lemons JE. *Grain boundary hardening in alpha brass*. STP 839. Philadelphia: ASTM Publications, 1984:3–28.
19. Roberts VL, Huiskies R. Special issue on bone biomechanics. *J Biomech* 1987:20(11/12).
20. St. John K, ed. *Particulate debris from medical implants*. STP 1144. Philadelphia: ASTM Publications, 1992.
21. Syrett BC, Acharya A, eds. *Corrosion and degradation of implant materials*. STP 684. Philadelphia: ASTM Publications, 1978.
22. Transactions, Society for Biomaterials Symposium. Retrieval and analysis of surgical implants and biomaterials. Snowbird, UT, 1988.
23. Transactions, Society for Biomaterials Workshop 10. New bone cement. Berlin, Germany, 1992.
24. von Recum A, ed. *Handbook of biomaterials evaluation*. New York: Macmillan, 1986.
25. Williams DF, Roaf R. *Implants in surgery*. London: WB Saunders, 1973.

Biological, Material, and Mechanical Considerations of Joint Replacement, edited by B. F. Morrey. Raven Press, Ltd., New York © 1993.

3

Keynote Address: Biological Implications

*Barbara D. Boyan, *†Zvi Schwartz, *†Jona Sela, ‡Jeffrey Hambleton, *Bryan Brooks, *Monica Luna, and *Stefan Kreuzer

*Department of Orthopaedics, University of Texas Health Science Center at San Antonio, San Antonio, Texas 78284-7774; †Hebrew University Hadassah Faculty of Dental Medicine, Jerusalem 91-010, Israel; ‡Wilford Hall Medical Center (USAF), Lackland Air Force Base, Lackland, Texas 78236

GENERAL CONSIDERATIONS

Biological implications for orthopaedic implants begin the moment the initial surgical incision is made (7). All subsequent events develop as a consequence of the wound-healing response. The success of the process is tightly regulated in space and time by the cascade of factors synthesized and secreted by the succession of cells populating the wound (9,11,18). These critical early events include the release of inflammatory mediators that attract polymorphonuclear cells (PMNs) to the wound site. Factors released by the PMNs stimulate migration of monocytes and macrophages, which in turn release factors into the wounded region. Fibroblastic mesenchymal cells migrate to the wound site, first using fibronectin and hyaluronic acid, and later collagen, as a scaffold for movement. Once at the site, these cells differentiate, assuming a more mature phenotype. Following the formation of a scar-like fibrous connective tissue, the type III collagen matrix is ultimately remodeled.

In the case of bone, physical forces promote the remodeling of the tissue to its original morphology. However, introduction of implants into the bone causes a shift in the applied forces and a resultant shift in the response of the affected cells. This can alter the balance between bone formation and bone resorption, thereby compromising the clinical success of the implant.

The situation is further complicated by the fact that implant materials elicit a biological response due to their chemical composition and surface texture. This response will vary, depending on the adsorption of serum proteins onto the surface of the material; the ability of cells to attach, proliferate, differentiate, and repair the tissue; the presence of appropriate growth factors; and the type of tissue in apposition to the implant, itself. For orthopaedic implants, this is minimally bone and marrow but may also include cartilage and other connective tissues, such as muscle and skin, as well as epithelia.

The majority of studies concerning the biological response to orthopaedic implants has been at the light microscopic level. These studies have relied on polished sections for visualizing the adaptation of the tissue to the implant. Because of the differences in the physical properties of the material and the tissue, fine detail is often lost. As technology has improved, the quality of the microscopy has also improved. Little is known, however, concerning the mechanisms of cellular response. Some of this is due to the availability of a limited number of suitable animal models. Cell biologists have shied away from the field because of the difficulties in working with the kinds of materials commonly used as implants. Recently, scientists have begun to look at the cellular response to the materials using innovative methodology. Some of this research will be described briefly below.

OSTEOGENESIS ASSOCIATED WITH MARROW ABLATION: EFFECTS OF IMPLANTS

Injury to marrow initiates endosteal bone formation. In rats, when the marrow is ablated, as it would be for joint replacement, new woven bone fills up the marrow cavity. During the osteogenic phase, bone-promoting factors are released by the regenerating bone marrow (15). We have examined the process with respect to early events involved in mineralization of the osteoid (38,40). These ultrastructural and biochemical studies have provided a quantitative assessment of events associated with matrix vesicle production, maturation, and degradation not only in the ablated bone (Table 1), but also in the contralateral limb (data not shown).

Ultimately, the newly formed bone is remodeled and the bone returns to its normal morphology. Thus, for long-term assessments of normal bone healing, the effects of subtle alterations in the wound-healing cascade may not be evidenced at later time points. However, the ability of bone cells to rapidly synthesize and mineralize osteoid may be critical to the long-term acceptance and retention of an implant material, whether it be titanium, titanium alloy, stainless steel, a bioceramic, or polymer.

This hypothesis led us to examine the effects of implant materials on the osteogenic response of ablated marrow (31,37,39). The results of these studies show that the morphology of matrix vesicles and the number produced by the osteogenic cells is altered by the presence of implants. Materials described as "bonding" promote matrix vesicle production (number of matrix vesicles per square micrometer of matrix) at early time points, whereas those that are "nonbonding" do not. Maturation

TABLE 1. *Changes in matrix vesicle structure and function during endosteal healing*

	Days of healing				
Parameter	0	3	6	14	21
Number/μm^{2a}	N.P.	1.7 ± 0.0	1.9 ± 0.0	1.7 ± 0.0	1.6 ± 0.1
Alkaline phosphatase[b]	0.5 ± 0.1	3.0 ± 0.8	10.7 ± 1.5^c	8.2 ± 1.8^c	2.2 ± 0.9
Phospholipase A_2[d]	1.6 ± 0.3	2.8 ± 0.4	11.5 ± 2.1^c	11.4 ± 1.8^c	2.9 ± 0.4
Phosphatidylserine[e]	0.1 ± 0.1	0.2 ± 0.1	5.5 ± 1.4^c	8.5 ± 0.8	0.8 ± 0.4

[a]Number of matrix vesicles per square micrometer of matrix measured on transmission electron microscope micrograph as part of the morphometric analysis.

[b]Specific activity of alkaline phosphatase expressed as micromoles of inorganic phosphate per protein/minutes.

[c]Signifies the difference versus time 0.

[d]Specific activity of phospholipase A_2 expressed as percentage of hydrolysis per milligram of protein per minute.

[e]Phosphatidylserine content expressed as micrograms of phospholipids per leg.

Each point is the mean $\pm$ SEM.

of matrix vesicle morphology is delayed, however. In addition, the matrix vesicles differ biochemically from those isolated from normally healing bone. There are several explanations for these observations: (a) adherent serum proteins have altered the attachment of cells to the material and/or their maturation, thereby altering the apparent cellular response (5); (b) ions leached from the materials affect the cells, regulating cellular function (8,33); (c) ions from the materials directly affect the matrix vesicles in the matrix, altering their activity; (d) other cells present in the healing bone are affected, releasing factors that affect the osteogenic cells.

SYSTEMIC EFFECTS OF IMPLANT MATERIALS

Injury to bone is known to promote an osteogenic response in other bones in the body (2,22). Although this observation is used empirically in clinical practice, the biology of the effect is not well understood. Animal models, particularly the rat, have provided the first quantitative assessments of the systemic effects of bone injury (4,13,28). The mechanism of the systemic effect is unclear. Investigators have hypothesized release of a unique bone-wound–healing factor, but there is little evidence to support such an entity. A more likely possibility is that injury to bone causes systemic release of a mixture of factors that target bone preferentially. It may also be that the systemic effects of bone injury result from a perturbation of the general wound-healing response that is detected in bone because the researchers have looked for it there.

One might presume that biocompatible implant materials would not interfere with such a generalized systemic response. However, recent studies in our laboratory have shown that this is not the case (37,39). Changes in the biochemistry of matrix vesicles in the contralateral limb following marrow ablation and implantation are altered from those observed during normal healing (Fig. 1). Moreover, the changes

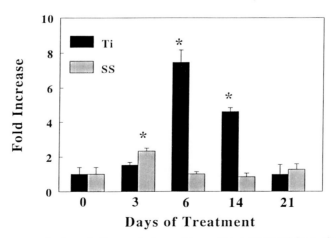

FIG. 1. Fold increase of phospholipase A_2 in matrix vesicles isolated from the unimplanted, contralateral limb following marrow ablation and implantation of rat tibia with titanium (Ti) or stainless steel (SS). Values are derived from the means of six samples, where each sample represents the matrix vesicles isolated from the endosteal bone of six rats. *$p < 0.05$, each day versus time 0. Rats were killed on days 0, 3, 6, 14, and 21 following marrow ablation.

are dependent on the nature of the implant. For nonbonding implants, there may even be suppression of matrix vesicle enzyme activity below that seen in normal bone.

Two possible mechanisms can be proposed to account for this. It is likely that the presence of the implant in the treated bone has altered the release of wound-healing factors by the cells at the wound site and this implant-specific mix of factors has entered into the general circulation. In addition, leached ions from the implant will also be present in serum (25), thereby affecting not only contralateral bone but other tissue as well. It is clear that mechanical forces alone cannot account for this systemic response because the changes observed for each material are distinct and unlike those of marrow-ablated, nonimplanted animals.

UNDERSTANDING CELLULAR RESPONSE
TO ORTHOPAEDIC IMPLANT MATERIALS

In vitro studies of cellular response to implants have been limited by the physical characteristics of the materials used. Conventional cell culture relies on the ability

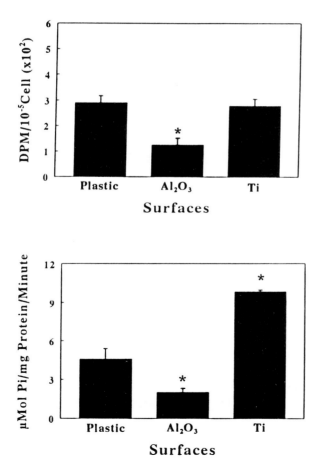

FIG. 2. Alkaline phosphatase specific activity and [³H]-thymidine incorporation in growth zone chondrocytes cultured on sputter-coated titanium (Ti) or aluminum oxide (Al₂O₃) surfaces. Values are the means ± SEM of six confluent, fourth-passage cultures of rat costochondral chondrocytes. *$p < 0.05$ for culture surface versus tissue culture plastic. DPM, disintegrations per minute; Pi, inorganic phosphate.

of the investigator to monitor cell morphology by phase contrast microscopy. Unfortunately, the density of the implant materials prevents this; as a consequence, many of the analyses using cells cultured on thin disks of the material of interest are indirect. Biochemical data are expressed as a function of cell number or protein or DNA content (17), but it is not possible to know whether the cultures are confluent or if nodules have formed. Visualization of cell morphology has been by scanning electron microscopy, after the fact (5,10,29). Even with these difficulties, there have been advances in our understanding of matrix synthesis by connective tissue cells, including chondrocytes, osteoblast-like cells and marrow cells, cultured on various implant surfaces (17). These studies indicate that connective tissue cells show distinct differences in their response to orthopaedic materials.

Recently, scientists at the University of Texas Health Science Center at San Antonio developed culture plates that have been sputter coated with transparent films of various orthopaedic materials (41). Although the surfaces that result are not comparable to the implant surfaces seen by cells *in vitro,* they do permit analysis of cell response to a material using conventional cell culture techniques. These culture plates have been used to study the response of osteoblasts, osteoclasts, and epithelial cells to titanium, among other materials. The results demonstrate that these cells exhibit phenotypic differences depending on the surface on which they were cultured.

We have used growth plate chondrocytes to determine whether growth on sputtered titanium or aluminum oxide alters their phenotypic expression. Growth on titanium had no effect on proliferation, but enhanced differentiation when compared to tissue culture plastic. In contrast, growth on the aluminum oxide surface resulted in inhibition of both parameters (Fig. 2). These data show that cells other than osteoblasts are affected by implant materials and that the effects are material specific.

BONE RESORPTION

Bone is continuously remodeling; therefore, the implant is exposed to osteoclasts and the factors that activate them throughout its life in the patient (14,30). The surface properties of the implant, including any surface coatings or cement, can markedly affect osteoclastic activity. This is particularly true for implants with hydroxyapatite coatings. One reason for this is that osteoclasts and their precursors are attracted to osteocalcin, a protein synthesized by bone-forming cells, which adsorbs onto hydroxyapatite (12) and is postulated to coat bone mineral. Hydroxyapatite is an excellent material for chromatographic separation of proteins *in vitro* due to its ability to bind proteins with varying affinity. *In vivo,* it is rapidly coated with osteocalcin as well as with other serum proteins, such as fibronectin (34), which regulate bone formation. Although osteoblasts may be encouraged to form bone more readily on a hydroxyapatite surface, resorption of the newly formed bone, and the implant's hydroxyapatite coating, may be enhanced as well. Once the coating is gone, the resident cells must interact with the underlying material under circumstances that are no longer stimulated by the critical inflammatory response needed for bone healing. Regulation of the osteoclast precursors by the implant may play as important a role as regulation of the osteoclast itself.

Bone resorption around an implant can occur via other mechanisms as well. Septic loosening is a major problem. Adsorption of serum proteins to the surface of the implant can have marked effects on the binding of osteolytic bacteria and their eventual colonization (24,26,35). Proteolytic enzymes produced by the bacteria can cause tissue destruction directly. In addition, toxins released by the bacteria activate local bone resorbing cells (16).

Aseptic loosening of components for joint replacement is still an unsolved problem. The focus of much research has been on the pseudomembrane structure that forms at the bone-cement interface (1,36). This tissue has the histological characteristics of a foreign body reaction due, presumably, to repeated microtrauma-associated release of methacrylate cement and polyethylene wear debris (3). One role of the macrophages and giant cells present in aseptic loosening may be to degrade matrix proteins, thereby exposing the mineral phase to osteoclasis. The membrane produces prostaglandins (PGE_2) as well as growth factors (interleukin-1, tumor necrosis factor), which stimulate bone resorption (6,21,23). Inflammatory mediators, like the prostaglandins, are retained in the fibrous membrane that separates cemented implants from the bone surface, thereby exacerbating the resorptive response (20).

Progress in understanding the effects of particulates on the immune response has been slow, due to the need for well-characterized materials. Polymer cement particles in rabbit tibias have been shown to produce a foreign body histological reaction that is similar to that associated with prosthetic loosening in humans. For example, the membrane surrounding the particulate cement exhibited high PGE_2 production (19). Studies have also shown that monocytes and macrophages are activated by particulates and release cytokines, which stimulate bone resorption (32).

The role osteoblasts play in loosening prostheses is also not understood. Solubilization of hydroxyapatite by osteoblasts is two to 10 times greater than by fibroblasts (27). Studies on the toxicity of the leading ion (8,33) suggest that inhibition of osteogenic activity may also play a role.

SUMMARY

The studies described in this brief review demonstrate that the success of orthopaedic implants depends on maximizing biological responses to them. To accomplish this, it is necessary to understand the basic underlying mechanisms of tissue and cellular response. New models, both *in vivo* and *in vitro,* are required. Issues include the adsorption of serum proteins on the implant surface; the attachment, proliferation, and differentiation of appropriate cells; autocrine, paracrine, juxtacrine, and endocrine regulation of the cells; and mechanisms of septic and aseptic loosening. A more thorough understanding of the systemic effects of implant materials is critical.

ACKNOWLEDGMENTS

The authors thank Ms. Sandra Messier for her assistance in the preparation of the manuscript. We are indebted to our laboratory research team, particularly Ruben Gomez, Stephanie Scheele, and Roland Campos. This research is supported by PHS grants DE-05937 and DE-08603, the Biomedical Development Corporation, the US/Israel Binational Science Foundation, and the State/Industry/University Cooperative Research Center for the Enhancement of the Biology/Biomaterials Interface at the University of Texas Health Science Center at San Antonio.

REFERENCES

1. Amstutz HC, Campbell P, Kossovsky N, Clark IC. Mechanisms and clinical significances of wear debris induced osteolysis. *Clin Orthop* 1992;76:7–18.
2. Andersson SM, Nilsson BE. Changes in bone mineral content following tibial shaft fracture. *Clin Orthop* 1979;144:226–229.
3. Appel AM, Sowder WG, Siverhus SW, Hopson CN, Herman JH. Prosthesis associated with pseudomembrane-induced bone resorption. *Br J Rheumatol* 1990;29:32–36.
4. Bab I, Gazit D, Massarawa A, Sela J. Removal of tibial marrow induces increased formation of bone and cartilage in rat mandibular condyle. *Calcif Tissue Int* 1985;37:551–555.
5. Bagambisa FB, Joos U, Schilli W. Interaction of osteogenic cells with hydroxylapatite implant materials *in vitro* and *in vivo*. *Int J Oral Maxillofac Implant* 1990;5:217–226.
6. Bell RS, Schtzker J, Fornasier VL, Goodman SD. Study of implant failure in the Wagner resurfacing arthroplasty. *J Bone Joint Surg* 1988;67:1165–1174.
7. Binderman I. Bone and biologically compatible materials in dentistry. *Curr Opin Dentistry* 1991; 1:836–840.
8. Blumenthal NC, Posner AS, Cosma V, Gross U. The effect of glass ceramic bone implant materials on the in vitro formation of hydroxyapatite. *J Biomed Mater Res* 1988;22:1033–1041.
9. Bonewald LF, Mundy GR. Role of transforming growth factor beta in bone remodeling. *Clin Orthop* 1990;250:261–276.
10. Brook IM, Craig GT, Lamb DJ. *In vitro* interaction between primary bone organ cultures, glass-isonomer cements and hydroxyapatite/tricalcium phosphate ceramics. *Biomaterials* 1991;12:179–186.
11. Canalis E, McCarthy TL, Centrella M. Growth factors and cytokines in bone cell metabolism. *Annu Rev Med* 1991;42:17–24.
12. Defranco DJ, Glowacki J, Cox KA, Lian JB. Normal bone particles are preferentially resorbed in the presence of osteocalcin deficient bone particles *in vivo*. *Calcif Tissue Int* 1991;49:43–50.
13. Einhorn JA, Simon G, Devlin VJ, Warman J, Sidhu SP, Vigorita VJ. The osteogenic response to distant skeletal injury. *J Bone Joint Surg [Am]* 1990;72:1374–1378.
14. Galante JO, Jacobs J. Clinical performance of ingrowth surfaces. *Clin Orthop* 1992;276:41–49.
15. Gazit D, Karmish M, Holzman L, Bab I. Regenerating marrow induces systemic increase in osteo- and chondrogenesis. *Endocrinology* 1990;126:2007–2013.
16. Gillespie WD, Allardyce RA. Mechanisms of bone degradation in infection: a review of current hypotheses. *Orthopedics* 1990;13:407–410.
17. Goldring SR, Flannery MS, Petrison KK, Evins AE, Jasty MJ. Evaluation of connective tissue cell responses to orthopaedic implant materials. *Connect Tissue Res* 1990;24:77–81.
18. Goldring MB, Goldring SR. Skeletal tissue response to cytokines. *Clin Orthop* 1990;258:245–278.
19. Goodman SB. Suppression of prostaglandin E_2 synthesis in the membrane surrounding particulate polymethylmethacrylate in the rabbit tibia. *Clin Orthop* 1991;271:300–304.
20. Goodman SB, Chin RC. Prostaglandin E_2 level in the membrane surrounding bulk and particulate polymethylmethacrylate in the rabbit tibia: a preliminary study. *Clin Orthop* 1990;257:305–309.
21. Goodman SB, Chin RL, Chiou SS, Schurman D, Woolson ST, Masada MP. A clinical pathologic biochemical study of the membrane surrounding loosened and nonloosened total hip arthroplasties. *Clin Orthop* 1989;244:182–187.
22. Guzel I, Muller WA. Bone mineral metabolism in mice after fracture of tibia. Double labeling with Ca and Ra. *Biophysics* 1973;10:262–272.
23. Herman JH, Sowder WG, Anderson D, Appel AM, Hopson CN. Polymethylmethacrylate induced release of bone resorbing factors. *J Bone Joint Surg [Am]* 1989;71:1530–1541.
24. Holt SC, Bramanti TE. Factors in virulence expression and their role in periodontal disease pathogenesis. *Crit Rev Oral Biol Med* 1991;2:177–281.
25. Jacobs JJ, Skipor AK, Black J, Urban RM, Galante JO. Release and excretion of metal in patients who have a total hip-replacement component made of titanium-base alloy. *J Bone Joint Surg [Am]* 1991;73:1475–1486.
26. Keogh BS, Triplett RG, Aufdemorte TB, Boyan BD. The effect of local antibiotics in treating chronic osseous Staphylococcus aureus infection. *J Oral Maxillofac Surg* 1989;47:2–7.
27. Kwong CH, Burns WB, Cheung HS. Solubilization of hydroxyapatite crystals by murine bone cells, macrophages and fibroblasts. *Biomaterials* 1989;10:577–584.
28. Lowe J, Bab I, Stein H, Sela J. Primary calcification in remodeling haversian systems following tibial fracture in rats. *Clin Orthop* 1983;176:291–297.
29. Malik MA, Puleo DA, Bizios R, Doremus RH. Osteoblasts on hydroxyapatite, alumina and bone surfaces *in vitro*: morphology during the first 2 h of attachment. *Biomaterials* 1992;13:128.
30. Maloney WJ, Jasty M, Harris WH, Galante JO, Callaghan JS. Endosteal erosion in association with stable uncemented femoral components. *J Bone Joint Surg [Am]* 1990;72:1025–1034.
31. Marshall TS, Schwartz Z, Swain LD, et al. Matrix vesicle enzyme activity in endosteal bone

following implantation of bonding and non-bonding implant materials. *Clin Oral Implant Res* 1991;2:112–120.

32. Murray DW, Rae T, Rushton N. The influence of the surface energy and roughness of implants on bone resorption. *J Bone Joint Surg [Br]* 1989;71:632–637.

33. Pappas AM, Cohen J. Toxicity of metal particles in tissue culture. *J Bone Joint Surg [Am]* 1968;50:535–556.

34. Pearson BS, Klebe RJ, Boyan BD, Moskowicz D. Comments on the clinical application of fibronectin in dentistry. *J Dent Res* 1988;67:515–517.

35. Sanderson PJ. Infection in orthopaedic implants. *Hosp Infec* 1991;18:367–375.

36. Schmalzried TP, Kwong LM, Jasty M, et al. The mechanisms of loosening of cemented acetabular components in total hip arthroplasty: analysis of specimens retrieved at autopsy. *Clin Orthop* 1992;274:60–78.

37. Schwartz Z, Amir D, Boyan BD, et al. Effect of glass ceramic and titanium implants on primary calcification during rat tibial bone healing. *Calcif Tissue Int* 1991;49:359–364.

38. Schwartz Z, Sela S, Ramirez V, Amir D, Boyan BD. Changes in extracellular matrix vesicles during healing of the rat tibial bone: a morphometric and biochemical study. *Bone* 1989;10:53–60.

39. Schwartz Z, Swain LD, Marshall T, et al. Modulation of matrix vesicle enzyme activity and phosphatidylserine content by ceramic implant materials during endosteal bone healing. *Calcif Tissue Int* 1992;51:429–437.

40. Sela J, Amir D, Schwartz Z, Weinberg D. Changes in the distribution of extracellular matrix vesicles during healing of rat tibial bone: computerized morphometry and electron microscopy. *Bone* 1987;8:245–250.

41. Windler AS, Bonewald L, Khare AG, Boyan BD. The influence of sputtered bone substitutes on cell growth and phenotypic expression. The Bone-Biomaterials Interface and International State of the Art Workshop. Toronto, Canada, 1990.

Biological, Material, and Mechanical
Considerations of Joint Replacement,
edited by B. F. Morrey.
Raven Press, Ltd., New York © 1993.

4

Device Function and Retrieval

Classification of ASTM/AAOS Bioengineering Committee

Bernard F. Morrey

Department of Orthopaedics, Mayo Clinic, Rochester, Minnesota 55905

The value of implant retrieval has long been recognized. The importance of standardizing terminology, retrieval expectations, methods, analysis, and communication of findings in a reliable and timely fashion to the orthopedic community has been a particular concern of the American Academy of Orthopaedic Surgeons (AAOS) for a number of years.

The ultimate goal of any intervention following a prosthetic implant is to improve the functional life of the extremity or joint. Typically this is accomplished by the successful realization of several factors: patient selection, technical implantation, compliance by the patient, and implant integrity. The realization of such goals is determined by the effectiveness as well as the duration of the implant device, specifically as it relates to improved joint or unit function. The corollary of this is that analysis of the failure mode is helpful to further delineate the success of the implant and provide data that may enhance its longevity or optimize its function.

In spite of the frequent occurrence of revision surgery, the precise incidence, analysis, and interpretation of retrieved implanted material remain difficult to determine and assimilate. One problem in the past has been confusion regarding the discrete differences in the need to remove implants. Removal of an intramedullary rod after fracture healing, revision of a loose prosthetic device 20 years after implantation, and removal of a prosthesis 3 years after insertion because of debris all constitute instances of implant retrieval. However, the implications are dramatically different.

It is obvious that this complex issue cannot be effectively addressed by attributing a single cause of failure or considering in the same fashion all clinical circumstances. The Bioengineering Committee of the AAOS and the F-4 section of ASTM have recognized this discrepancy. In 1987 a symposium was cosponsored by the ASTM and AAOS Bioengineering Committee to help to clarify and define a classification of retrieved implants. As a result of this discussion, consideration of the features under which a surgical implant might be revised was classified in three broad categories: (i) patient-related factors, (ii) elements that relate to surgical judgment or technical execution, and (iii) features involving the integrity of the implant itself (Table 1).

TABLE 1. *Implant retrieval*

I. Planned
    A. Routine—open reduction and internal fixation
        1. Avoids complications of the implant or the effect of its presence
II. Unplanned factors
    A. Patient
        1. Disease: Paget's disease, osteogenesis imperfecta
        2. Compliance: impact loading, obesity
        3. Accidents: fracture, dislocation
    B. Procedure
        1. Implant selection: cemented, uncemented; constrained, unconstrained
        2. Technique: malalignment
    C. Implant
        1. Design
        2. Manufacture
           a. Fabrication
           b. Quality control

Factors determining the types of implant retrieval based on the AAOS-ASTM Workshop, 1987.

PATIENT-RELATED FACTORS

The physical, physiologic, and biomechanical effects of some disease states may influence the host in such a way as to compromise the short- or long-term functional success of an implanted device. All physicians recognize that osteogenesis imperfecta is a condition that may not allow the long-term success of a joint replacement. Underlying medications such as steroids may also have a systemic effect that influences the survival of some device replacements. Dietary problems, the consumption of alcohol, and even smoking may also adversely affect the results of joint replacement surgery. In addition to these disease states, compliance with instructions, maintenance of an ideal body weight, and physical activity can also directly affect the longevity of the prosthetic device. Finally, aspects that are beyond the patient's control, such as accidental events that disrupt the reconstructed part, may result in failure that cannot be reversed by improved technique, patient selection, or implant design.

SURGICAL JUDGMENT

It is well recognized that in all elective surgery, patient selection is an important consideration. It is also well recognized that high-risk factors such as youth, activity, obesity, and catabolic medication can adversely affect the longevity of an implant. The surgeon's selection of the type of fixation for a given prosthesis and for certain conditions may affect the long-term success of the device more so than the activity of the disease, the patient, or implant design.

SURGICAL TECHNIQUE

The insertion of prosthetic or reconstructive devices is typically very technically demanding. Evidence suggests that a successful outcome is directly related to the technical competence or precision of device insertion. In some instances, due to deformity brought about by the disease state, it may be difficult to attain the desired technical goals. Nonetheless, this particular variable and patient selection tend to be factors relating to implant failure that are within the control of the surgeon.

DEVICE INTEGRITY

Finally, a failed device may be directly associated with the integrity of the device. This takes three broad forms: (i) the design, (ii) materials, and (iii) manufacturing process.

Design

Design failure is known to all; one obvious example of a design failure is that due to a stress riser. Inadequate substance or configuration to accommodate the loads carried by the joint is a generic description of implant failure. The reason for such failure is a lack of awareness of the normal kinematics and force transmission required of the device or frank error in the design parameters. This type of failure was particularly prevalent in the early years of joint replacement when the comprehension of normal joint biomechanics was lacking.

Material Selection

Deficiencies in material selection may take two forms. One is that the material is inappropriate for the intended application. An example of this is the early attempts to use Teflon as a bearing surface. The adverse reaction to particulate debris rendered this substance inappropriate for consideration of any joint replacement arthroplasty. The second is that the material is inappropriate for the specific use intended. This type of deficiency was seen when high-density polyethylene was used to fashion the intramedullary component of artificial joints. The strength of this material was simply inadequate to withstand the loads imparted to it, and a high fracture rate and subsequent debris formation were common.

Manufacturing Process

The manufacturing industry typically follows ASTM standards when fabricating artificial implants. However, the standards do not govern the intended use of the device. The discrepancy is added to by the inadequate understanding of the kinematics or kinetics of the replaced part. For example, the manufacturing process of high-density polyethylene for knee joint replacement with a thin tibial component becomes vulnerable to wear.

IMPEDIMENTS

The study of retrieved devices is an invaluable resource to understand implant success and failure modes. Unfortunately the transmission and implementation of insights gained from the study of retrieved implants have been significantly hampered by potential litigious actions stemming from the publication of such material. It is unlikely that this circumstance will change in the near future. This reality places a significant burden on other methods of communication, such as the Bristol-Myers Squibb/Zimmer Orthopaedic Symposium.

*Biological, Material, and Mechanical
Considerations of Joint Replacement,*
edited by B. F. Morrey.
Raven Press, Ltd., New York © 1993.

5

Cemented and Hydroxyapatite-Coated Hip Implants

An Autopsy Retrieval Study

Archie J. Malcolm

*University Department of Pathology, Royal Victoria Infirmary,
Newcastle-upon-Tyne NE1 4LP, United Kingdom*

The most frequent serious long-term complication of all joint prostheses is aseptic loosening (2,15). Because of an increasing problem of loosening of cemented prostheses with time, there was a rapid growth in the design and use of uncemented prostheses in an effort to reduce the failure rate. Many of these newer designs, however, have similarly failed. It is now apparent that osseointegration of cement and bone can occur and remain stable for many years (9). Many implant retrieval studies have shown that there is limited bone ingrowth into porous-coated implants, much of the implant being secured by fibrous tissue (3). Although there has been a return to the use of cemented prostheses, at least on the femoral side, some investigators have introduced hydroxyapatite coatings (HAC) onto press-fit and porous-coated implants in the hope that this might accelerate and assure bone ingrowth, following animal models that demonstrated the osteoinductive properties of hydroxyapatite (4).

However, it is not just implant materials, methods and quality of fixation, and mechanical factors that are implicated in aseptic loosening. Biological factors, such as tissue response to implants and the response of bone to the new stresses placed on it by the implant and osteoporosis, have been investigated in the context of loosening. The tissue response to wear particles has been particularly scrutinized in recent years (7). Many of these biological factors are problems common to all of the prostheses currently available.

This report, which includes autopsy-retrieved Charnley prostheses studies, emphasizes the fixation that cement can confer on the femoral side of hip arthroplasty. It describes the pathology of nine autopsy-retrieved hydroxyapatite-coated prostheses that have withstood up to 26 months of use—a unique collection. The study also reemphasizes the potential problems caused by wear debris.

MATERIALS AND METHODS

Cemented Prostheses

Seventy-eight Charnley hip joint replacements were retrieved at autopsy from 62 patients who had good or excellent clinical results. The specimens had been functioning from 7 months to 20 years with an average of 14.2 years. Sixty-four hip joint replacements were in females, 14 in males, and 16 patients had bilateral replacements. At the time of implantation the ages ranged from 46.7 to 80 years (average 68.6 years). Fifty-six patients underwent hip joint replacement for osteoarthritis, 15 for rheumatoid arthritis, three for protrusio, two for congenital dislocation of the hip, and two for Paget's disease of bone. Fifty-two of the 78 specimens were in the form of a cemented stem and cemented, high-density polyethylene cup. Nineteen patients had cemented stems with press-fit, metal-backed cups, and there were six patients who had cemented stems with cemented cups as revisions from previous arthroplasties in which a Teflon cup had been inserted. All the specimens had been sliced longitudinally and the metal femoral component removed. It was therefore not possible to examine the metal-cement interface. All the acetabular cups were still seated within the pelvic bone and all specimens had a soft-tissue capsule. A minimum of three cross-sections from every femoral component were taken to correspond to the lines of Gruen et al. (5), namely, zones 1 and 7, 6 and 2, and 5 and 3. A few cases also had sections taken from zone 4. All the sections were subjected to specimen radiography prior to being processed undecalcified using a technique that prevents dissolution of the bone cement (10). All the blocks were then cut at 7 μm using a Reichert-Jung motorized microtome, and the sections were stained using hematoxylin-eosin and the Masson-Goldner method. This method allows differentiation between mineralized bone, osteoid, fibrous tissue, and cellular tissue. The sections retained the cement, and therefore the bone-cement interface could be examined at a microscopic level. Sections through the center of the cemented acetabulae were prepared in the same way. In addition, some of the more interesting cases were subjected to microradiology using 50-μm thick sections, and some specimens from both the femoral bone-cement interface and the acetabular bone-cement interface were prepared for scanning electron microscopy. The capsular soft tissues were subjected to routine histology together with some immunostaining for the demonstration of macrophages using antibodies to alpha$_1$-antitrypsin and muramidase. Some of the capsular tissues were also subjected to transmission electron microscopy.

Forty-nine cemented femoral and 39 acetabular cases had their postoperative radiographs and the radiographs nearest to the date of death reviewed by three clinicians. The findings in the last radiograph were correlated with the pathology.

Hydroxyapatite-Coated Prostheses

Nine autopsy-retrieved hydroxyapatite-coated Furlong femoral prostheses from eight patients (ages 46–85 years, average 69.2 years) were available for study. These prostheses had been inserted 1 to 26 months (average 6.9) prior to death. Three patients had metastatic carcinoma to the femoral neck, three had osteoporotic femoral neck fracture, one suffered bilateral osteoarthritis, and the last patient suffered unilateral osteoarthritis. There were six hydroxyapatite-coated Furlong acetabular components.

All specimens were subjected to gross radiology, sectioned transversely by a diamond-edged circular saw operated by a stepper motor. Sections were taken at the top, middle, and bottom of the specimen through bone and metal to correspond with the radiological zones of Gruen et al. (zones 1 and 7, 2 and 6, and 3 and 5). The resultant 10-mm-thick blocks were embedded in the same plastic as that used for the cemented prostheses. The same saw was used to cut 1-mm sections that were radiographed and then had both surfaces polished. Sections were glued to large, clear plastic mounts and surface stained. The acetabular specimens were embedded in their entirety in plastic and sections were prepared from each quadrant as for the femoral component. Capsular tissue was processed using routine procedures.

RESULTS

Cemented Prostheses

Femoral Aspects

Sixty of the 78 femoral specimens showed an intact bone-cement interface throughout the length of the femoral component. The sections showed mineralized bone pegs integrated intimately with the bone cement and that the intervening tissue between these bone pegs contained fatty and hematopoietic marrow (Fig. 1). In a small number of cases there was a single cell layer of foreign-body giant cells between the cement and fatty marrow. A few of the bone pegs showed caps of osteoid. The specimen radiographs showed multiple voids within the cement layer, but the majority of cases showed an intact bone-cement interface even at the microradiological level. No microfractures of cement were found. When the bone-cement interface was examined microscopically, it could be seen that in places the cement indented the mineralized bone, thus outlining spherules of cement. This bone was viable and of lamellar type (Fig. 2). Scanning electron microscopy of the bone-cement interface showed the bone arranged in a coral-like fashion with irregular bone indentations into the corresponding irregular cement indentations. When a cross section of the femur in the area immediately beneath the lesser trochanter was examined, it could be seen that a neocortex of bone had formed at the bone-cement interface, and this neocortex was strutted onto the endosteum of the femur by radiating mineralized bone trabeculae (Fig. 3).

However, 18 of the 78 specimens examined showed a radiolucent line as thick as 2 mm between the bone cement and mineralized bone. This lucent area corresponded to a fibrous membrane interposed between the cement and bone. The fibrous membrane was relatively acellular but contained many tiny wear particles and scattered macrophages. Polarizing microscopy showed these macrophages to contain numerous medium- and small-size shards of high-density polyethylene wear particles. In addition, eight of these 18 cases showed a severe degree of thinning of the bone trabeculae between the neocortex and endosteum of the femur. These thin cross struts occasionally showed microfractures that were healing by cartilaginous rather than osteoblastic tissues. These areas were not avascular. Transmission electron mi-

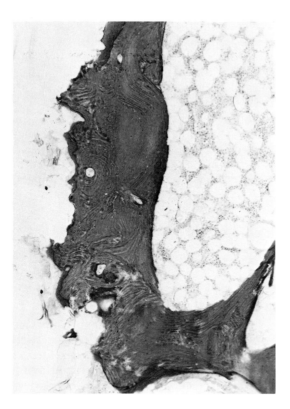

FIG. 1. Cement (*left*) in intimate contact with mineralized viable lamellar bone. Hematopoietic and fatty marrow are present on the *right*. Undecalcified section with Masson-Goldner stain.

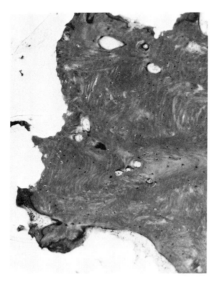

FIG. 2. Viable lamellar mineralized bone with irregular outline in tight apposition to cement with no cellular or fibrous interface. Undecalcified section with Masson-Goldner stain.

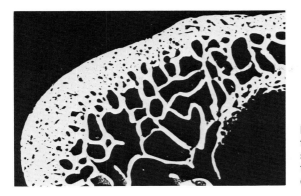

FIG. 3. Microradiograph through section of femur below lesser trochanter showing thin neocortex, bone interdigitation, and radial bone cross struts to cortex.

croscopy showed minute particles of metal and high-density polyethylene in macrophages within the fibrous membranes.

Acetabular Component

All the acetabular components, whether cemented or metal backed, demonstrated a significant lucent line between the cement or prosthesis and the acetabular bone. This lucency could be up to 5 mm. Histological examination showed a thick, relatively acellular fibrous layer interposed between the cement and bone. Within this fibrous layer there were numerous large-, medium-, and small-size wear particles of high-density polyethylene together with some metal particles. The bone beneath the fibrous layer showed both active and previous osteoclastic resorption (Fig. 4). There

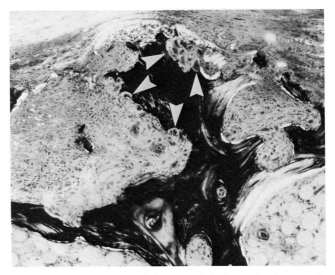

FIG. 4. Partially polarized photomicrograph from acetabulum showing small and tiny birefringent wear particles in macrophages (*left*), fibrous membrane (*top*), and intense osteoclastic activity (*arrows*). Undecalcified section with Masson-Goldner stain.

were numerous macrophages that occasionally aggregated together to form small foreign-body granulomas. The intact bone-cement interface, as seen in most of the femoral components, was not found in any of the acetabular specimens.

Soft Tissues

All the capsular soft tissues showed variable degrees of histiocytic infiltrate with foreign-body giant cells. There were very numerous large, medium, and small wear particles of high-density polyethylene together with a moderate number of tiny metal wear particles. Some, but not all, of the specimens contained islands of cement surrounded by giant cells. The small- and medium-size high-density polyethylene wear particles were contained within macrophages, whereas the very large particles were surrounded by giant cells. There was a mild inflammatory reaction composed predominantly of lymphocytes with a few plasma cells.

Immunoperoxidase staining with alpha$_1$-antitrypsin and muramidase showed that the vast majority of cells present were macrophage in type. Transmission electron microscopy showed that many of these macrophages contained numerous minute particles of both high-density polyethylene and metal, these particles being as small as 0.01 μm.

The six cases that previously had a Teflon acetabular cup showed very large, irregular particles of Teflon still trapped within the soft tissues. These particles were too large to be ingested by macrophages and instead were surrounded by numerous, huge, multinucleated foreign-body giant cells.

Radiological-Pathological Correlation

Each case available for radiological review had the appearances in Gruen zones 1 and 7, 2 and 6, and 3 and 5 on the femoral side of the last clinical radiographs compared to the appropriate histology. Thus, there were 147 areas for comparison. No lucency between bone and cement was found in 131 areas despite histological evidence of fibrosis at the interface in 24. Interestingly, of the 16 areas that showed clinical radiographic lucency, nine had fibrosis as expected, but seven had an intact bone-cement interface.

On the acetabular side of the 39 cases, nine showed no radiological demarcation, but these all had incomplete or complete thin fibrous membranes. The 13 cases that had radiological demarcation of the outer third showed a complete thin or moderately thick fibrous membrane. The seven acetabula that showed demarcation of two-thirds all had a moderate or thick complete fibrous membrane. Nine cases showed complete demarcation, one showed migration, and all had grossly thick fibrous membranes. All membranes, irrespective of thickness, contained wear particles.

Hydroxyapatite-Coated Prostheses

Femoral Components

Irrespective of the underlying disease, age of the patient, or length of the postoperative period, all the implants showed a remarkable degree of osseointegration of the HAC by thin layers of mature lamellar bone. The lamellar bone was found parallel to the HAC and this thin layer often totally encircled the implant. This bone did not appear to be formed in response to stress. In contrast, there were thick new bone trabeculae arranged at right angles to the prosthesis between the implant and endosteum of the cortex, clearly reflecting the new stresses created by the implant. Occasionally new bone encased preexisting bone (Figs. 5 and 6). This cross strutting was seen best in the bone adjacent to the proximal-medial and distal-lateral aspects of the implant, reflecting areas of greatest stress. Fatty and hematopoietic marrow were present near the HAC suggesting that it was not cytotoxic. In one case (retrieved at 26 months), some of the HAC was being resorbed by giant cells, and there were a few areas in the proximal part of the prosthesis where the HAC had disappeared, leaving bare metal. The two most recently inserted cases showed a small amount of marrow fibrosis. A foreign-body reaction was not seen in any of the specimens, and wear particles were not present.

Acetabular Components

All six acetabular components showed some osseointegration with the HAC. Four cases had thick new bone laid down around the screw threads of the cup in response

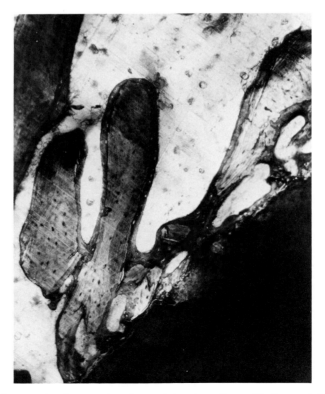

FIG. 5. Photomicrograph of ground surface-stained section with the metal implant (*bottom right*) and new bone trabeculae radiating from the HAC.

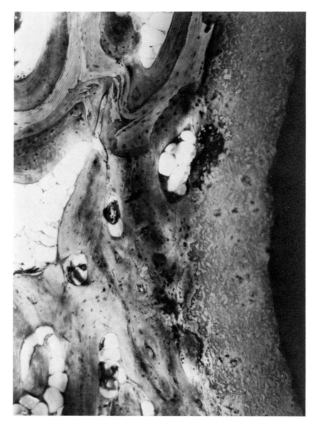

FIG. 6. Photomicrograph of a ground surface-stained section showing the intimate association of bone and HAC (to the *right*). The pale bone is preexisting trabeculae encased in darker staining new bone.

to stress, whereas two cups had clearly migrated after insertion. The latter two showed a thick fibrous layer around the screw threads in the gap between the metal and new bone. The nonthreaded roof of all the cups showed some new bone formation encasing the HAC, and much of this bone did not appear to be stress related. One acetabular specimen showed that the HAC had separated from the metal and viable bone was interposed between the HAC and metal. The acetabular specimen that had been inserted only 2½ months prior to death, showed some fibrosis of adjacent marrow. A foreign body reaction was not seen in any of the specimens and there were no wear particles.

Capsular Tissues

The capsule was fibrotic in all cases, and in seven of the nine specimens, small fragments of HAC were found in relation to foreign-body giant cells. There was no significant inflammation, and a few wear particles were found only in the case that had survived the longest (26 months).

DISCUSSION

Sixty of the 78 femoral specimens showed an intact bone-cement interface with no fibrous layer. Some of these cases had been implanted and used for as long as 20 years. The presence of bone cement within 1 μm of hematopoietic tissue would suggest that toxins from intact cement do not leach and cause cell damage in the long term. The presence of mineralized viable bone integrated with the cement indicates that a true bone-cement osseointegration is possible. The arrangement of this bone within the medullary canal of the femur showed a neocortex with cross struts to the endosteum of the femur. This arrangement, the amount of bone present, and its viability indicate that all of this bone is new and has formed following insertion of the prosthesis. Indeed, when the arrangement of this new bone is examined, it would appear to reflect the new stresses and strains placed on the bone by the insertion and use of the prosthesis. This would be in keeping with Wolff's law (18) that bone is laid down along the line of stress.

In the 18 cases in which the osseointegration was not present throughout the femoral component, a fibrous membrane had formed between the bone cement and bone. Wear particles could be found in this fibrous layer. It seems that these wear particles, having been generated within the joint cavity, migrated into the fibrous membrane. This migration could either be "active" within macrophages or "passive" within the fluid flux that takes place between the fibrous membrane and joint cavity when the prosthesis is cyclically loaded. In either case activated macrophages can release numerous factors including proteinases, collagenases, prostaglandins, interleukin-1, and tumor necrosis factor. Some or all of these factors are known to be potent stimulators of osteoclasts (16). The presence of wear particles will activate macrophages, which will stimulate osteoclasts, causing further bone loss. Indeed it has been suggested that macrophages per se can resorb bone (1). It is therefore possible that one method of fibrous layer formation would be erosion of the proximal femur by activated osteoclasts stimulated by the presence of macrophages containing wear particles and bone resorption perhaps being enhanced by the direct action of the macrophages. As the bone-cement interface is eroded at the proximal end of the femur or around the margin of the acetabulum, more particles can then enter and travel between the cement and bone. As this progresses there will come a time when the cement-bone interface has been sufficiently eroded over its length so that excessive micromotion will take place at the bone-cement interface. This will further enhance wear particle migration around the prostheses. The micromotion will result in increased fibrous membrane formation. With increasing micromotion, there will be increased loosening of the prostheses.

It could be expected that a thin fibrous layer on microscopy may not be detectable on clinical radiographs, as was the case in this study. However, it is more difficult to explain the seven radiolucent areas on clinical radiographs on the femoral side, which did not have a fibrous membrane. These cases had significant osteoporosis of the medullary bone. It is likely that the radiolucency between cement and cortex in these cases is due to osteoporosis.

In eight of the 18 cases in which a fibrous membrane had formed on the femoral side, there were microfractures of the supporting medullary trabeculae. It is known that with increasing age the medullary canal enlarges as the result of endosteal removal of bone and periosteal new bone formation (12). This occurs at a time or age when patients are liable to develop a degree of osteoporosis. The enlargement of the canal would place more reliance on the medullary bone to stabilize the implant, yet that medullary bone is likely to be thinner and weaker than in a younger patient. Sudden stress placed on the supporting trabeculae could result in microfractures. If there were sufficient microfractures occurring at one particular site, then the bone-cement interface would no longer be supported, and with further cyclical loading, the interface would move. The continuous cyclical movement of this interface could result in nonunion of the microfractures and cause a fibrous membrane to form between the bone and cement. Once this fibrous membrane has extended, wear particles could then enter this fibrous membrane and cause further bone erosion. Although fracturing of the cement was not seen in any of the femoral components, despite numerous voids, it is possible that cement mantle fracture could result in micromovement with fibrous membrane formation and loosening.

Sixty of the 78 specimens showed an intact bone-cement interface many years after implantation. All of these patients had wear particles within their soft tissues around the capsule. It would seem that an intact bone-cement interface, with the spaces between the bone pegs being filled by viable fatty or hematopoietic marrow, may act as a biological barrier preventing migration of wear particles.

All the cemented acetabular cups had a fibrous interface between prosthesis/cement and bone and these contained wear particles. They all showed active osteoclastic resorption of the underlying bone. The stresses and strains in the acetabular region are different than those within the femoral component, and it is known that the pelvic bone repairs differently compared to long bones. A combination of these may explain in part the lack of osseointegration. It should be noted that despite the absence of osseointegration in all specimens, none of the patients complained of pain, discomfort, or difficulty in the use of their implant, and only one of the cups had migrated. This confirms previous reports indicating that a fibrous membrane around the acetabular component can be asymptomatic (6), yet the same changes around the femoral component would be symptomatic. It would seem that with the low-friction torque design a fibrous membrane can maintain the position of the socket until factors related to socket wear come into play. It would also appear that for the long-term clinical success, maintenance of the socket position is essential and that osseointegration on the socket side is not necessarily essential.

The presence of wear particles associated with a vigorous macrophage response has been well reported previously, and the findings in these cases are not new (11,17). The size of the wear particles may play an important role in any pathology they may cause. Large particles are unable to be ingested by macrophages and therefore remain at the site of production. It is the medium-size and smaller particles that are able to be transported to sites distant from their production. There is some evidence that transportation of wear particles within macrophages may initiate bone resorption at the interface, particularly in the acetabulum (13). It has been shown that both cement particles and fresh bone fragments are capable of causing scratching, not only of the high-density polyethylene but also stainless steel femoral heads (8). Entrapment of these particles within the joint space following surgery may increase the wear rate, particularly generating small particles, hence hastening prosthesis loosening.

The early results of hydroxyapatite-coated femoral implants suggest that the HAC has strong bone morphogenic properties, thus the advantage of genuine early osseointegration and early fixation, hence early mobilization of the patient (14). There is no evidence of cellular toxicity, and the bone around the prosthesis remodels along lines of stress in keeping with Wolff's law. Early osseointegration has already been reported, but this study indicates that osseointegration persists. However, the HAC can be resorbed, resulting in uncovered metal after 26 months implantation, and this uncovered metal is completely smooth. It may be that, over a period of a few years, the entire coating may be removed, leaving the prosthesis like a smooth press-fit type. In addition, loss of bonding between the HAC and metal has occurred, and this may similarly cause loss of osseointegration.

The early results of hydroxyapatite-coated acetabular threaded components are encouraging in that the components appear secure with good bone ingrowth. However, it is likely that the coating on the acetabular side may also be lost, resulting in loss of fixation. The presence of HAC particles in the capsular tissues even 1 month after insertion suggests that tiny fragments of HAC may be dislodged during insertion of one or another of the components. These HAC particles could interpose between head and cup, resulting in scratching the head and scoring of the cup. This would generate numerous small wear particles, which may lead to failure as proposed in the cemented prostheses.

SUMMARY

It would seem that osseointegration between bone and cement in the femur can occur and remain stable for many years. Hydroxyapatite-coated prostheses also demonstrate rapid osseointegration. Loosening may be caused by a variety of factors and, in many cases, may be of a multifactorial nature. Enlargement of the medullary canal and loss of bone stock may both conspire to cause loosening through fracturing of supporting bone. However, in a significant number of cases the presence of wear particles may either initiate or contribute to loosening on the femoral side. The lack of osseointegration on the cemented acetabular side has been suspected for a long time and this study confirms this. Again it is likely that small wear particles play a major role in acetabular loosening. The initial response of the bone to a hydroxyapatite-coated prosthesis is encouraging, but loss of the HAC through resorption or HAC-metal separation could precipitate failure in the longer term. The presence of HAC fragments in the joint space might cause increased wear particle production analogous to that of cement particles.

ACKNOWLEDGMENTS

I would like to thank the John Charnley Trust for allowing me to examine the specimens in the Charnley collection and James Buchanan for providing me with the HAC specimens. The Charnley study was kindly supported by a grant from Action Research.

REFERENCES

1. Athanasou NA, Quinn J, Bulstrode CJK. Resorption of bone by inflammatory cells derived from the joint capsule of hip arthroplasties. *J Bone Joint Surg [Br]* 1992;74B:57–62.
2. Charnley J. Low friction arthroplasty of the hip. In: *Theory and practice*. New York: Springer, 1979.

3. Engh GA, Bobyn JD, Petersen TL. Radiographic and histologic study of porous coated tibial component fixation in cementless total knee arthroplasty. *Orthopedics* 1988;11:725–738.
4. Geesink RGT, de Groot K, Klein CPAT. Chemical implant fixation using hydroxyl-apatite coatings: the development of a human total hip prosthesis for chemical fixation to bone using hydroxyl-apatite coatings on titanium substrates. *Clin Orthop* 1987;225:147–154.
5. Gruen TA, McNeice GM, Amstutz HC. "Models of failure" of cemented stem-type femoral components. A radiological analysis of loosening. *Clin Orthop* 1979;141:17–27.
6. Hodgkinson JP, Shelley P, Wroblewski BM. The correlation between the roentgenographic appearance and operative findings at the bone-cement junction of the socket in Charnley low friction arthroplasties. *Clin Orthop* 1988;228:105–113.
7. Howie DW, Cornish BL, Vernon-Roberts B. Resurfacing hip arthroplasty. Classification of loosening and the role of prosthetic wear particles. *Clin Orthop* 1990;255:144–153.
8. Isaac GH, Atkinson JR, Dowson D, Kennedy PD, Smith MR. The causes of femoral head roughening in explanted Charnley hip prostheses. *Eng Med* 1987;16:167–173.
9. Malcolm AJ. The bone-cement interface in longstanding prosthetic implants. In: Langlais F, Tomeno B, eds. *Limb salvage*. Berlin: Springer-Verlag, 1991:319–328.
10. Pallet CD, Mawhinney WHB, Malcolm AJ. Plastic processing of cemented hip joint replacement specimens. *J Clin Pathol* 1986;39:339–342.
11. Revell PA. Tissue reactions to joint prostheses and the products of wear and corrosion. *Curr Top Pathol* 1982;71:73–101.
12. Ruff CB, Hayes WC. Subperiosteal expansion and cortical remodelling of the lumen femur and tibia with ageing. *Science* 1982;217:945–951.
13. Schmalzried TP, Kwong LM, Jasty M, et al. The mechanism of loosening of cemented acetabular components in total hip arthroplasty. *Clin Orthop* 1992;274:60–78.
14. Soballe K, Gotfredsen K, Brockstedt-Rasmussen H, Nielsen PT, Rechnagel K. Histologic analysis of a retrieved hydroxy-apatite-coated femoral prosthesis. *Clin Orthop* 1991;272:255–258.
15. Sutherland CJ, Wilde AH, Borden LS, Marks KE. A ten-year follow-up of one hundred consecutive Muller curved stem total hip arthroplasties. *J Bone Joint Surg [Am]* 1982;64:970–983.
16. Thomson BM, Saklatvala J, Chambers TS. Osteoblasts mediate interleukin-1 stimulation of bone resorption by rat osteoclasts. *J Exp Med* 1986;164:107–112.
17. Willert HG, Ludwig J, Semlitsch M. Reaction of bone to methacrylate after hip arthropathy. A long-term gross, light microscopic and scanning electron microscope study. *J Bone Joint Surg [Am]* 1974;56:1368–1382.
18. Wolff J. *Das Gesetz der Transformation der Knochen*. Berlin: Hirschwald, 1892.

Biological, Material, and Mechanical Considerations of Joint Replacement, edited by B. F. Morrey.
Raven Press, Ltd., New York © 1993.

6

The Cement Interface

Retrieval Studies

*William J. Maloney, †‡Thomas P. Schmalzried, §Murali Jasty,
†Louis M. Kwong, and ¶‖William H. Harris

*Palo Alto Medical Clinic, Palo Alto, California 94301-2794; †Harbor-UCLA Medical
Center, Torrance, California 90509; ‡Joint Replacement Institute,
Los Angeles, California 90007; §Orthopaedic Biomechanics Laboratory,
¶Hip and Implant Unit, Massachusetts General Hospital, Boston, Massachusetts 02114;
‖ Department of Orthopaedics, Harvard Medical School, Boston, Massachusetts 02114*

Late aseptic loosening, prosthetic failure, and bone resorption are major problems associated with cemented total hip arthroplasty. In order to gain insight into the initiating events of aseptic loosening and implant failure, it is important to delineate the mechanical and biological response of the implant-cement-bone construct to repetitive *in vivo* loading. Clinical and radiological features of prosthetic failure are discussed in detail elsewhere in this text.

Extensive research has been performed *in vitro* analyzing the behavior of cemented components after acute implantation (6–9,11,15,18,39,41,48,59). These studies have measured strain in the bone and cement and implant stability. Analytical models (14,33,38,58) have been used to evaluate the mechanical behavior of cemented total hip replacement and have improved our understanding, leading to improvement in implant design, surgical technique, and long-term results (44,46,51,52).

As is noted in other sections of this text, these studies are limited in that they model only the conditions that exist immediately after implantation. Joint loading is simulated in a limited number of positions and does not take into account multidirectional forces and loading at the hip joint (16,27,29). By design, they cannot take into account biological processes such as skeletal remodeling and fibrous tissue formation, which cannot only occur at the interface between implant and bone but between implant and cement. In addition, it is difficult to model in the laboratory the effect of fatigue loading on implant and cement.

In vivo animal studies (21,22,25,32,40), as well as *in vitro* tissue culture studies (21,24,28,47), have been used to examine issues of biocompatibility and cellular response. Isolated tissue cultures provide a practical way to study specific aspects of cellular response and overt toxicity. Particulate and bulk materials have been implanted in animals to evaluate both local and systemic responses to bulk and particulate implant materials. Both methods provide valuable information, but isolate biological and mechanical factors.

Finally, much of the information to date on aseptic loosening has come from clinical and radiographic studies (1,10,12,56,57). Conclusions from these studies concerning the mechanism of implant loosening are limited because they are analyzing failed replacements. They delineate the state of the reconstruction at the time of failure, but do not elucidate the events leading up to failure.

For these reasons, analysis of autopsy specimens prior to clinical failure is essential. In addition, although knowledge of the clinical status of the patient is important with reference to hip replacement function, only instrumented mechanical testing allows quantitative assessment of implant stability. These measurements allow placement of the implant along a continuum of implant stability or loosening. This further enhances the interpretation of the findings at the interfaces between bone and cement and cement and implant by permitting correlation of these findings with the mechanical stability of the implant. In this chapter, we review our findings concerning the interface between bone and cement as well as implant and cement with both cemented femoral and acetabular components and correlate these findings to implant stability (35–37,42,53). In addition, our insights into the mechanisms of aseptic loosening based on a detailed analysis of autopsy-retrieved specimens are discussed (36,53).

SPECIMEN ANALYSIS

Implant stability has traditionally been evaluated based on clinical radiographs or gross mechanical testing at the time of revision surgery. A radiolucency between cement and bone has been widely thought to represent fibrous tissue and be associated with aseptic loosening. On the acetabular side, Hodgkinson et al. (30) and Wroblewski et al. (62) have shown that 94% of the acetabular components with a complete radiolucency at the cement-bone interface, regardless of width, were loose at revision surgery. Comparable clinical studies on the femoral side have not been done; however, radiographic grading systems of femoral component stability have emphasized the presence or absence of a radiolucency at the cement-bone interface as well as evidence of implant subsidence or change in position (49).

At revision surgery, push-pull testing has been used to evaluate implant stability. Intraoperative mechanical testing of this type has several inherent problems. The force applied to the implant cannot be quantitated nor applied in sufficient magnitude to mimic *in vivo* conditions. Davy et al. (16) have shown that out-of-plane forces on the femoral component can reach 200 inch-pounds in activities such as rising from a chair or stair climbing. Moreover, intraoperatively, it is not possible to use instrumentation sensitive enough to reliably detect displacement on the order of 20 μm or less. Although these types of analyses are beneficial clinically, they are not adequate to accurately assess implant stability or define a stable implant. Since it is critically important to have an accurate assessment of implant stability to be able to interpret the findings at the interface between implant and host bone, more sensitive testing is required. Therefore, in addition to performing an in-depth radiographic analysis of these autopsy specimens, a detailed biomechanical analysis was performed to assess implant stability (42).

Technique

More than 40 hemipelvi and whole cadaveric femora were harvested at autopsy from patients who had previously undergone cemented total hip replacements. The duration of implantation of these components ranged from 15 days to 17 years. The specimens were radiographed in several planes. The methods of radiographic analysis have been previously reported in detail (37,42,53). Removal of the soft tissues improved the resolution of specimen radiographs as compared to clinical radiographs. Further, it has been demonstrated that multiple views of the acetabulum are necessary in order to visualize both the full extent and maximal width of acetabular radiolucencies. In our experience, the standard anteroposterior view underrepresents the degree of cement-bone interface radiolucencies that are present. For the purpose of this study, a radiolucency was defined as any radiolucent area between bone and cement regardless of the presence or absence of demarcation lines.

Using specially designed loading jigs, the specimens were loaded in a servohydraulic testing machine using physiologic loads. Extensometers, which are electrical displacement transducers, were used to detect motion between implant and bone. By changing the orientation of the extensometers, displacement of the femoral components could be measured in the axial, transverse, and rotational directions. Similarly, acetabular displacement could be determined in several planes.

Mechanical testing of the femoral and acetabular components was performed separately (42,53). The femoral components were loaded in both simulated single-limb stance and stair-climbing positions. The parameters for single-limb-stance loading were based on the data of McCleish and Charnley (44). A 100-lb spinal load was used, resulting in a joint reaction force of 250 lb and an abductor force of 180 lb. The loading parameters for simulated stair climbing were taken from the data of Burke et al. (8). The load was applied to the femur in 30° of flexion. This resulted in a joint reaction force of 400 lb and an abductor muscle force of 100 lb. Rotational stability was also tested using a specially designed torque wrench micrometer that could apply a known torsional load to the femoral component. The acetabular components were tested in the single-limb-stance position using similar loading parameters. In addition, the acetabular components were tested in torque by applying a rotational force to the mouth of the component. The surfaces of the acetabular components were also assessed for surface damage. The acetabular bearing surfaces were examined grossly and analyzed with a dissecting microscope for surface damage and wear mechanisms. Casts were then made of the acetabular bearing surface, and linear wear and the wear angle were measured using a variation of the shadowgraph technique (53). By performing this type of detailed mechanical analysis, the stability of both cemented femoral and acetabular components could be accurately assessed.

After the nondestructive mechanical testing, the autopsy specimens were embedded in potting cement using a coordinate system enabling accurate orientation of the specimens. A high-speed, water-cooled saw with a ceramic blade was used to section the specimens. The femora were sectioned in the transverse plane and the hemipelvi in the coronal plane. Contact radiographs were made of each section. All sections were examined grossly as well as under a dissecting microscope. The integrity of the implant-cement and cement-bone interface and the presence and distribution of the intervening soft tissue were noted. Representative sections were examined using a scanning electron microscope or ground thin for routine histology.

FINDINGS

Radiographic and Biomechanical Analysis

Femoral Component

Only two of the femoral components met the radiographic criteria for definitely loose. One had obviously subsided and one was graded loose based on a new metal-cement radiolucency. Although there were radiolucent lines between the cement and bone in all specimens, only four had complete bone-cement radiolucencies, and in two cases the radiolucencies were complete on both the anteroposterior (AP) and lateral radiographs.

The femoral component with radiographic evidence of subsidence noted above was loose with manual testing. This implant was not tested further mechanically. The remainder of the femoral and acetabular components did not demonstrate motion between implant and bone using manual push-pull tests. Axially, the femoral components were remarkably stable in both single-limb stance and stair-climbing loading (37,42). Only two implants demonstrated axial displacement of more than 30 μm. This stability is comparable to *in vitro* studies testing the stability of acutely cemented femoral components. The greatest micromotion for the cemented femoral components was routinely noted in the transverse plane in stair-climbing loading or in pure rotation with torque testing. In the simulated stair-climbing loading, micromotion ranged from 32 to 249 μm. Using the torque wrench, rotational displacement ranged from 10 to 300 μm with an applied torque of 200 inch-pounds. As expected, the implant with the greatest micromotion on mechanical testing was the implant graded as radiographically loose. In the stair-climbing position, the maximal micromotion of the loose femoral component was 249 μm. These data emphasize the importance of understanding the out-of-plane forces acting on the femoral component.

Acetabular Component

All of the acetabular specimens that we examined have had cement-bone interface radiolucencies. In some cases these radiolucencies were thin (0.5 mm) and limited to the periphery of Charnley zones 1 and/or 3. Other cases have had more extensive radiolucencies including four specimens that had a continuous radiolucent line over the entire cement-bone interface. Although the maximal width of a radiolucent line was seen on the AP projection in only two cases, the obturator oblique projection has proved to be particularly sensitive. When the acetabular component is inserted in anteversion, the obturator oblique projection rotates the mouth of the component into a plane that is nearly parallel with the plane of the x-ray film. Viewing in this projection indicates that the radiolucencies are not linear in Charnley zones 1 and 3, but are in fact circumferential, with their greatest extent and thickness generally at the periphery (intra-articular margin) of the implant. This has been confirmed by computed tomography (CT) scanning in two planes and analysis of the specimen coronal sections.

The results of mechanical testing of the acetabular components from both loading conditions were similar and revealed a continuum of loosening from well fixed to grossly loose. Eight specimens moved less than 100 μm under physiologic loading and a maximum of 114 μm under torque load. These specimens are considered to be well fixed (55). None of these components had a radiolucent line wider than 1 mm. Similar to the clinical results of Hodgkinson et al. (30), the four specimens with a continuous radiolucent line (loose by radiographic criteria) demonstrated the greatest displacements (greater than 250 μm of displacement under torque loading). Thus, in this small series, there is a relationship between the radiographic appearance of the cement-bone interface and the measured mechanical stability of the component. No correlation was found between the results of biomechanical testing and any of the following: age, sex, months of service, type of implant, or inner or outer diameter.

Polyethylene Changes

Analysis of the polyethylene revealed a brown discoloration indicative of oxidation in many cases. Of note, sometimes the oxidation occurred in the loaded portion of the socket and sometimes in the unloaded portion. We have no explanation for this variance at this time. The most common finding on analysis of the acetabular bearing surface was wear polishing (loss of the machining marks from manufacturing) in the loaded portion of the component. Randomly oriented scratches were found in all cases. In general, larger scratches were found in the unloaded portion of the components. Evidence of impingement wear was found on the anterosuperior rim of four all-polyethylene components. The surface of this worn area was not as smooth as the polished areas of the load-bearing surface. In the mechanical testing, motion was observed to occur at the cement-bone interface of these acetabular specimens and not at the polyethylene-cement or metal-cement interface. Deformation of the outer hemisphere or other gross evidence of outer bearing wear was not observed on these components. More subtle, microscopic degrees of wear cannot be excluded at this time.

Wear

In retrieval studies, the shadowgraph technique has been used as an indirect measure of polyethylene wear. The initial internal geometry of the component is assumed to be a hemisphere. Over the life of the patient and the implant, the hard metallic femoral head bores a path into the relatively soft polyethylene acetabular bearing surface. A cast of the internal surface (bearing surface) of the retrieved acetabular component reveals portions of two hemispheres: the original machined hemisphere in the unloaded area and the acquired hemisphere in the load-bearing area. The difference in the center points of the two hemispheres is the linear wear. Volumetric wear is calculated using geometric relationships. The accuracy of the technique is improved by adding a correction factor for the direction of wear (53). The technique actually measures the cumulative deformation of the polyethylene and includes any component that may be due to creep.

All the components that we examined had sufficient deformation of the bearing surface to be measured using this technique. Volumetric wear of the primary components ranged from 130 to 682 mm³. There was a great variation in the volumetric wear rate, ranging from 14 to 71 mm³ per year (a fivefold variation). The highest volumetric wear was in a revision component at 1,280 mm³ over 12.5 years. Despite the great number of variables involved, a rough correlation was found between the volumetric wear of PE and the mechanical stability of the implant (53).

Bone-Cement Interface

The remarkable finding at the cement-bone interface on the femoral side was the paucity of fibrous tissue seen at this interface (35–37,42) (Fig. 1). Despite the frequent occurrence of radiolucencies noted on clinical and specimen radiographs, fibrous tissue at this interface was seen only rarely, with the exception of the implant that was grossly loose on manual testing. This implant had multiple fractures in the cement mantle and extensive fibrous tissue formation at the cement-bone interface. When fibrous tissue was present in the remaining specimens, it most commonly occurred in the proximal 1 to 2 cm and was an extension of particulate-induced membrane formed at the hip joint. In addition, on direct examination of the transverse sections, there was no evidence that the cement-bone interface had failed or was in the process of failing.

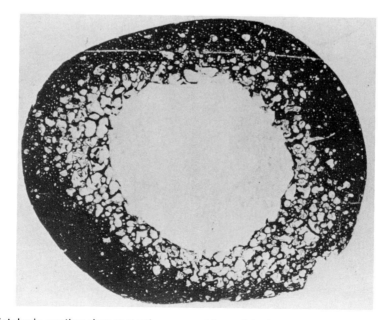

FIG. 1. Histologic section demonstrating cement-bone interface 3.5 years after surgery. The metal has been removed, but the cement remains in place. Note the lack of soft-tissue interposition.

In these specimens, the bone was in intimate contact with the cement with no intervening fibrous tissue over the majority of the surface area. Osseointegration with the bone cement was a common finding. Only one specimen retrieved at 101 months following surgery had any significant fibrous tissue present distal to the proximal 2 cm of the femur, and even in this specimen, the fibrous tissue was thin and sporadic. Occasional areas of fibrous tissue could be found in the other sections; however, they were never more than 5 to 10 cell layers thick or more than a few millimeters long. Normal marrow elements were commonly seen at the cement-bone interface. Foreign-body giant cells were not seen at this interface, and there were no areas of macrophage aggregates commonly seen in the membrane around loose cemented components.

Intimate apposition of bone with cement was also noted in the acetabulum after many years of *in vivo* service (53). However, as suggested by the plain radiographs, the coronal sections and contact radiographs of these sections revealed soft-tissue interposition between cement and bone to varying degrees in every specimen. In all of the implants examined, a soft-tissue layer was universally present, and was generally thickest, in the intra-articular margin. The histologic composition of the pseudo capsule and that of the peripheral interface membrane was essentially identical. This tissue was characterized by plump macrophages containing multiple particles of polyethylene. The joint pseudo capsule was in continuity with the soft tissue between the bone and cement at the intra-articular margin (Fig. 2). In the well-fixed implants this soft-tissue layer was thin (not greater than 1 mm), and it diminished in thickness and extent with increasing distance from the intra-articular margin. To-

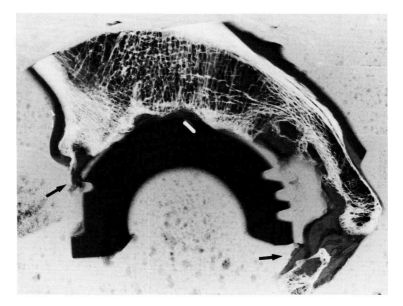

FIG. 2. Contact radiograph of an acetabular coronal section. Note the continuity of the joint pseudo capsule with the peripheral interface membrane (*arrows*). Consistent with the poor mechanical testing results of this specimen, the majority of the cement-bone interface has been disrupted. Note also the obvious deformation of the polyethylene bearing surface.

ward the dome of the implant at a variable distance from the intra-articular margin, transition zones from areas with membrane interposition between the bone and cement to areas of intimate apposition of bone and cement without any intervening soft tissue were identified. The three-dimensional extent of the soft-tissue interposition was directly related to implant stability.

With regard to the mechanism of loosening of acetabular components, the most important and revealing information was the histology of the transition zones. These regions were characterized by a cutting wedge of bone resorption that appears to progressively disrupt the cement-bone interface. This cutting wedge consists of collections of plump macrophages laden with submicron polyethylene wear debris in association with evidence of active bone resorption (53). A metal backing on the acetabular component did not appear to have any effect on this process (55). The presence of polyethylene debris in these locations, which are remote from the articular surfaces in specimens that move less than 50 μm, is the critical evidence indicating the central role of polyethylene debris in the initiation of late aseptic loosening of acetabular components. Further, the presence of polyethylene in these locations demonstrates the potential expanse and practical importance of the effective joint space (4). What was not observed in the transition zones was equally important. There was no evidence of mechanical failure; cement fragmentation and particulate polymethylmethacrylate were distinctly absent in these regions. Moreover, this active resorptive process was seen aggressively involving healthy trabeculae, which showed no evidence of trabecular microfracture.

In addition to progressive disruption of the hemispherical contour of the cement-bone interface due to the cutting wedge, a similar mechanism of bone resorption is involved in the widening of cement-bone interface radiolucencies. Regions with soft-tissue interposition between cement and bone, corresponding to the linear radiolucencies on the specimen radiograph, were generally composed of a superficial layer directly apposed to the cement mantle with variable amounts of fibroblasts and organized collagen and occasional macrophages containing polyethylene debris. In some regions, however, there was a deeper layer directly apposed to the bone with local accumulations of plump polyethylene debris-laden macrophages in association with active bone resorption (4,55).

Implant-Cement Interface and Bone Cement

In spite of the intact femoral cement-bone interface, partial separation of the cement-prosthesis interface (debonding) and fractures in the cement mantle were ubiquitous findings (36,42). A continuum existed in the pattern of debonding seen. Debonding started proximally and distally around the tip of the implant. In some specimens this had progressed to involve the entire metal-cement interface. Circumferential fractures were noted in the cement mantle associated with a debonded interface. In addition, radial fractures initiating at the metal-cement interface, often at sharp corners on the femoral component, were common findings. Cement fractures most commonly occurred in areas where the cement mantle was thin or in association with adjacent mantle defects. Fractures in the cement were also associated with pores in the cement. Cement fractures rarely occurred in mantles that were 2 mm or greater in thickness. In addition, fractures in the cement mantle that appeared to initiate at the cement-bone interface were rare.

The femoral component, which was radiographically loose as defined by a radiolucency at the cement-metal interface, had been retrieved at 156 months. It showed that the prosthesis was completely debonded from the cement mantle and was surrounded by a layer of fibrous tissue at the cement-metal interface (Fig. 3). There were numerous radial fractures within the cement mantle, and the prosthesis had rotated into retroversion. Despite this, the cement-bone interface was intact, and the patient was not experiencing pain at the time of death. Based on this information, the micromotion detected on mechanical testing for this specimen was likely occurring at the metal-cement interface and not the cement-bone interface, which was intact.

While cement fractures were not apparent on any of the whole specimen radiographs of the cemented acetabular components, they were seen in the coronal sections, although not commonly. Cement fractures were occasionally noted at the junction of the hemispherical cement mantle with cement pseudopods and in regions where the mantle was less than 2 mm thick. Cement fractures were notably absent from regions of predicted high stresses such as at the periphery of the acetabular component. The relationship between bone resorption, membrane interposition, and cement fractures was of interest. There were many areas of bone resorption and membrane formation without any cement fractures (such as at the intra-articular margin of the components). When acetabular cement fractures were observed, they were generally seen in association with extensive loss of bony support. Based on these observations, it is our interpretation that cement fractures occurred after there was a loss of bony structural support. Cement fracture has been observed with a metal-backed component. However, we have not examined enough metal-backed components to make any statements about the effect of this addition on the occurrence of cement fractures.

Local Osteolysis

Two of the femoral specimens in this series demonstrated focal cortical osteolysis despite being graded radiographically stable as well as being stable on mechanical testing (43). In one of these specimens, focal osteolysis at the tip of the implant was noted. Localized debonding of the tip of the prosthesis from the cement mantle had occurred. This combined with a thin cement mantle in this region led to numerous fractures through the voids in the cement and generation of particulate debris. In both specimens, the area of focal osteolysis was restricted to areas of localized acrylic fragmentation.

Skeletal Remodeling

Femoral bone remodeling was extensive (35). As described by Charnley (10), a second medullary canal frequently formed between the endosteal surface and outer cortex in these specimens (Fig. 4). Endosteal bone initially present around the cement mantle was preserved. This bone appeared to have remodeled into circumfer-

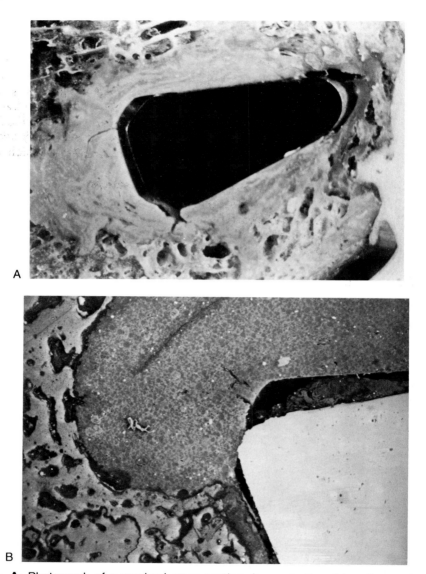

FIG. 3. A: Photograph of a proximal cross section demonstrating debonding at the metal-cement interface with fibrous tissue at this interface. Note fractures in the cement mantle laterally and a mantle defect medially. The cement-bone interface remains intact. **B:** Scanning electron micrograph demonstrating similar findings in a distal section. Note that the implant has rotated into retroversion.

ential lamellae, which were frequently osseointegrated with the cement mantle, forming a so-called "inner cortex." This inner cortex interdigitated with the cement and often grew into areas of mantle defects. The inner and outer cortices were connected by a series of radial struts of trabecular bone. This remodeling pattern was the basis for most of the radiolucencies seen on clinical and whole-specimen radiographs (37). Because of the presence of barium in the cement in most of these specimens, the inner cortex was indistinguishable from the bone cement on clinical or

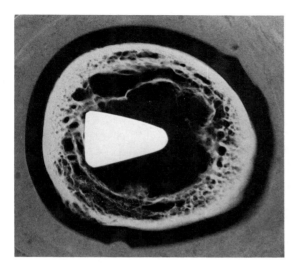

FIG. 4. Cross-section slab radiograph demonstrating neocortex around the cement mantle (barium-free cement) 17 years after surgery.

whole-specimen radiographs, emphasizing the inadequacies of these modalities in evaluating bone remodeling. The second medullary canal that forms appears as a radiolucency between the cement and outer cortex on radiographic analysis. These radiolucencies have been incorrectly interpreted as representing fibrous tissue in the past.

When available, the contralateral intact femur could be compared to evaluate cortical remodeling. As expected, the most extensive cortical remodeling occurred in the proximal femur and was more extensive in women than in men. In addition, the

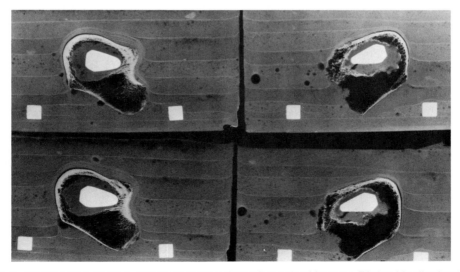

FIG. 5. Serial cross-section slab radiographs through a pair of femora. **Right:** Mueller implant that had been implanted 15 years earlier. **Left:** Implantation had been performed in the laboratory after death. Note on the right, the densification of bone around the cement mantle, loss of bone in the calcar region and thinning of the cortex circumferentially.

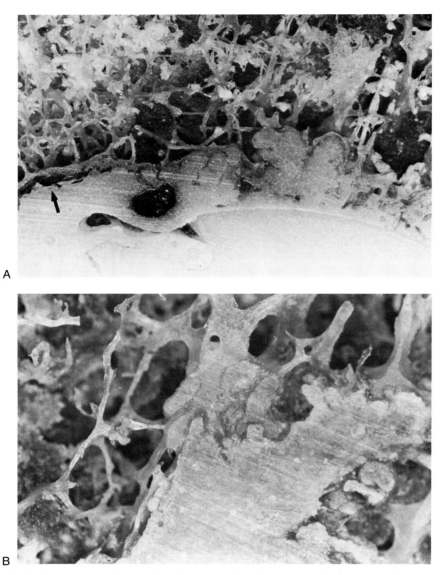

FIG. 6. A: Photograph of an acetabular coronal section demonstrating cancellous bone that has grown into and remodeled around the irregular contours of the cement mantle. A thin soft-tissue membrane is interposed between the cement and bone at the intra-articular margin is present near the intra-articular margin (*arrow*). **B:** Bone ingrowth and remodeling around a cement pseudopod in the same specimen at higher magnification. This specimen has been *in vivo* for 58 months.

remodeling was not limited to the calcar region, but occurred circumferentially (Fig. 5). Both thinning of the outer cortex and an increase in cortical porosity in the remaining cortex were noted in the proximal third of the femur in these specimens. Similar changes, to a lesser extent, were seen around the distal two-thirds of the implant.

Bone remodeling in the pelvis was less dramatic. There were numerous areas where bone and cement appeared osseointegrated in which the bone followed the smooth contours of the cement and interdigitated with the irregular contours of cement pseudopods that extended into the cancellous bone of the pelvis (Fig. 6). New bone formation appeared in these areas of direct contact. In addition, there was no evidence of microfracture of the trabeculae supporting these implants.

DISCUSSION AND INTERPRETATION OF DATA

The stability offered by bone cement over the long term in these specimens was remarkable (42). As noted, the greatest micromotion seen in the femoral components was rotational. This agrees with previously published work that suggests that torsional forces on the femoral component and rotational stability are important factors in femoral component failure. Mjoberg et al. (45), using stereophotogrametric techniques, demonstrated that rotational displacement was the most sensitive measure of femoral loosening. Wroblewski (61) concluded that torsional loading was responsible for femoral component fracture based on an analysis of the fracture surfaces. Burke et al. (8) have shown that significant rotational movement of the femoral component occurs during stair climbing. Mechanical testing of the femoral components in this autopsy study demonstrates similar results.

Analysis of the interface between bone and cement provided valuable information concerning the biological response to cemented components in terms of both skeletal remodeling and compatibility. The extensive femoral remodeling appears to play a critical role in long-term implant stability. Past clinical reports have addressed the issue of endosteal enlargement in the role of femoral component failure (13,31,50). However, these studies are based on clinical radiographic reviews. Although much valuable information has been obtained from radiographic reviews, there are several inherent difficulties in performing retrospective clinical radiographic studies to assess architectural change in the proximal femur. Radiographs are not sensitive enough to detect even moderate changes in cortical density. Subtle rotation of the femur leads to significant differences in the radiographic measurement of the canal diameters and cortical thicknesses. Barium in the bone cement makes it impossible to distinguish the neocortex around the cement mantle. Finally, once the loosening process begins, associated bone resorption could lead to an overestimation of remodeling changes secondary to aging or mechanically induced bone loss (stress shielding). Thus, only by direct examination of autopsy specimens can the skeletal remodeling that occurs after total hip replacement be adequately characterized.

After insertion of a femoral component, the transfer of load from the hip joint to the proximal femur changes markedly, now with partial load transfer occurring at the endosteal surface (42,48). The skeleton responds to this alteration in load transfer by creating a neocortex surrounding the cement mantle. The new bone at the cement-bone interface condenses and remodels around the cement mantle forming what Charnley (10) termed the *inner cortex*. This is the exact opposite of the normal process of endosteal enlargement. Between this inner cortex and the outer cortex trabecular struts develop similar to what was observed by Draenert (17) in animal experiments. This densification of bone or inner cortex surrounding the cement mantle is connected to the outer cortex by a series of trabecular struts and provides excellent stability for these cemented femoral components, even in female patients over the age of 90 with advanced skeletal atrophy.

The findings with respect to the presence of fibrous tissue at the cement-bone interface were also surprising. It has generally been accepted that fibrous tissue invariably forms at the cement-bone interface (5,19,20). Goldring et al. (23) examined the thick fibrous membrane found at revision surgery, noting that it contained numerous macrophages and giant cells. In addition, it contained particulate polymethylmethacrylate and polyethylene, suggesting that particulate debris may have been a causative factor in membrane formation. Aseptic loosening of cemented acetabular components has been attributed to this phenomenon, incorrectly referred to as cement disease, and was one of the driving forces behind the development of cementless implants.

This work (35–37,42) has demonstrated that with stable cemented femoral components, fibrous tissue does only not necessarily form at the cement-bone interface, but that it is not a common occurrence. In contrast, osseointegration frequently occurs with intimate contact between the bone and cement with no intervening fibrous tissue or gaps. There was no evidence of a deleterious effect as a result of the long-term presence of bulk cement. This agrees with previous work examining the tissue around loose and well-fixed cemented femoral components (34) as well as *in vivo* studies examining the difference between the cellular response to bulk and particulate polymethylmethacrylate (25). Similarly, osseointegration can and does occur with cemented acetabular components (53). However, there are two distinct differences between the femoral and acetabular side. First, the patchy areas of an organized collagenous membrane were distinctly more common around the acetabulum. Second, the acetabular cement-bone interface was more prone to invasion of the polyethylene-induced membrane. This finding has implications concerning the initiation of loosening of these components.

As discussed elsewhere in this volume, there has been a long-standing controversy over the relative role of biological and mechanical factors in aseptic loosening of cemented components. Charnley (10) maintained loosening was primarily mechanical, whereas others (23,60) have postulated that biological reaction to implanted materials leads to fibrous tissue, bone resorption, and failure. Both are obviously important. The studies to date have focused on findings at revision surgery, which is late in the process of loosening and does not provide information on the initiating events.

On the femoral side, the initiating events appear mechanical. Debonding between the metal and cement is the earliest detectable event in the failure of these components. The location of early debonding, proximally along the anterolateral surface of the implant and at the tip of the stem, has been predicted by finite element studies (26). In addition, finite element studies have predicted that debonding at the cement-metal interface may lead to high focal stresses in the cement capable of causing mechanical failure of the cement mantle (15,26). Review of these autopsy-retrieved specimens supports those conclusions. Debonding was associated with fractures in the cement mantle most commonly proximally and distally.

As the integrity of the cement mantle is compromised, at least three deleterious events may occur. First, motion may increase. The more the cement mantle was compromised in terms of debonding and cement fracture, the greater the implant micromotion on mechanical testing. In these specimens, motion was probably not occurring between cement and bone, but between cement and implant, as the cement-bone interface was intact. Second, particulate debris may be generated. High focal stresses within the cement as a result of debonding can lead to fragmentation of the cement. Cement fragmentation can lead to focal osteolysis, as we have previously demonstrated. In addition, debonding allows a fibrous tissue layer to form between the metal and cement, as we and others (3,19) have demonstrated. This in turn may act as a conduit for polyethylene debris to gain access to the endosteal surface through mantle defects as well as fractures in the cement mantle. Motion and particulate debris can stimulate the pseudo membrane formation that is a late finding with aseptic loosening of cemented femoral components.

Mechanism of Femoral Implant Loosening

As a result of review of autopsy-retrieved material, we have been able to elucidate the mechanism of failure of cemented femoral components. Failure is a continuum that begins prior to clinical or radiographic evidence of failure. The initiating events are mechanical. Debonding at the cement-metal interface occurs early and is associated with fractures in the cement mantle. Most fractures occur proximally and commonly occur in deficient cement mantles or are associated with mantle defects. This leads to increased motion and fragmentation of cement, which can subsequently lead to fibrous tissue formation. Biological processes then begin to play an important role. Particulate polymeric debris can gain access to the endosteal surface and stimulate cells to produce mediators of bone resorption. A progressive radiolucency and demarcation lines between the bone and cement may develop as a result, leading to clinical failure. The rate of progression of this process probably depends on several factors including the activity level and weight of the patient, the design of the femoral component, as well as the surgical technique (4,46,51,52).

Mechanism of Acetabulum Loosening

In contrast, the initial events in the loosening of well-fixed acetabular components appear to be biological (53). Willert and Semlitsch (60) focused on the adverse effects of particulate debris on the femoral side. With regard to loosening, however, our studies indicate that particulate wear debris plays a greater role on the acetabular side. In these specimens, a soft-tissue membrane between the cement and bone was invariably present at the intra-articular margin on the implant. This membrane was histologically similar to and in continuity with the pseudo capsule containing numerous macrophages laden with polyethylene debris. Three-dimensional bone resorption immediately adjacent to the cement mantle noted in association with this membrane appeared to result in acetabular component loosening. This process appears to be driven by very small particles of polyethylene wear debris and does not appear to be affected by the presence of a metal backing on the acetabular component. Once fixation has been compromised, any additional motion can only be detrimental. This is further supported by the mechanical testing, which showed a correlation between the amount of fibrous tissue present and implant micromotion.

As suggested by the concept of the effective joint space (54), a similar process of bone resorption was noted in the proximal 1 to 2 cm of the femur. However, due to the anatomical differences between the femur and acetabulum and the relative differences between the ratio of the circumference of the mouth of the femur and acetabulum to the total surface area of the cement-bone interface around these two components, 1 to 2 cm of circumferential bone resorption in the proximal femur does not compromise femoral component stability. However, if 2 cm of the acetabular cement-bone interface is circumferentially disrupted, the majority of the interface has been compromised, resulting in an unstable implant.

Significance of Radiolucent Lines

Special mention should be made concerning the etiology of radiolucent lines seen on clinical radiographs. The discussion of radiolucent lines around cemented implants is usually done in generic terms, and the presence of a radiolucent line at the cement-bone interface has traditionally been interpreted to mean the presence of fibrous tissue. Our studies, however, indicate that the histologic constituents, and therefore the etiology, of radiolucent lines can be quite variable. The majority of radiolucencies around our well-fixed femoral components did not contain any fibrous tissue and were in fact a result of endosteal remodeling, discussed above. Radiolucent lines at the most proximal femoral cement-bone interface contained numerous debris-laden macrophages and appear to be the result of particulate-induced bone resorption. In these specimens the extent of this process was limited and did not result in femoral loosening. The soft-tissue constituents of acetabular radiolucencies were variable and location dependent. Radiolucencies near the intra-articular margin were in continuity with the joint pseudo capsule and contained a predominance of polyethylene debris-laden macrophages in association with active bone resorption (2). A relatively greater proportion of collagen and fibroblasts could be found in radiolucencies located closer to the apex of the implant.

CONCLUSIONS

In summary, in contrast to Charnley's proposal, we have not found any evidence indicating that frictional torque plays a role in either femoral or acetabular component loosening. Further, our studies indicate that the initiating events in the loosening of cemented femoral and acetabular components are distinctly different. These differences are at least in part due to differences in the loading environments and the differences between femoral and acetabular anatomy and the shapes of the corresponding components. Because of high stresses in shear and retroversion, mechanical forces dominate femoral-side loosening. In contrast, the acetabulum experiences relatively benign compressive stresses, but the soft and porous cancellous bone of the acetabular interface appears to be more susceptible to resorption by the adverse biological reaction to polyethylene wear debris. This likely accounts for the differences observed clinically in the rates of loosening of femoral versus acetabular components (56,57,62) and the differences in the clinical function of loose components (62).

REFERENCES

1. Amstutz HC, Markolf KL, McNeice GM, Gruen TA. Loosening of total hip components: cause and prevention. In: *The Hip. Proceedings of the 4th open meeting of the Hip Society.* St Louis: CV Mosby, 1976:102.
2. Athanasou NA, Quinn J, Bulstrode CJK. Resorption of bone by inflammatory cells derived from the joint capsule of hip arthroplasties. *J Bone Joint Surg [Br]* 1992;74:57.
3. Anthony PP, Gie GA, Howie CR, Ling RM. Localized endosteal bone lysis in relation to the femoral components of cemented total hip arthroplasties. *J Bone Joint Surg [Br]* 1991;72:971.
4. Barrack RL, Mulroy RD, Harris WH. Improved cementing techniques and femoral component loosening in young patients with hip arthroplasty. *J Bone Joint Surg [Br]* 1992;74:385.
5. Bullough PG, DiCarlo EF, Hansraj KK, Neeves MC. Pathologic studies of total joint replacement. *Orthop Clin North Am* 1988;19:611.
6. Burke DW, Davies JP, O'Connor DO, Harris WH. Experimental strain-analysis in the femoral cement mantle of simulated total hip arthroplasties. *Orthop Trans* 1984;9:296.
7. Burke DW, Gates EI, Harris WH. Centrifugation as a method of improving tensile and fatigue properties of acrylic bone cement. *J Bone Joint Surg [Am]* 1985;66:1265.
8. Burke DW, O'Connor DO, Zalenski EB, Rubash HE, Harris WH. Biomechanics of femoral total hip replacement in simulated stair climbing. *Orthop Trans* 1988;13:345.
9. Burke DW, O'Connor DO, Zalenski EB, Jasty M, Harris WH. Micromotion of cemented and uncemented femoral components. *J Bone Joint Surg [Br]* 1991;73:33.
10. Charnley J. *Low Friction Arthroplasty of the Hip.* New York: Springer-Verlag, 1979.
11. Charnley J, Kettlewell J. The elimination of slip between prosthesis and femur. *J Bone Joint Surg [Br]* 1965;47:56.
12. Collis DK. Long-term (twelve–eighteen-year) follow-up of cemented total hip replacements in patients who were less than fifty years old: a follow-up note. *J Bone Joint Surg [Am]* 1991;73:593.
13. Comadoll JL, Sherman RE, Gustillo RB, Bechtold JE. Radiographic changes in bone dimensions in asymptomatic cemented total hip arthroplasties. *J Bone Joint Surg [Am]* 1988;70:433.
14. Crowninshield RD, Brand RA, Johnston RC, Milroy JC. An analysis of femoral component design in total hip arthroplasty. *J Bone Joint Surg [Br]* 1965;47:56.
15. Crowninsheild RD, Tolbert JR. Cement strain measurement surrounding loose and well-fixed femoral component stems. *J Biomed Mat Res* 1983;17:819.
16. Davy DT, Kotzar GM, Brown RH, et al. Telemetric force measurements across the hip after total arthroplasty. *J Bone Joint Surg [Am]* 1988;70:45.
17. Draenert K. Histomorphology of the bone-to-cement interface: remodeling of the cortex and revascularization of the medullary canal in animal experiments. In: Salvati EA, ed. *The Hip. Proceedings of the Ninth Open Scientific Meeting of The Hip Society.* St. Louis: CV Mosby, 1981:71.
18. Fischer KJ, Carter DR, Maloney WJ. In vitro study of initial stability of a conical collared component. *J Arthroplasty (in press).*
19. Fornaiser VL, Cameron HU. The femoral stem/cement interface in total hip replacement. *Clin Orthop* 1976;116:248.
20. Freeman MAR, Bradley GW, Revell PA. Observations upon the interface between bone and polymeric cement. *J Bone Joint Surg [Br]* 1982;64B:489.
21. Galante JO, Lemmons J, Spector M, Wilson PD, Wright TM. The biologic effects of implant materials. *J Orthop Res* 1991;9:760.
22. Goldring SR, Jasty M, Paiement G. Tissue response to bulk and particulate biopolymers in a rabbit wound chamber model. *Orthop Trans* 1986;11:288.
23. Goldring SR, Jasty M, Roelke MS, Rourke CM, Bringhurst FR, Harris WH. Formation of a synovial-like membrane at the bone-cement interface: its role in bone resorption and implant loosening after total hip replacement. *Arthritis Rheum* 1986;29:836.
24. Goldring SR, Schiller AL, Roelke M, Rourke CM, O'Neill DA, Harris WH. The synovial-like membrane of the bone-cement interface in bone lysis. *J Bone Joint Surg [Am]* 1983;65:575.
25. Goodman SB, Fornaiser VL, Kei J. The effects of bulk versus particulate polymethylmethacrylate on bone. *Clin Orthop* 1988;232:255.
26. Harrigan TP, Harris WH. A three dimensional non-linear finite element study of the effect of cement-prosthesis debonding in cemented femoral total hip components. *J Biomech* 1991;24:1047.
27. Harris WH, Hodge WA, Fijan RS, Carlson KL, Burgess RG, Mann RW. Contact pressures in the human hip joint measured in vivo. *Proc Natl Acad Sci USA* 1986;83:1.
28. Herman JH, Sowder WG, Anderson D, Appel AM, Hopson CN. Polymethylmethacrylate-induced release of bone-resorbing factors. *J Bone Joint Surg [Am]* 1989;71:1530.
29. Hodge WA, Carlson KL, Fijan RS, et al. Contact pressures from an instrumented hip endoprosthesis. *J Bone Joint Surg [Am]* 1989;71:1378.
30. Hodgkinson JP, Shelley P, Wroblewski BM. The correlation between roentgenographic appear-

ance and operative findings at the bone-cement junction of the socket in Charnley low friction arthroplasties. *Clin Orthop* 1988;228:105.

31. Hoffman AA, Wyatt RB, France EP, Bigler GT, Daniels AU, Hess WF. Endosteal bone loss after total hip arthroplasty. *Clin Orthop* 1989;245:138.

32. Howie DW, Vernon-Roberts B, Oakeshott R, Manthey B. A rat model of resorption of bone at the cement-bone interface in the presence of polyethylene wear particles. *J Bone Joint Surg [Am]* 1988;70A:257.

33. Huiskes R. Stress patterns, failure modes, and bone remodeling. In: Fitzgerald RH Jr, ed. *Noncemented total hip arthroplasty.* New York: Raven Press, 1988:283.

34. Jasty M, Goldring SR, Harris WH. Comparison of bone cement membrane around rigidly fixed versus loose total hip implants. *Orthop Trans* 1980;9:125.

35. Jasty M, Maloney WJ, Bragdon CR, Harie T, Harris WH. Histomorphological studies of the long-term skeletal responses to well fixed cemented femoral components. *J Bone Joint Surg [Am]* 1990;72:1220.

36. Jasty M, Maloney WJ, Bragdon CR, O'Connor DO, Harie T, Harris WH. The initiation of failure in cemented femoral components of hip arthroplasties. *J Bone Joint Surg [Br]* 1991;73:551.

37. Kwong LM, Jasty M, Mulroy RD, Maloney WJ, Bragdon CR, Harris WH. The histology of the radiolucent line. *J Bone Joint Surg [Br]* 1992;74:67.

38. Lewis JL, Askew MJ, Wixson RL, Kramer GM, Tarr RR. The influence of prosthetic stem stiffness and of a collar on stresses in the proximal end of a femur with a cemented femoral component. *J Bone Joint Surg [Am]* 1984;66:280.

39. Lewis JL, Nicola T, Keer LM, Clech JP, Steege JW, Wixson RL. Failure processes at the cancellous bone-PMMA interface. Transactions of the 31st Annual Meeting of the Orthopaedic Research Society, Las Vegas, NV 1985, p. 144.

40. Maguire JK, Coscia MF, Lynch MH. Foreign body reaction to polymeric debris following total hip arthroplasty. *Clin Orthop* 1987;216:213.

41. Maloney WJ, Burke DW, O'Connor DO, Harris WH. Cement strain profile in cemented acetabular components: the effects of metal-backing. Transactions of the 16th Annual Meeting of the Society for Biomaterials, Charleston, SC, 1990.

42. Maloney WJ, Jasty M, Burke DW, et al. Biochemical and histological investigation of cemented total hip arthoplasties: a study of autopsy-retrieved femurs after in vivo cycling. *Clin Orthop* 1989;249:129–140.

43. Maloney WJ, Jasty M, Rosenberg AS, Harris WH. Bone lysis in well-fixed cemented femoral components. *J Bone Joint Surg [Br]* 1990;72:966.

44. McCleish RD, Charnley J. Abduction forces in the one-legged stance. *J Biomech* 1970;3:191.

45. Mjoberg B, Hansson LI, Selvik G. Instability of total hip prosthesis at rotational stress. *Acta Orthop Scand* 1984;55:504.

46. Mulroy RD, Harris WH. The effect of improved cementing techniques on component loosening in total hip replacement. *J Bone Joint Surg [Br]* 1990;72:757.

47. Murray DW, Rushton N. Macrophages stimulate bone resorption when they phagocytose particles. *J Bone Joint Surg [Br]* 1991;72:988.

48. Oh I, Harris WH. Proximal strain distribution in the loaded femur: an in vitro comparison of the distributions in the intact femur and after insertion of different hip replacement femoral components. *J Bone Joint Surg [Am]* 1978;60:75.

49. O'Neill DA, Harris WH. Failed total hip replacement: assessment by plain radiographs, arthrograms and aspiration of the joint. *J Bone Joint Surg [Am]* 1984;66:540.

50. Poss R, Staehlin P, Larson M. Femoral expansion in total hip arthroplasty. *J Arthroplasty* 1987;2:259.

51. Roberts DW, Poss R, Kelly K. Radiographic comparison of cementing techniques in total hip arthroplasty. *J Arthroplasty* 1986;1:241.

52. Russotti GM, Coventry MB, Stauffer RN. Cemented total hip arthroplasty with contemporary techniques: a five-year minimum follow-up study. *Clin Orthop* 1988;235:141.

53. Schmalzried TP, Kwong LM, Jasty M, et al. The mechanism of loosening of cemented acetabular components in total hip arthroplasty: analysis of specimens retrieved at autopsy. *Clin Orthop* 1992;274:60.

54. Schmalzried TP, Jasty M, Harris WH. Periprosthetic bone loss in total hip arthroplasty: the role of polyethylene wear debris and the concept of the effective joint space. *J Bone Joint Surg (in press).*

55. Schmalzried TP, Maloney WJ, Kwong LM, Jasty M, Harris WH. Autopsy studies of the cement-bone interface of well-fixed cemented total hip replacements. *J Arthroplasty (in press).*

56. Stauffer RN. Ten year follow-up study of total hip replacement. *J Bone Joint Surg [Am]* 1972;64:983.

57. Sutherland CJ, Wilde AH, Borden LS, Marks KE. A ten year follow-up of one hundred consecutive Mueller curved-stem total hip replacement arthroplasties. *J Bone Joint Surg [Am]* 1982;64:970.

58. Vasu R, Carter DR, Harris WH. Stress distributions in the acetabular region. I. Before and after total joint replacement. *J Biomech* 1982;15:155.
59. Walker PS, Schneeweis D, Murphy S, Nelson P. Strain and micromotions of press-fit femoral stem prosthesis. *J Biomech* 1987;20:693.
60. Willert H-G, Semlitsch J. Reactions of the articular capsule to wear products of artificial joint prostheses. *J Biomed Mater Res* 1977;11:157.
61. Wroblewski BM. The mechanism of failure of the femoral prosthesis in total hip replacement. *Int Orthop* 1979;3:137.
62. Wroblewski BM, Taylar GW, Sined P. Charnley low-friction arthroplasty: 19–25 year results. *Orthopaedics* 1992;15:421.

Biological, Material, and Mechanical Considerations of Joint Replacement, edited by B. F. Morrey. Raven Press, Ltd., New York © 1993.

7

Experimental Studies of the Cement Interface

Peter S. Walker

Department of Biomedical Engineering, University College London, Royal National Orthopaedic Hospital, Stanmore, Middlesex HA 74LP, United Kingdom

The nature of the interface between the cement and bone and between the cement and implant components affects the stresses and strains occurring not only in the vicinity of the interface itself, but in the system as a whole. There are several factors that affect these interfaces. The surface of the implant, whether smooth, macro-rough, or porous, will determine the extent to which shear, tensile, and compressive stresses can be transmitted. The same applies to the bone interface due to the bone itself, whether trabecular, slightly rough, or almost smooth as in many revision situations. The cleanliness of the surfaces, pressure applied to the cement at surgery, and viscosity of the cement will determine the intimacy of contact between the cement and bone. The integrity of the cement layer itself will depend on its thickness and uniformity, and the presence of inclusions or cracks. Laboratory testing has included investigations of most of these factors. Although this chapter concentrates mainly on the knee, with some references to the hip, most of the methods are applicable to both.

PENETRATION OF CEMENT INTO TRABECULAR BONE

Studies were carried out to investigate the variables controlling the amount of cement penetration into trabecular bone on the proximal tibial surface and the resulting strengths of the interface (10). The upper tibia was resected and the trabecular bone was prepared in several ways including as cut, placement of blood clot, towel brushing, plastic brushing, and low- and high-intensity lavage. Cement was then applied by either finger packing or a syringe that pressurized at 0.17 MPa. Samples were tested in tension, obtaining values of 1.8 to 5.4 MPa for finger packing and 6.4 to 8.5 MPa for pressure injection. The highest values were obtained for plastic brushing and high-pressure lavage. Failures were observed to occur either within the trabecular bone itself or within the cement, depending on the bone quality. Shear strengths were 9.6 to 20.7 MPa for finger packing and 25.2 to 42.0 MPa for pressure injection. The depths of penetration were 1 to 15 mm, and a trend of increased tensile strength with depth was found. An upper limit of 5-mm penetration was suggested for clinical application based on their data and thermal considerations.

In a similar study (21) tibial surfaces were resected, cement applied to the surface, the tibias inserted into a pressure chamber, and, when the cement had hardened, the depth of penetration was measured. The variables were the time of cement mixing, the pressure (0.17–0.52 MPa), and the mean pore size of the trabecular bone, covering the range expected in surgery. The depths of penetration were from 0.5 to 4.0 mm. The depth was proportional to pore diameter and applied pressure, and inversely proportional to the time of mixing. Based on Poiseuille's equation, most of the penetration would be reached soon after pressure application, the more so because of the increase of viscosity with time. When surgical conditions were simulated, by applying a force to the tibial component, the penetration showed a U shape, consistent with the theoretical pressure distribution, maximal at the center and zero at the periphery (Fig. 1). Tensile strengths of the cement-bone interface were in the range of 0.5 to 3.5 MPa. There was no strong correlation of strength with depth. This was because low penetration occurred mostly in dense cancellous bone where the cement tended to pull out of the bone, whereas higher penetration occurred in less dense and weaker bone, where the failure was primarily in the bone itself. The overall conclusion was that 3- to 4-mm depth was the ideal in order to engage sufficient transverse trabeculae, but that to achieve that clinically, some means of achieving peripheral penetration was needed.

In a further study on this subject, distal femoral and proximal tibial bone samples were prepared and mounted in a pressure chamber (1). Pressures up to 0.17 MPa were applied to cement mixed for 90 sec and held for 5 to 30 sec. The mean depths of penetration for the different applied pressures were 1 to 7 mm, but with a wide range at each pressure. An increase in the time of pressure application from 5 to 30

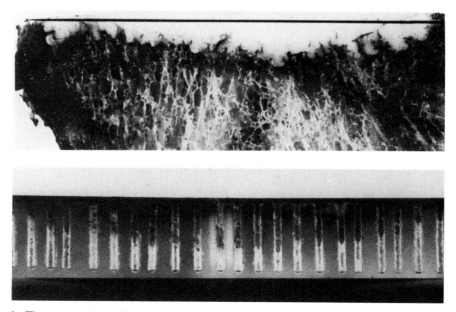

FIG. 1. The penetration of cement into the upper tibia under clinical conditions by pressing the tibial component onto the bone. The low penetration at the sides is typical. This is simulated in a test with tubes (*bottom*). (From ref. 21.)

sec made little difference to depth. Penetration was inversely dependent on compressive strength. The failure load in tension increased with pressure up to 0.08 MPa and then leveled off. Weak bone gave the lowest values of failure load for the highest applied pressure values. A plot of failure load against penetration depth showed no correlation, but with the highest values in the range of 3 to 5 mm. The magnitude of the pressure was the largest single determinant of penetration. Time of pressure application had little effect, indicating that most of the penetration occurred early. The authors suggested that 4-mm depth was the optimum for clinical application, a value beyond which little further increase in tensile load could be obtained.

Clinical Relevance

The above studies are generally consistent in their findings and recommendations. The subject is likely to be important from a clinical point of view. A critical review of radiographs (19) showed that the depth of penetration varied widely between cases, that the depths around pegs were high, and that the depths at the sides of the plateau were low. There was an association of radiolucent lines with low penetration (which may be due to factors other than low penetration) and vice versa. Other authors have shown that penetration of at least several millimeters resulted in a low incidence of radiolucent lines. In clinical practice, a variety of methods are widely used, presumably because the clinical results are not believed to vary substantially as a function of method and because the available surgical equipment for achieving uniform penetration is not generally accepted.

Pressurized Cement Techniques

Sustained pressurization to achieve high penetration has been investigated in an animal model (15). Canine proximal tibias were used to compare the effects of applying cement to the surface by sustained pressurization at 0.69 MPa, compared with finger packing. The tests were done *in vivo,* and then after sacrifice. Transverse slices 5 mm thick were taken and push-out tests performed. Failure forces were significantly higher for the pressurized samples *in vivo* and *in vitro.* The *in vitro* results were around 30% higher than *in vivo* results, probably due to blood flow effects. The lowest strengths were obtained for finger packing in the *in vivo* tests, emphasizing the advantage of pressurization from the strength point of view.

Continuing these studies (7), total knee replacements were performed on goats, cementing by sustained pressurization of 0.69 MPa and by finger packing. The animals were sacrificed at 3 and 6 months, at which time another total knee replacement was performed to obtain immediate surgery data. Thin sections were prepared to observe the interfaces. Surprisingly there was a significantly larger area of the interfaces showing fibrous tissue interposition in the pressurized group. This fibrovascular membrane had replaced trabecular bone away from the cement border. The authors attributed the finding to heat injury and devascularization of the encased bone. These results can be compared with those of another study (13). Hemitibial metal plateaus with a fixation peg were fixed to the upper tibia using cement or had a porous surface for press fit. After certain periods of time in the body, sagittal slices were made and observations made through a stereomicroscope under cyclic loading conditions. For the cemented interfaces with good penetration, little cement-trabecular bone micromotion was seen, although overall trabecular deflections were apparent. In contrast, the porous surface showed trabecular movements, except around the peg, which was well fixed. Fibrous tissue was seen beneath the plateau but not around the peg. The authors concluded that micromotion and microfracture of trabecular bone at the interface were the initiators of subsidence.

Clinical Experience and Retrieval Studies

Certainly, changes in morphology at the cement-bone interface over time have been shown by many authors. For example, in a roentgenstereophotogrammetric study, Marmor tibial components were shown to be stable after 3 years. Yet on removal of three cases, all of the interfaces were found to be primarily fibrous (17). Although such findings may well reflect the initial cement technique used, as well as the design of the implant, they do illustrate that the mechanical properties of the interface are likely to change over time. A possible mechanism whereby an initially interlocked interface can change to one where the cement and bone become separated was suggested by Steege et al. (18). The hypothesis was that gradual failure of the interlocking bond at a cement-cancellous bone interface was primarily due to mechanical effects, in particular, that a crack was initiated at a point in the interface and then gradually propagated through the interface. Sections of interfaces were prepared, viewed in a stereomicroscope and the crack behavior studied. Apart from the gradual progress of a primary crack through the interface, and often a secondary crack remote from the first, micromotion between cement and bone was observed. Fluid was pumped into and out of the crack regions a great deal more than in the more rigidly bonded regions. Both of these phenomena could result in resorption of bone and replacement by fibrous tissue. There was considerable variation in the crack propagation rate between specimens. High cement penetrations usually resulted in low rates, whereas the interposition of fixation posts across the interface greatly slowed down crack growth.

Remodeling

A possibly important factor relating to the stability of a cement-bone interface is the remodeling of the bone that occurs. In the knee, correction of the deformity is expected to result in a redistribution of the relative forces on the lateral and medial condyles. In total knee patients, transverse computed tomography (CT) 3-mm slices were taken of the proximal tibia before and after surgery (9). A sampling technique was used to obtain a map of CT number, from which was calculated the linear attenuation coefficient (LAC), a function of the Hounsfield number. The LAC was shown to be closely related to the yield strength (and other mechanical properties) of the trabecular bone. The patients, with both varus and valgus deformities, were scanned preoperatively and then postoperatively at 6 or 25 months. The strength data across selected sections were displayed in a similar way to that shown in Fig. 2. At follow-up, the high strength on the side of the deformities had considerably decreased, whereas on the opposite side, only a slight increase in strength had occurred. Such changes would be associated with a change in trabecular pattern and density. Around intramedullary stems, remodeling can be caused not by a realignment, but by a change in bone stresses due to the presence of the stem. General trabecularization

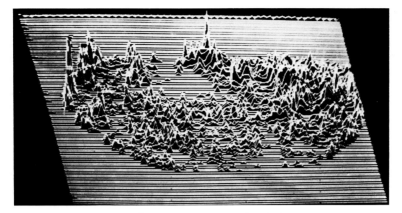

FIG. 2. The pressure distribution of a tibial component loaded onto the upper tibia. The differences in pressure are due partly to variations in trabecular density.

of the inner part of the cortex has been observed by several authors (4). In this case, a dense layer of bone has been observed encircling the cement, joined to the compact outer cortex by the intervening region of trabecular bone. In such circumstances, the question arises as to whether the trabeculae entering the cement itself, of the morphology prevailing at the time of operation, will be still compatible in terms of the new local stresses.

Interface Strength

A final subject in this section is that of measurement of the strength of the cement-bone interface itself. For the proximal tibia, tensile or shear strength has usually been measured. However, for intramedullary fixation of hip stems, the shear strength has usually been measured as being the most clinically relevant parameter. Measurements are most often made by push-out tests of transverse slices. The method has a number of drawbacks, however, not the least of which is the geometric irregularity of the slice. An analytical approach to an assessment of the method was made (8). The standard push-out test was analyzed using finite element analysis, where a rod was pushed through an annulus, and the annulus was supported circumferentially around the base, with a radial clearance between the rod and interface. Substantial variations in interface shear stress were calculated. This variation changed with material and interface strength properties. Hence comparative testing was only valid between specimens of generally similar nature, and it is preferable to quote failure forces as opposed to failure shear stresses. A preferable method may be to adopt the approach of cutting segments across the interface, eliminating a number of the problems (2). The cement-bone interface in the proximal femur was evaluated by cutting transverse cylindrical slices and then cutting these into quadrants. These quadrants were mounted in special holders and subjected to a shear force in a direction parallel to the interface until failure. Significant regional variations in average shear stress were found, with the medial quadrant giving values of 2.5 times that of the lateral (15.0 vs 6.0 MPa). This method was considered to be less subject to errors and inconsistencies compared with testing complete cylindrical slices.

STRESSES, STRAINS, AND RELATIVE MOTION

These mechanical factors have been variously used to evaluate cement-bone interfaces and the influence of component designs. There is considerable evidence that relative motion between the implant and bone should be minimized in order to avoid bone resorption and fibrous tissue formation. There is also evidence that excessive compressive stresses will lead to gradual sinkage of the component into the bone, a process that can take several years. On the basis of these two aspects, measurements of relative interface motion (often called micromotion) can be used as a basis of comparison between components of different design.

Displacement Studies

In one study, 12 different tibial component designs were compared, including one-piece central peg, one-piece two peg, one-piece anteriorly joined, and unicompartmental with two pegs; all in all plastic or metal backed (20). They were cemented into cadaveric bones and into foam polyurethane bones. The advantage of the latter is that large numbers of closely consistent samples can be produced, suitable for comparative studies provided there is a reasonable simulation of mechanical properties and shape. A metal ring was clamped around the upper tibia on which were mounted displacement transducers used to measure the distance to targets mounted on the periphery of the tibial component (Fig. 3). This gave a measure of the distraction or compression at the cement-bone interface. Using a bicondylar roller, loads and torques resembling physiological values were applied to the plastic tibial surface and the peripheral displacements were recorded. On the foam bones (values for actual bones were approximately half those of the foam), for direct loading of

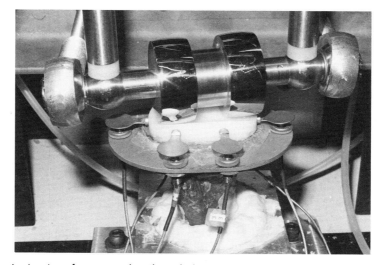

FIG. 3. The test set-up for measuring the relative motions between the periphery of the tibial component and the bone. The vertical and horizontal cylinders apply forces and moments. The noncontact eddy current transducers measure displacements. (From ref. 20.)

2,250 N, the medial and lateral compressions were 0.1 to 0.4 mm. For varus or valgus loading (1,500 N on one condyle 24 mm from center), there was 0.2- to 0.5-mm compression on the loaded side and zero compression on the opposite side. An anterior shear force of 450 N produced compression anteriorly and distraction posteriorly, torque resulting in twisting of the components, the amount depending on rigidity. Overall, the least deflections occurred for one-piece metal-backed components with one or two pegs. The largest deflections occurred for the unicompartmentals, metal or plastic.

Similar methods of measuring implant-bone motions at interfaces have been widely used to investigate tibial components, femoral stems, acetabular components, and other constructs. The method is not without possible misinterpretation, however. Although components are often rigid, to which transducer attachments can be rigidly fixed, the same cannot be said for bone, particularly trabecular. Hence, local elastic deflections can distort the results obtained. The attachment points of the transducers can also give misleading results. If the distance between the two points of measurement spans a region of bone, the axial deflection of the bone will affect the readings. The interface relative motion of hip stems is particularly prone to such error because of the small distances involved, usually in the range of 10 to 100 μm. Even if the two measurement points are close together, elastic deformations of cement and bone can still be significant. Direct observation of the interface (13,18) may be a preferred method for accurately measuring small interface motions.

Strain Measurement

Strain gages have provided useful information about the behavior of different components and allowed inferences to be made about the interfaces. The purpose of several investigations has been to determine the changes in strain in the proximal tibia after insertion of tibial components. In one study, the variables were all plastic versus a metal tray; short, medium, and long central post; and complete versus incomplete surface coverage of the upper tibia (16). Strain gauges were attached to the outer surface of the proximal tibia at different heights from the surface. The central post was strain gauged at three levels (Fig. 4). A load rig was used to apply compression, varus-valgus, anteroposterior, and rotational forces to the femur. Strains on the intact knee before the introduction of components were used as a baseline. For incomplete surface coverage, the proximal strains on the bone were considerably reduced. This effect was greatest for the 60-mm metal post, implying stress protection. The low axial stiffness of the plastic post prevented this effect. For complete coverage, the strains were restored to normal for plastic but higher than normal for the metal component because of its high rigidity. For varus-valgus bending loads, the strains on the proximal part of the plastic post were 10 times higher than for the metal, threatening the integrity of the surrounding cement. However, the proportion of the applied bending moment carried by the plastic post was calculated to be negligible, whereas it was 25% for the 40-mm metal post.

Analytical Studies

Analytical approaches to a problem similar to the above have been reported by a number of authors. Finite-element analysis was used to study a metal-backed tibial

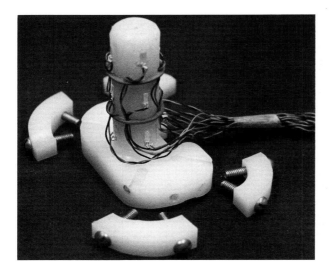

FIG. 4. A test tibial component instrumented with strain gauges to determine the strain under different test conditions. The rubber washers are to wall off different amounts of cementing around the stem. (From ref. 16.)

component with four short metal posts (5). High stresses were calculated to occur in the cement and trabecular bone immediately beneath the posts, due to load transfer to the cortical bone in that vicinity. Reducing the surface area of the metal tray had little effect on overall stresses, except for an obvious reduction in the proximal peripheral bone. Overestimation of the stiffness of the cortical shell led to a significant overestimate of shell stresses and underestimate of cancellous bone stresses. Cement-bone interface stresses were calculated at 32% of failure stress for 2,000-N force, but higher stresses occurred if the cement penetration was greater. Tilting in response to a medial load was not predicted, which is at variance with some experimental and theoretical studies. However, the location of the force is important. In some total knee designs, if the frontal geometry is flat and conforming, varus-valgus moments are likely to lead to contact at the sides, leading to a greater likelihood of distraction at the opposite condyle.

Considering these studies of stress and strain, with those of cement penetration, can be useful. Complete coverage of the upper tibia may not be important so much because it produces cortical contact, but because it avoids understressing the peripheral bone, which has important soft-tissue attachments. On the other hand, a small amount of no coverage is unlikely to have a significant effect, because of the lack of any real cortex (Fig. 5). Cement penetration should not be overdone because a strength limit is reached, the heating effects are likely to be detrimental, the stresses may start to increase anyway, and too much bone is invaded. Ultimately, it is necessary to obtain some clinical manifestation of the various interface conditions, such as relative motion and stresses. As already noted, adverse conditions are likely to lead to bone resorption and gradual sinkage. The roentgenstereophotogrammetry technique is ideal for such an evaluation. Originated by Selvik, the method has been applied in many studies of component stability at the knee and hip. One example was provided by Nilsson et al. (14). At surgery, tantalum beads were inserted into the proximal tibial metaphysis and in the plastic of the tibial component. At follow-up, a Plexiglas calibration cage with beads embedded was placed around the knee and simultaneous anteroposterior and mediolateral radiographs were taken. By dig-

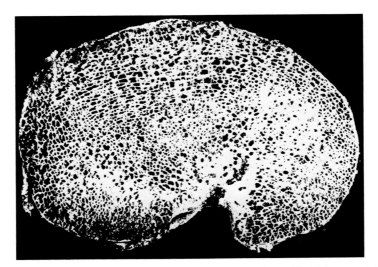

FIG. 5. The resected surface of the upper tibial after cleaning with high-speed lavage. The variations in trabecular density and the absence of a cortex are noted.

itizing the x-rays and utilizing a computer program, the relative three-dimensional orientation of the tibial component to the tibia could be determined. At a 99% confidence level, the calculations were accurate to 0.5° and 0.2 mm. Cemented and porous-coated data were similar. Over a 2-year period, the maximal distal motion of any point was 1.2 mm, but the migration of the center of the component was only 0.3 mm. However, there was lift-off in some regions of 0.4 mm. Rotations about any of the three axes was less than 1°. It must be recognized that the data are both design and technique dependent, but the accuracy of the method makes it a valuable tool. Other simpler methods have recently been introduced that provide less extensive data but more convenience and will no doubt also prove useful.

Determination of the stresses in the cement mantle itself are important for predicting integrity. The stresses will be determined to a great extent by the adjacent implant, less the greater the rigidity. However, bonding also will play a large role. The strain at the center of a 2-mm thick sandwich of cement between a tibial component and bone was measured with strain gauges in a direction parallel to the tibial surface (6). The strains were almost all tensile, due to bending and Poisson effects. The highest principal strains were found under the condylar loading points, being around 1,000 microstrain for an 8-mm all-plastic component. This strain value has been measured as the fatigue limit for noncentrifuged cement, indicating that the cement is at risk of fracture. Metal backing dramatically reduced the strains to under 500 microstrain for 2-mm thick metal. Varus deformity increased strains, but the application of torque or removal of cortical rim support had little effect.

The drawbacks of the measurement of two-dimensional strains were pointed out by other researchers (12). The goal of their investigation was to determine the three-dimensional strains in the cement layer. However, because of the small size of the actual construct, a large-scale model was made with material properties and loading so as to represent the actual situation by use of dimensional analysis. Three-dimensional rosette gauges were mounted on carriers and cemented into the simulated cement layer. The data could be used to calculate the maximal shear stresses and principal stresses. Although their data were of limited value in the tests performed, they demonstrated that the additional data would be of more significance than just two-dimensional data, which could be misleading. Such a method, that of applying strain gauges to a carrier and then cementing the carrier into a cement mantle, has been successfully applied to studies of cemented hip stems in other laboratories.

The Cement-Implant Interface

The importance of the cement-implant interface has been recognized in terms of integrity of the cement mantle, generally by reducing tensile stresses. Some implant designs have a thin precoat of cement applied for secure bonding of the cement applied at surgery. One of the first reports that discussed the interface stresses, taking into account the friction coefficient at the stem-cement interface, was by Berme and Paul (3). The forces on the femoral head were described for different points in the loading cycle of normal gait, forces in the frontal and sagittal planes being considered. By making a number of simplifying assumptions, the stresses at the interface of the stem and cement were calculated. In particular, the differences in these distributions due to friction at the interface were determined. For example, a vertical force could be carried by friction or a wedging action, which would develop tensile hoop stresses in the cement mantle. The static coefficient of friction was measured at 0.32 and dynamic friction at 0.18, values high enough to resist considerable forces. Some of the highest stresses were due to the torsional component of force because of the short distance to the stem surface from the neutral axis.

In most studies, the time-dependent properties of the cement are not accounted for, and yet this could have most important effects on the results. At body temperature, which is just below the glass transition temperature, cement behaves as a viscoelastic solid, which had previously been demonstrated by several researchers. In a series of experiments, the creep rate was found to vary with time after mixing, temperature, and time of immersion in fluids (11). The much higher creep rate at 37°C compared with 20°C was notable. However, the tensile strength was not affected after specimens had been subjected to periods of creep. A tapered rod, representing a stem, was cemented into a tube, surrounded by saline at 37°C, and loaded for a sustained time period. Flow of the cement from the bottom and into grooves cut into the tube was noted, together with gradual sinkage of the stem. Unfortunately no values were given, but the phenomenon of a gradual change in shape of the cement mantle over time allowing a change in stem position was highlighted.

SUMMARY

Laboratory studies of the cement-bone and cement-component interfaces have provided valuable information about the mechanical conditions acting, allowed comparisons to be made among different components, and given guidelines for surgical technique. The experimental methods have included the measurement of cement penetration, shear and tensile strengths of the interfaces, relative motion between cement and bone, even on a microscopic scale, and strains on the various parts of the system including bone, cement, and components. The rationale for the methods themselves has been based on evidence of biological responses to mechanical conditions, such as the resorption of bone in response to relative interface motions and the compressive failure of trabecular bone. Experimental methods are ideally carried out in conjunction with theoretical analysis, such that if good agreement is reached between them, more extensive data can be obtained with the analysis. Further refinements of experimental methods would certainly be beneficial, not only for studying cement-bone interfaces, but uncemented interfaces as well. Experimental measurements carried out in the laboratory on cadaveric specimens are limited, however, in that they represent the state at time of surgery at best. Methods that can be applied during surgery, and after different time periods in the patient, will inevitably yield more valuable data.

REFERENCES

1. Askew MJ, Steege JW, Lewis JL, Ranieri JR, Wixson RL. Effect of cement pressure and bone strength on polymethylmethacrylate fixation. *J Orthop Res* 1984;1:412–420.
2. Bean DJ, Convery FR, Woo SL, Lieber RL. Regional variation in shear strength of the bone-polymethylmethacrylate interface. *J Arthroplasty* 1987;2:293–298.
3. Berme N, Paul JP. Load actions transmitted by implants. *J Biomed Eng* 1979;1:268–272.
4. Blunn GW, Wait ME. Remodelling of bone around intramedullary stems in growing patients. *J Orthop Res* 1991;9:809–819.
5. Cheal EJ, Hayes WC, Lee CH, Snyder BD, Miller J. Stress analysis of a condylar knee tibial component: influence of metaphyseal shell properties and cement injection depth. *J Orthop Res* 1985;3:424–434.
6. Finlay JB, Hardie WR, Bourne RB, Chris AD. Deformation of the cement mantle of tibial components following total knee arthroplasty: a laboratory study. *Proc Inst Mech Eng* 1991;205:211–217.
7. Hadjari M, Reindel ES, Kitabayashi L, Convery FR. The effects of cement penetration on the bone-cement interface. *Proc Orthop Res Soc* 1990;15:439.
8. Harrigan TP, Kareh J, Harris WH. The influence of support conditions in the loading fixture on failure mechanisms in the push-out test: a finite element study. *J Orthop Res* 1990;8:678–684.
9. Hvid I, Bentzen SM, Jorgenson J. Remodelling of trabecular bone at the proximal tibia after total knee replacement. A CT scan study. *Eng Med* 1986;15:89–93.
10. Krause WR, Krug W, Miller J. Strength of the cement-bone interface. *Clin Orthop* 1982;163:290–299.
11. Lee AJC, Perkins RD, Ling RSM. Time-dependent properties of polymethylmethacrylate bone cement. In: Older J, ed. *Implant-bone interface*. London: Springer-Verlag, 1990.
12. Little EG, O'Keefe D. An experimental technique for the investigation of three-dimensional stress in bone cement underlying a tibial plateau. *Proc Inst Mech Eng* 1989;203:35–41.
13. Manley MT, Stulberg BN, Stern LS, Watson JT, Stulberg SD. Direct observation of micromotion at the implant-bone interface with cemented and non-cemented tibial components. *Proc Orthop Res Soc* 1987;12:436.
14. Nilsson KG, Karrholm J, Ekelund L, Magnusson P. Evaluation of micromotion in cemented vs uncemented knee arthroplasty in osteoarthritis and rheumatoid arthritis. *J Arthroplasty* 1991;6:265–278.
15. Ober NS, Lavernia CJ, Reindel ES, Woo SL, Convery FR. Sustained pressurisation of PMMA—a biomechanical study of the bone-cement interface. An in vitro and in vivo comparison. *Proc Orthop Res Soc* 1989;14:395.
16. Reilly DT, Walker PS, Ben-Dov M, Ewald FC. Effects of tibial components on load transfer in the upper tibia. *Clin Orthop* 1982;165:273–282.
17. Ryd L, Linder L. On the correlation between micromotion and histology of the bone-cement interface. *J Arthroplasty* 1989;4:303–309.
18. Steege JW, Lewis JL, Keer LM, Wixson RL. Crack propagation at the bone-cement interface. *Proc Orthop Res Soc* 1987;12:54.
19. Uematsu O, Hsu HP, Kelley KM, Ewald FC, Walker PS. Radiographic study of kinematic total knee arthroplasty. *J Arthroplasty* 1987;2:317–326.
20. Walker PS, Greene D, Reilly DT, Thatcher J, Ben-Dov M, Ewald FC. Fixation of tibial components of knee prostheses. *J Bone Joint Surg [Am]* 1981;63:258–267.
21. Walker PS, Soudry M, Ewald FC, McVickar H. Control of cement penetration in total knee arthroplasty. *Clin Orthop* 1984;185:155–164.

Biological, Material, and Mechanical Considerations of Joint Replacement, edited by B. F. Morrey. Raven Press, Ltd., New York © 1993.

Discussion of the Cement Interface

Richard Coutts

San Diego, California 92123

Fifteen participants of the symposium attended the session on cement. These individuals were a combination of orthopaedic surgeons, who represented varying philosophies with regards to the use of cement and cementless techniques, basic scientists, and pathologists. The discussion was lively and participatory by all members attending with a number of issues discussed. Consensus was reached on many of these issues, which are summarized below.

AGREEMENTS

1. It was agreed that cement is here to stay and that it will remain a significant component of total joint replacement with indications and contraindications yet to be clarified completely. On the basis of retrieval and long-term survival studies, it is clear that cement has the capacity to provide fixation of components for a long period of time in a very high percentage of cases. In this circumstance, long term is defined as 15 to 20 years. This statement presumes that cement will be used properly, reflecting the results of research on how the qualities of cement can be maximized in clinical usage.

2. The optimal performance of cement is technique dependent. This means that an appropriate cement mantle with optimal bone intrusion and minimization of entrapped contaminants or voids will give the best results. A number of variables at the time of usage are under the control of the surgeon and require an understanding of the principles of appropriate usage.

3. In bulk form, cement is well tolerated in the body. It is agreed that in bulk form, cement does not elicit an inflammatory response and is capable of maintaining a symbiotic relationship with the host bone.

4. Cement provides rigid mechanical fixation of joint replacement components. The definition of "rigid" is relative, but in this circumstance implies satisfactory fixation for good clinical function.

5. There does not appear to be any loss of component fixation provided by cement due to aging, with or without progressive osteoporosis. Fixation remains intact through the elaboration of an osseous cortical shell around the cement, which maintains connection with the host cortex through transverse struts. Because of the development of a neocortex, the weakening of the bone with age is not thought to be a cause of implant loosening.

6. A well-cemented stem does lead to stress shielding. Retrieval studies clearly demonstrate a process of cancellization of cortical bone with thinning of the cortices. This, however, has not been demonstrated to be a cause of fixation failure.

7. Polymethylmethacrylate (PMMA) cement in particulate form will cause osteolysis. Both basic research and clinical experience support the contention that particulate PMMA elicits a giant-cell reaction with the stimulation of osteolytic cytokines. This can occur independent of the presence or absence of any other particulate material from a different material source.

8. Cracks in cement will not heal over time. This, of course, is self-evident since one is not dealing with a living tissue when considering PMMA cement. Still, it is important to conceptualize the fact that once a crack occurs in cement, it is likely that it will progress and could contribute to a failure process. The clinical expression of cracks is activity dependent.

9. The radiographic appearance of the interface between cement and bone or between cement and prosthesis is not necessarily a reflection of the clinical status of the patient. This conclusion is related to findings that x-rays that show radiolucent lines of varying width and extent can exist in a patient who is fully functional and without pain.

10. At this point in time, there is no evidence that PMMA cement has a carcinogenic effect. There are no reported cases nor is there anecdotal evidence that tumors have arisen as a result of the presence of PMMA.

There were some issues of a contentious nature that also were discussed, for which there is either insufficient information to resolve or a clear difference of opinion.

ISSUES LACKING CONSENSUS

1. In addition to its function as a stabilizer of implants, cement acts as a seal or barrier to the migration of debris and thereby blocking the effects of the debris on biologic behavior. Although it is clear that the particulate debris, particularly polyethylene particles, will have no effect on the properties of the cement, debris is capable of generating an osteolytic process by virtue of its ability to stimulate the secretion of cytokines that promote osteolysis. Whether the cement-bone interface is more resistant to this action than a bone-prosthesis ingrowth interface, or even a fibrous membrane, remains an unresolved issue.

2. It is thought by some that debonding of the cement-prosthetic interface will lead to failure in all circumstances. This differs from the theory that states that prosthetic-cement debonding can restabilize and continue to function satisfactorily. This remains an unresolved issue as to the degree or importance of prosthetic/cement "debonding."

3. A difference of opinion exists as to the indications and contraindications for the use of cement, particularly with regards to femoral components. There are those who think that cement should be restricted to use only in those individuals who, by virtue of age and activity, are unlikely to outlive the current expected life of the cemented prosthesis. Others think that the use of cement should be broadened to almost all circumstances. The opinion was also articulated that acetabular components should be cemented in some cases. The same dispersion of opinion exists with regards to cementing of total knee components. Upper extremity components, particularly the

glenoid, have a history of loosening in the long term, and a difference between cemented and uncemented components has been noted.

It was thought that the circumstance with cement is not perfect or ideal, and certain improvements would be welcome. These are listed below.

Desired Improvements

1. Improve the characteristics of the cement. This basically means that the fatigue strength should be improved, while at the same time making sure that the cement remains the same or more ductile than it is currently configured. A benefit of these changes in material properties would be an improved ultimate yield strength. Strategies for achieving these goals were not defined, but it is known that the addition of other materials to produce a composite cement might ultimately prove feasible in the future. Work continues in the area of adding allogeneic bone particles or demineralized bone to cement to act as a template for bone ingrowth into the PMMA. Likewise, the addition of fibers to the cement may prove technically feasible in the future as the technological details of this addition are better defined. Basic improvement in the chemistry of the cement might also be used to achieve the goal of a mechanically superior product.

2. A greater emphasis of the importance of technique in the use of cement should be undertaken. There are methods that have been defined that improve the strength and fatigue life of the cement, but only if used in the manner prescribed and implanted in such a way as to avoid inclusions, such as blood and marrow debris.

3. It is important that the nature of different cements be defined, not only in terms of both description of the materials and their mechanical properties, but also in terms of the differences between clinical series already published that have used different types of cement.

SUMMARY

In summary, it was the opinion of this study group that the goal of hip replacement is a "stable" implant. Although there is no definition of stability, a joint replacement would be considered as such if it were painless and functional. Cement is a proven and reliable method for achieving clinically satisfactory stability in almost all circumstances and as such continues to have wide applicability. Cement can still be improved and, combined with improvements in other areas that are known to lead to implant failure, could result in extended longevity of joint replacement.

Biological, Material, and Mechanical Considerations of Joint Replacement, edited by B. F. Morrey. Raven Press, Ltd., New York © 1993.

8

Particle Disease Due to Wear of Ultrahigh Molecular Weight Polyethylene

Findings from Retrieval Studies

Hans-Georg Willert and Gottfried H. Buchhorn

Orthopaedic Department, University Hospital of Goettingen, D-3400 Goettingen, Germany

Ultrahigh molecular weight polyethylene (UHMW-PE) is still used today as bearing material in the majority of joint endoprostheses. This undoubtedly results from the fact that UHMW-PE seems to be destined for this application due to a relatively high impact strength and a low friction coefficient, properties that are clearly superior to other polymers (35). Furthermore, alternatives such as metals and ceramics lack of any shock absorbing properties.

Yet, the application of UHMW-PE in artificial joints also gives rise to certain problems, especially with respect to long-term function and durability. These problems originate from other attributes of UHMW-PE, such as the limited resistance to wear, which is acceptable only under ideal conditions, as well as from its creep and fatigue behavior. In addition, effects of aging and degradation reduce the resistance to wear and cause embrittlement (13).

ORIGIN OF UHMW-PE PARTICLES

Wear of UHMW-PE is naturally combined with the liberation of particles. The mechanism of wear includes abrasive, adhesive, and fatigue wear. Three-body wear caused by fragmented or abraded bone cement (22) and occasionally bone fragments is frequently observed in retrieved polyethylene components. This is discussed both to increase the wear rate by roughening the articulating metal ball head by means of the content of very hard contrast medium of the cement or, in contrast, once embedded and worn in, to protect the polyethylene against further penetration of the ball head.

Particle abrasion may occur at different sites and/or levels (Table 1) (Fig. 1).

From the site of origin, the particles are released into the joint fluid and/or adjacent tissues. Tissues from the surrounding of artificial joints often contain particles of all the materials of which the endoprostheses are made, including polymethylmethacrylate (PMMA) in the cemented ones. Because of this, the morphology of the par-

TABLE 1. *Modes of polyethylene particle origin*

Mode	Site	
	Cemented hip joints	Noncemented hip joints
I	Articulating surface	Articulating surface
a	UHMW-PE/metal/ceramic	UHMW-PE/metal/ceramic
b	UHMW-PE/cartilage and bone (soft top prosthesis)	
II	Anchoring surface	Anchoring surface
a	UHMW-PE/PMMA-bonding	
b	UHMW-PE/bone-interface (cementing defects)	UHMW-PE/bone-interface

ticles and the tissue reaction becomes more complicated. Whereas metallic and ceramic particles are relatively easy to recognize, it is much more difficult to differentiate small particles of UHMW-PE from PMMA. The differentiation between UHMW-PE and PMMA is often necessary, since in cemented endoprostheses particles are frequently liberated, not only from the joint implants but also from the bone cement, especially if the cement fixation is about to become loose and the cement disintegrates. Furthermore entrapment of bone cement particles between the articulating surfaces increases the abrasion of material due to three-body wear. Thus, if the area surrounding an artificial joint is already flooded with wear products of different implant materials, it is difficult, if not impossible, to determine where and at which point the process has started. Nevertheless, to ascertain whether polyethylene debris is incorporated in fluids or tissues, we have several identification methods available (34).

IDENTIFICATION OF UHMW-PE PARTICLES

Macroscopically, in contrast to metallic debris in metallosis, the presence of UHMW-PE, like other polymers, cannot be recognized. Analytically, UHMW-PE can be determined qualitatively and quantitatively by pyrolytic gas chromatography (17,39) and differentiated from PMMA (3) or polyethyleneterephthalate (4). For this analysis, only small quantities of fluid or tissue are required.

Under the light microscope, in sections from decalcified frozen or paraffin-embedded tissue stained by routine methods, polyethylene particles are colorless and transparent to normal white light and hence not, or barely, visible. However, because of their strong birefringent property, they shine brightly in polarized light (Fig. 2). This light effect is almost evenly distributed over the whole area of small- and medium-size particles. Large polyethylene particles sometimes show irregular internal patterns, which possibly correspond to boundary surfaces within the crystalline structures. In order to detect polyethylene particles in the tissue, we prefer to examine the routinely stained histological sections under polarized light, with full-power illumination and the polarization filters crossed at 90°. However, in cases in which the material combination of the endoprosthesis is unknown, it can be quite difficult to identify the polymer from which the particles are derived.

Staining of polyethylene particles has been tried repeatedly. Although PMMA in frozen sections can be stained orange well with Sudan III (41), we were not able to

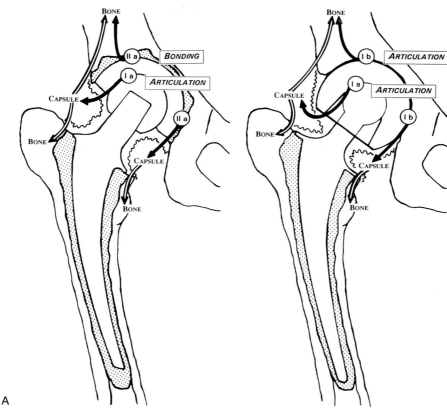

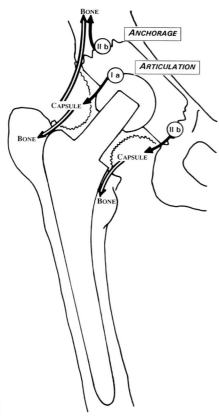

FIG. 1. Modes of polyethylene particle origin and transportation routes. **A:** Cemented polyethylene socket. Mode Ia: Particles originate from the articulating surface, spread first to the joint capsule, and from there to bone marrow and implant-bone interface. Mode IIa: Particles originate from the bonding to bone cement, spread in the case of cement defects first to the cement-bone interface and from there to the other regions such as bone marrow, joint capsule, and remote implant-bone interfaces. In the case of intact cement mantle, particle spreading follows mode Ia. **B:** Polyethylene (soft top) ball head. Mode Ia: Particles originate from the articulating surface with a metal or ceramic head, spread first to the joint capsule, and from there to bone marrow and implant-bone interface. Mode Ib: Particles originate from the articulating surface with cartilage or bone in the acetabulum, spread first to the bone, and from there to the other regions such as bone marrow, joint capsule, and remote implant-bone interfaces. **C:** Noncemented polyethylene socket. Mode Ia: Particles originate from the articulating surface, spread first to the joint capsule, and from there to bone marrow and implant-bone interface. Mode IIb: Particles originate from the anchoring surface at the implant-bone interface, spread from there to the bone and joint capsule, and from there to other regions like bone marrow and remote implant-bone interfaces.

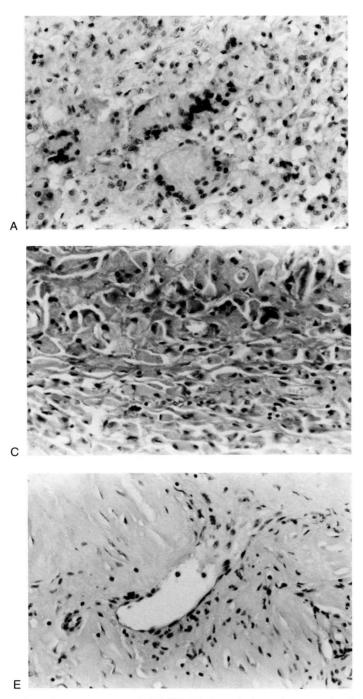

FIG. 2. Loosening of a noncemented UHMW-PE threaded cup 6 years after implantation in a 68-year-old woman. At revision tissue was taken from the implant-bone interface and joint capsule. **A–D:** Histological specimen from a foreign-body granuloma at the implant-bone interface. UHMW-PE particles of various sizes are phagocytosed by multinucleated giant cells and mononuclear macrophages. Microphotographs, hematoxylin-eosin, ×406. (*Figure continues.*)

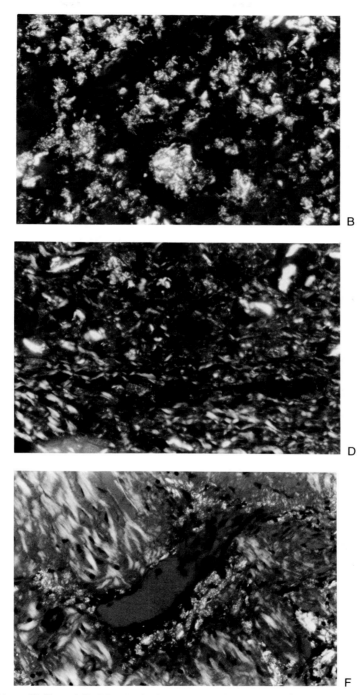

FIG. 2. (*Continued.*) **E** and **F:** Histological specimen from the joint capsule. Macrophages laden with UHMW-PE particles are accumulated next to a vessel in perivascular lymph spaces. Microphotographs, hematoxylin-eosin, ×329. A, C, E: normal bright transmitted light; B, D, F: polarized light.

TABLE 2. *Melting point of polymers used as bearings*

Material	Melting point	
	°C	°F
UHMW-PE	130–140	266–284
Polyoxymethylene	164–167	327–333
Polyethyleneterephthalate	255–258	491–497

demonstrate a clear stainability for polyethylene by this method. In contrast to our own experience, Lintner and co-workers (16) maintained that not only PMMA but also polyethylene and polyester particles show definite sudanophilia and orange-red coloration in Sudan III stained frozen sections.

Recently, a method based on oil red O was described to stain UHMW-PE (7,23,27). Schmalzried et al. (27) and Campbell et al. (7) intend to stain not only particles visible with light microscopy but also those of submicroscopic dimensions. Our experiments, using their exact recipe show that UHMW-PE particles are not always and not regularly homogeneously stained in our material. PMMA, however, is stained homogeneously and intensely (in frozen sections) as well. Thus, it still remains uncertain whether the tiniest and submicroscopic elements within the cytoplasm of macrophages are particles of UHMW-PE, PMMA, or lipid-like organic compounds not dissolved during the degreasing procedure. Nevertheless we regard this method as a helpful addition to the methods available up to now, although the method still lacks proof.

Several attempts have been made to describe cellular reactions to UHMW-PE by means of transmission or scanning electron microscopy (26). These investigations were always based on the thesis that the voids in the cells were occupied by UHMW-PE wear particles; nevertheless the chemical nature of these particles could not be proven.

Discrimination and identification of particles from different polymers used in bearings (or sutures and ligaments) are possible by the determination of their melting point. We used routine histological slides and applied heat to the particle being studied by means of a specially designed heating stage and polarized light microscopy (34). Independent of the temperature (see Table 2), the crystal orientation and thus the birefringency of the polymer particle are lost. Provided that a too-high temperature does not destroy the polymer chains, birefringency of the polymer returns due to recrystallization.

SIZE AND SHAPE OF UHMW-PE PARTICLES

The sizes of diameters of the UHMW-PE particles visible in the light microscopic range from 0.5 to 300 μm (30–47). Other authors report particles of submicron sizes (7,11,26,28) or confirm in principle our measurements (19,21,23). The tissue samples taken from hip joint replacements investigated by Lee and co-workers (14) contained only small particles measuring 2 to 4 μm by 8 to 13 μm, whereas McKellop and co-workers (18) described particles greater than 100 μm. Kilgus et al. (12) investigated tissues from a knee joint replacement and only mentioned particle sizes up to several millimeters. These references are good descriptions for different modes of particle production: adhesive, abrasion, and fatigue wear. Thus, it becomes obvious that the size distribution depends, at least in part, on the mechanism of particle production.

It appeared that wear particles from polyethylene surfaces that articulate with metals (mode Ia) or are rubbed against bone cement (mode IIa) are smaller (ranging mainly between 0.5 and 20 μm, respectively) (38,39), whereas those originating from the convex surfaces of heads in soft top prostheses (mode Ib) and from the anchoring surfaces of noncemented implants (mode IIb), which are in contact with bone or cartilage, are larger. In the latter case the polyethylene fragments are not simply wear products but are generated by a kind of a cutting mechanism, when the relatively soft polymer is scraped off by hard bone (Fig. 6A). Measurements by means of television image analysis (38) revealed that the majority of particles exhibit an area of 1 to 2 μm², the average being 15.2 μm², and an average circumference of 6.3 μm (39).

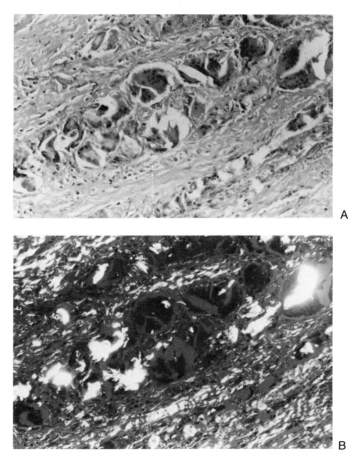

FIG. 3. Loosening of a noncemented UHMW-PE threaded cup 4.5 years after implantation in a 57-year-old woman. At revision tissue was taken from the implant-bone interface. **A** and **B:** Histological specimen from a thick soft-tissue membrane between the polyethylene cup and acetabular bone. Large UHMW-PE particles are incorporated or surrounded by multinucleated giant cells. Microphotographs, hematoxylin-eosin, ×259. A, normal bright transmitted light; B, polarized light.

The shapes of the very small and small polyethylene particles appear as grains or oblong platelets, the larger ones resembling needles, threads, splinters, or plates with irregular boundaries, whereas large chunks present as plump, oval, or elongated, and often as sharp-edged fragments.

TISSUE REACTION TO UHMW-PE PARTICLES

UHMW-PE particles released into the surrounding of artificial joints will be phagocytosed by cells of the adjacent tissues with which they come in contact and induce a foreign-body reaction. Very small and small particles are usually phagocytosed by mononuclear histiocytes; larger particles are incorporated in multinuclear giant cells (Fig. 2), whereas the large chunks of polyethylene are surrounded by several to many giant cells (Fig. 3). The giant cells likewise may also sometimes contain very small and small particles. Ratio and distribution of mononuclear macrophages and multinuclear giant cells are related to the size distribution of particles. Mono- and/or multinucleated phagocytes are mostly densely packed to layers and nodules, forming granulomas, often embedded in strands of fibrous tissue. Because any release of particles necessitates a supply of phagocytes, the extent of granulomatous-tissue formation depends on the amount of particle production.

Like Agins and co-workers (1) and Murray and Rushton (20) by light microscopy we did not see any changes in the cells and tissues, which would have to be attributed to toxic effects of the UHMW-PE inclusions. We would have taken as toxic effects necroses of individual cells laden with debris as well as pronounced inflam-

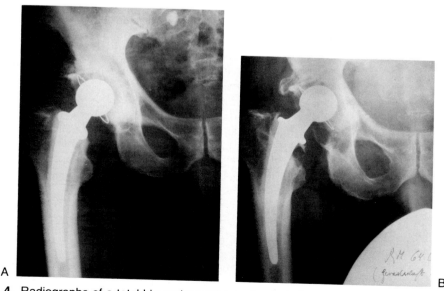

FIG. 4. Radiographs of a total hip endoprosthesis, implanted 1974 (**A**) in a 69-year-old man, with a cast cobalt-chromium-molybdenum femoral component and a UHMW-PE cup. The marked penetration of the metal head into the cup developed over a period of 15 years and the cup migrated in cranial and medial direction (**B**). Extensive osteolysis at the proximal femur (especially the calcar) and acetabulum.

matory reactions or damage to the vessels. The necroses, which are in accord with extensive granulomatous reactions, develop quite regularly in the center of large granulomas, probably due to disturbance of blood supply. The larger the granulomas grow, the more pronounced is their tendency to necrose.

The proliferation of foreign-body granulomas requires space. Consequently the joint capsule increases considerably in thickness (3,29,32,37,44,45), and, because bone is an obstacle for proliferating tissue, foreign-body granulomas developing in bone canals and marrow spaces induce bone resorption resulting in osteolyses (Fig. 4) (5,31,32,36). Recently, Murray and Rushton (20) also showed that macrophages become activated if they phagocytose over a certain amount of particles, although the particulated material (UHMW-PE and PMMA) itself is not toxic. The activated macrophages then release a soluble mediator, which stimulates bone resorption. This seems to be a strong argument in support of our opinion that it is the excessive amount of particles, rather than chemical effects, that causes the adverse effects to bone and other tissues surrounding an artificial joint.

AMOUNT OF RELEASED UHMW-PE PARTICLES

In some cases only very few polyethylene particles can be seen, and they appear more as a secondary finding. In other cases extensive amounts of polyethylene particles are present and dominate the histological picture.

Polyethylene wear undoubtedly correlates with the duration of function of the artificial joint. With the course of time effects of aging can increase the wear rate of UHMW-PE.

The amount of released polyethylene particles probably also depends on the mechanism of origin and articulating material (6,37,48) as well as the type (e.g., hip, knee) and design (e.g., diameter of ball head) of the artificial joint. Zichner and Willert (48) reported an examination that began in 1976 (by Scheier and Sandel (25)) and has been continued by the authors to date. Based on the design of the Müller acetabular cup, the penetration of the femoral ball head into the UHMW-PE socket could be measured by yearly routine anteroposterior radiographs (Fig. 4) over periods of implant function up to 90 months. Although articulations of Cobalt-Chromium- (CoCr) cast alloy or chromium-plated cobalt-nickel-chromium- (CoNiCr) forged alloy against UHMW-PE produced a shift of 0.20 to 0.15 mm per year, those made out of ceramic alumina (Al_2O_3) penetrated the UHMW-PE at a rate of 0.10 mm/year or less. Only 40% of the articulation CoCr cast/UHMW-PE showed a penetration rate less than 0.1 mm per year compared to 63% of hip joints with the articulation Al_2O_3/UHMW-PE.

Articulation of UHMW-PE ball heads or rubbing of loosened all-UHMW-PE sockets against bone liberated extensive amounts of UHMW-PE particles and chips (36). We had the chance to weigh 81 Endler all-polyethylene sockets retrieved at our hospital and compare them to nonimplanted devices (Table 3). During a time period of function of up to 7 years, the wear of the articulation Al_2O_3/UHMW-PE could be considered negligible in comparison to the damage on the outer surface. As an effect of shredding by hard bone tissues in extreme cases, more than 8 g of UHMW-PE had been worn off, mainly from the outer threaded surface.

Theoretically, two assumptions can be made to roughly calculate the volume of UHMW-PE wear of the socket: (i) the shift of the head is unidirectional and (ii) there

TABLE 3. *Weight loss of Endler polyethylene hip sockets at the time of revision (in grams)*

Size	Number of devices	Loss		
		Minimum	Maximum	Average
52	14	0.04	2.13	0.70
55	11	0.02	6.73	4.86
58	23	0.21	6.55	1.38
61	13	0.19	6.76	3.36
64	16	0.19	5.14	1.28
68	4	0.54	8.41	2.80

is no clearance between head and socket. The yearly shift of the head would wear out a volume of polyethylene represented by a cylinder. Its basis is equivalent to the largest circular area of the ball head; its height is equivalent to the shift of the head. For a shift of 0.1 mm and a head diameter of 32 mm, this would result in a volume of abraded polyethylene of 80.4 mm^3 per year.

Clinically, Engelbrecht and Hahn (8) investigated Buchholz total hip replacements with the coupling of CoCr cast alloy/UHMW-PE. The volume of polyethylene wear was described for two hip replacements: the one with a head diameter of 33 mm produced 55 mm^3 per year and the other with a 38-mm diameter released 77.7 mm^3 per year. Using the diagram of penetration given by these authors, we can roughly estimate that an annual shift of the head of 0.15 mm per year equals a volume of approximately 60 mm^3 per year.

The assumption that the average particle size would be approximately 1 to 6 μm^3 results in the conclusion that between 10^{10} and 6 × 10^{10} particles per year are liberated from the articulation. Assuming that a macrophage would be capable of incorporating 60 UHMW-PE particles, 10^9 macrophages would be necessary to store 60 × 10^9 particles. If a macrophage could be represented by a cube of 10 μm edge length, it would require a space of about 1,000 μm^3. Consequently 10^9 macrophages, densely packed, would fill a space of 1 cm^3. This would be the space required for a UHMW-PE particle storing macrophages during 1 year of hip function with a head shift of 0.15 mm per year, fibrous tissue and vessels not included. If the foreign-body granuloma spreads as a membrane in the pseudo capsule or at the implant-bone interface of approximately 0.2 mm thickness, an area of 5 cm^2 could be covered.

SPREAD OF PARTICLES TO TISSUES REMOTE FROM THEIR SITE OF ORIGIN

If one considers the volume of cells required to phagocytose the particles, it is easy to understand that, with continuous production of wear debris, the tissue directly adjacent to the site of origin can manage particle storage only to a limited extent (42,45,46). After this, the particles will spread to tissues remote from their site of origin. During the course of time, the UHMW-PE particles become distributed in the whole area surrounding the endoprosthesis, regardless of their site of origin. This, however, occurs only after a longer period of function and again depends on the amount of particles released. The transportation routes depend on the site of particle production (Fig. 1). In mode I of origin from an articulating surface, the UHMW-PE particles are released into the joint cavity. There they initially come into contact with the joint capsule from which they are subsequently phagocytosed. Further spreading proceeds from there to the bone marrow and the implant-bone interface.

In mode II of origin from an anchoring surface of noncemented and cemented components, in the case of cement defects, it is more likely that the released particles at first come in contact with the tissue at the implant-bone interface, which again starts phagocytosis. They then spread from here to other regions such as bone marrow, the joint capsule, and remote implant-bone interfaces. Free particles were found only in the joint fluid and fibrin exudations on the surface of the joint capsule or at the implant-bone interface. Within the tissues the particles always were incorporated by cells.

Transport of particles to the bone marrow results in granuloma formation in the marrow spaces of the bone, initially without connection to the implant-bone interface, but later also spreading to there and inducing osteolysis (33,40). On the other hand, direct transport of wear debris to the tissue at the implant-bone interface seems to be possible.

The following example is one of several similar cases that we observed recently (36) (Figs. 5 and 6). It illustrates the spread of UHMW-PE particles abraded from the anchoring surface of noncemented UHMW-PE threaded cups not only to the joint capsule but also to the implant-bone interface of the titanium-aluminum-vanadium (TiAlV) stem causing massive osteolysis (cf. Table 3). Abrasion of considerable amounts of polyethylene debris from the anchoring surface of the noncemented Endler threaded cup led to the formation of abundant granulomatous tissue at the implant-bone interface of the acetabulum. This resulted in expanding osteolysis of the

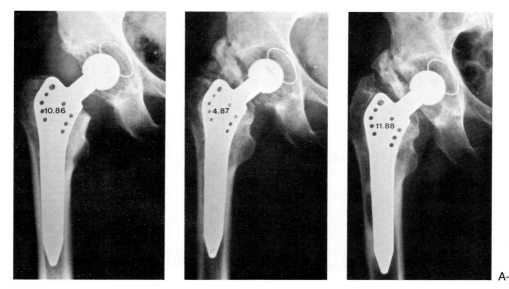

A–C

FIG. 5. Loosening of a noncemented UHMW-PE threaded cup 2.5 years after implantation in a very active 71-year-old woman. Radiographs taken 6 months (**A**), 1 year (**B**), and 2.5 years (**C**) after implantation show rapidly increasing osteolysis of the acetabulum with subsequent loosening of the polyethylene cup. Simultaneously with bone resorption in the acetabulum, scalloping endosteal osteolysis developed in the femur.

acetabulum with subsequent loosening of the polyethylene threaded-cup. Scalloping osteolysis also developed around the noncemented TiAlV stem in the femur. Here we found a thick membrane of granulomatous tissue incorporating large amounts of polyethylene particles at the implant-bone interface also, demonstrating that the polyethylene debris must have been transported from the implant-bone interface of the acetabulum to the implant-bone interface of the femur.

There are at least three different spreading mechanisms possible:

1. Transport via perivascular lymph spaces
2. Regional spread *per continuitatem*
3. Passive dissemination of free particles via open communicating spaces

1. Transport of wear particles by macrophages via the perivascular lymph spaces obviously occurs in the vast majority of cases, since we regularly see accumulations of particles containing mono- and multinucleated phagocytes around the vessels. This transport was also found quite distant from the site of particle production in the newly formed capsule around the joint, bone marrow, and tissue at the implant-bone interface (37,43,45,47). In this way wear debris is carried away centripetally from the surrounding of the implant and arrives in the regional lymph nodes.

2. Regional spread *per continuitatem*. Foreign-body granulomas may expand simply by continuous proliferation into the region. We see this in the form of particle-storing granulomatous tissue spreading from the joint capsule or implant-bone interface to the adjacent bone, along the bone canals and marrow spaces. Two examples of foreign-body granulomas spreading *per continuitatem* follow:

A. Calcar resorption can result from spreading of the granulomatous foreign body reaction from the joint capsule to the neighboring femur. We observed this in nine of 31 cases of a total series of 254 cemented Müller-type hip endoprostheses (Fig. 4). The 31 cases showed an extremely high penetration of the metallic head into the polyethylene cup, indicating a relatively high wear rate; nine of them (28.1%) developed pronounced bone resorption in the calcar region. In contrast to this, of 210 endoprostheses with normal penetration rates of the head, only seven endoprostheses (7.1%) showed calcar resorption. This difference is highly significant (6).

B. Cell-rich granulomatous tissue that stores wear debris at the implant-bone interface not only expands along this interface but also penetrates the marrow spaces and haversian canal of the adjacent bone. It is capable to infiltrate and perforate the entire width of the spongious and cortical bone and induce bone resorption in its vicinity, that results in osteolysis (32).

3. Passive dissemination of free particles via open communicating spaces is proposed by Ling et al. (2,15). This implies that the abraded particles remain free, mobile, and unbound by phagocytes, that there exist open spaces, for example, at the bonding between endoprosthesis and bone cement or at the interface between endoprosthesis and bone, and that a pumping mechanism moves the particles along these spaces. Passive dissemination could be a way of particle spreading. But, basing on the findings in our own studies, we have no positive proof yet for this mechanism and would therefore like to consider this an additional possibility for particle spreading, preferably in those cases in which the cement fixation is about to become loose or the cement has already started to disintegrate.

Production and spread of wear debris, the tissue reaction, treating the particles as foreign bodies, and even the development of osteolysis due to granuloma formation at the implant-bone interface in principle are not specific for UHMW-PE. We were able to show repeatedly that similar processes can be induced by almost every other material, such as Teflon, polyester, polyacetal, silicone rubber, metal alloys, alumina ceramic, and PMMA, regardless of the size of particles. Formation of granulomas and their adverse effects are not so much the result of a suspected behavior or toxicity of the material involved but depend first on the amount of particles released. Terms such as "cement disease" (10), "polyethylene disease" (9), or "metal disease" (24) seem inappropriate for the principle in general. We therefore propose that the clinical sequelae be called "particle disease."

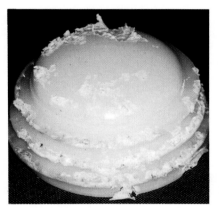

FIG. 6. Similar case as in Fig. 5, with loosening of a noncemented UHMW-PE threaded cup 3.5 years after implantation in a 69-year-old woman. **A:** At revision surgery the threaded cup was completely loose and showed considerable damage on the outer side, due to the heavy wear and tear of the polyethylene by the bone. Thick soft-tissue membranes were removed from the implant-bone interface of the acetabulum and the osteolytic areas in the femur. Histological specimen showed large amounts of UHMW-PE particles stored in huge granulomas that had developed in the acetabulum (**B** and **C**). (*Figure continues.*)

A

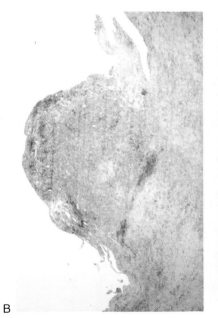

B

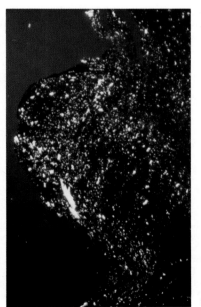

C

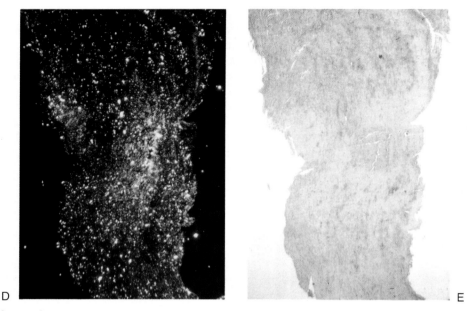

D   E

FIG. 6. (*Continued.*) **D** and **E**: Granulomas storing UHMW-PE particles (B and C) had also spread to the femur. Microphotographs, hematoxylin-eosin, × 31. B and D, normal bright transmitted light; C and E, polarized light.

ACKNOWLEDGMENTS

No benefits in any form have been received from a commercial party directly or indirectly to the authors of this chapter. Parts of this work were funded by the Deutsche Forschungsgemeinschaft (grant no. Wi 346). The assistance of Dr. Ingeborg Lang is gratefully acknowledged.

REFERENCES

1. Agins HJ, Alcock NW, Bansal M, et al. Metallic wear in failed titanium-alloy total hip replacements. *J Bone Joint Surg [Am]* 1988;70:347–356.
2. Anthony PP, Gie GA, Howie CR, Ling RSM. Localised endosteal bone lysis in relation to the femoral components of cemented total hip arthroplasties. *J Bone Joint Surg [Br]* 1990;72:971–979.
3. Buchhorn G, Luederwald I, Mueller K-E, Willert H-G. Detection of polymethylmethacrylate wear particles in capsule tissue surrounding endoprostheses by pyrolysis gas chromatography. *Fresenius Z Anal Chem* 1982;312:539–540.
4. Buchhorn G, Luederwald I, Mueller K-E, Willert H-G. Mass spectrometrical detection of polymer particles in capsule tissue surrounding joint endoprostheses of polyethyleneterephthalate. *Fresenius Z Anal Chem* 1982;312:331–334.
5. Buchhorn G, Willert H-G. Effect of plastic wear particles on tissue. In: Williams DF, ed. *Biocompatibility of orthopaedic implants.* Boca Raton, FL: CRC Press, 1982:249–267.
6. Buchhorn U, Willert H-G, Semlitsch M, Weber H. Dimensionsveränderungen der Polyäthylen-Hüftpfannen bei Müller-Hüftendoprothesen. Ein Bericht über die Messmethoden und ihre klinische Bedeutung. *Z Orthop* 1984;122:125–135.
7. Campbell P, Schmalzried T, Amstutz HC. Special staining supports the presence of submicron UHMWPE wear debris in periprosthetic tissues. Implant retrieval symposium of the Society for Biomaterials. Transactions, Society for Biomaterials, Minneapolis, 1992:31.

8. Engelbrecht E, Hahn M. Socket wear in the St. Georg hip prosthesis after long-term service. In: Willert H-G, Buchhorn GH, Eyerer P, eds. *Ultra-high molecular weight polyethylene as biomaterial in orthopaedic surgery.* Toronto, Lewiston, Bern, Goettingen, Stuttgart: Hogrefe & Huber, 1991:143–147.

9. Guttmann D, Schmalzried TP, Jasty M, Harris WH. Light microscopic identification of submicron polyethylene wear debris: specificity of "Willert's phenomenon." Implant retrieval symposium of the Society for Biomaterials. In: Transactions, Society for Biomaterials. Minneapolis, 1992:84.

10. Jones LC, Hungerford DS. Cement disease. *Clin Orthop* 1987;225:192–206.

11. Jones SMG, Pinder IM, Morran CG, Malcolm AJ. Polyethylene wear in uncemented knee replacements. *J Bone Joint Surg [Br]* 1992;74:18–22.

12. Kilgus DJ, Funahashi TT, Campbell PA. Massive femoral osteolysis and early disintegration of a polyethylene-bearing surface of a total knee replacement. *J Bone Joint Surg [Am]* 1992;74:771–774.

13. Kurth M, Eyerer P, Ascherl R, Dittel K, Holz U. An evaluation of retrieved UHMW-PE hip-joint cups. In: Willert H-G, Buchhorn GH, Eyerer P, eds. *Ultra-high molecular weight polyethylene as biomaterial in orthopaedic surgery.* Toronto, Lewiston, Bern, Goettingen, Stuttgart: Hogrefe & Huber, 1991:208–216.

14. Lee J-M, Salvati EA, Bets F, DiCarlo EF, Doty SB, Bullough PG. Size of metallic and polyethylene debris particles in failed cemented total hip replacements. *J Bone Joint Surg [Br]* 1992; 74:380–384.

15. Ling RSM, Anthony PP, Gie GA, Howie CR. Endosteal lysis. In: Older J, ed. *Implant bone interface.* Heidelberg, Berlin: Springer, 1990:117–121.

16. Lintner F, Boesch P, Brand G. The efficiency of the Sudan-III-staining to identify wear particles of PMMA-bone cement in tissues after total endoprostheses. *Arch Orthop Traumat Surg* 1982;100:79–81.

17. Luederwald I, Henkel M. Determination of poly(ethylene) and poly(methylmethacrylate) in human tissue by pyrolysis gas chromatography. In: Willert H-G, Buchhorn GH, Eyerer P, eds. *Ultra-high molecular weight polyethylene as biomaterial in orthopaedic surgery.* Toronto, Lewiston, Bern, Goettingen, Stuttgart: Hogrefe & Huber, 1991:114–118.

18. McKellop HA, Sarmiento A, Schwinn CP, Ebramzadeh E. In vivo wear of titanium-alloy hip prostheses. *J Bone Joint Surg [Am]* 1990;72:512–517.

19. Mirra JM, Amstutz HC, Matos M, Gold R. The pathology of the joint tissues and its clinical relevance in prosthesis failure. *Clin Orthop* 1976;117:211–240.

20. Murray DW, Rushton N. Macrophages stimulate bone resorption when they phagocytose particles. *J Bone Joint Surg [Br]* 1990;72:988–992.

21. Nasser S, Campbell PA, Kilgus D, Kossovsky N, Amstutz HC. Cementless total joint arthroplasty prostheses with titanium-alloy articular surfaces—a human retrieval analysis. *Clin Orthop* 1990; 261:171–185.

22. Nusbaum HJ, Rose RM, Paul IL, Crugnola AM, Radin EL. Wear mechanisms for ultra-high molecular weight polyethylene in the total hip prosthesis. *J Appl Polymer Sci* 1979;23:777–789.

23. Peters PC, Engh GA, Dwyer KA, Vinh TN. Osteolysis after total knee arthroplasty without cement. *J Bone Joint Surg [Am]* 1992;74:864–876.

24. Santavirta S, Hoikka V, Eskola A, Konttinen YT, Paavilainen T, Tallroth K. Aggressive granulomatous lesions in cementless total hip arthroplasty. *J Bone Joint Surg [Br]* 1990;72:980–984.

25. Scheier HJ, Sandel J. Wear affecting the plastic cup in metal-plastic endoprostheses. In: Gschwend N, Debrunner U, eds. *Total hip prostheses.* Bern: Hans Huber, 1976:186–190.

26. Schmalzried TP, Jasty M, Harris WH. Periprosthetic bone loss in total hip arthroplasty. *J Bone Joint Surg [Am]* 1992;74:849–863.

27. Schmalzried TP, Jasty M, Rosenberg A, Harris WH. Light microscopic identification of polyethylene wear debris using oil red O stain. *Trans Orthop Res Soc* 1992;17:346.

28. Schmalzried TP, Kwong LM, Jasty M, et al. The mechanism of loosening of cemented acetabular components in total hip arthroplasty—analysis of specimens retrieved at autopsy. *Clin Orthop* 1992;274:60–78.

29. Semlitsch M, Vogel A, Willert H-G. Kombination moderner Mikroanalysemethoden zur Untersuchung von Gelenkendoprothesen-Abrieb im Bindegewebe der Gelenkkapsel. *Medizinalmarkt/Medicotechnica* 1971;19:38–41.

30. Willert H-G. Tissue reactions around joint implants and bone cement. In: Chapchal G, ed. *Arthroplasty of the hip.* Stuttgart: Georg Thieme Verlag, 1973:11–21.

31. Willert H-G. Differences and similarities of osteolyses from particulate polyethylene and PMMA-bone cement. In: Willert H-G, Buchhorn GH, Eyerer P, eds. *Ultra-high molecular weight polyethylene as biomaterial in orthopaedic surgery.* Toronto, Lewiston, Bern, Goettingen, Stuttgart: Hogrefe & Huber, 1991:89–103.

32. Willert H-G, Bertram H, Buchhorn G. Osteolysis in alloarthroplasty of the hip—the role of UHMW polyethylene wear. *Clin Orthop* 1990;258:95–107.

33. Willert H-G, Buchhorn G. Pathogenese und Morphologie aseptischer und septischer Implantat-lockerungen. In: Ascherl R, Lechner F, Siebels W, Tensi HM, Blümel G, eds. *Die gelockerte Hüftprothese—Ursachen und therapeutische Konsequenzen.* Stuttgart/New York: Schattauer Verlag, 1990:161–180.
34. Willert H-G, Buchhorn G, Buchhorn U, Semlitsch M. Tissue response to wear debris in artificial joints. In: Weinstein A, Gibbons D, Brown S, Ruff W, eds. *Implant retrieval: material and biological analysis.* Washington, DC: US Department of Commerce, National Bureau of Standard, SP 601, 1981:239–267.
35. Willert H-G, Buchhorn GH, Eyerer P, eds. *Ultra-high molecular weight polyethylene as biomaterial in orthopaedic surgery.* Toronto, Lewiston, Bern, Goettingen, Stuttgart: Hogrefe & Huber, 1991.
36. Willert H-G, Buchhorn G, Hess T. Die Bedeutung von Abrieb und Materialermüdung bei der Prothesenlockerung an der Hüfte. *Orthopade* 1989;18:350–369.
37. Willert H-G, Buchhorn G, Luederwald I, Semlitsch M. Influences of special features of polymer wear particles on the reacting tissues near total joint replacements. International Conference on Biomaterial Polymers, July 12–15, 1982 (Proceedings, University of Durham), 1982:245–251.
38. Willert H-G, Buchhorn GH, Semlitsch M. Die Reaktion des Gewebes auf Verschleissprodukte von Gelenkendoprothesen der oberen Extremitäten. *Orthopade* 1980;9:94–107.
39. Willert H-G, Buchhorn G, Semlitsch M. Recognition and identification of wear products in the surrounding tissues of artificial joint prostheses. In: Dumbleton JJ, ed. *Tribology of natural and artificial joints.* Amsterdam: Elsevier, 1981:381–419.
40. Willert H-G, Lintner F. Morphologie des Implantatlagers bei zementierten und nichtzementierten Gelenkimplantaten. *Langenbecks Arch Chir* 1987;372:447–455.
41. Willert H-G, Puls P. Die Reaktion des Knochens auf Knochenzement bei der Alloarthroplastik der Hüfte. *Arch Orthop Unfall-Chir* 1972;72:33–71.
42. Willert H-G, Semlitsch M. Histo-pathology associated with polymers and metals in total hip replacement. Lecture at the Gordon Conference on Science and Technology of Biomaterials, Tilton USA, August 14–18, 1972 (reprint, Winterthur, Switzerland: Sulzer AG, 1972).
43. Willert H-G, Semlitsch M. Die Reaktion der periartikulären Weichteile auf Verschleissprodukte von Endoprothesenwerkstoffen. In: Cotta H, Schulitz K-P, eds. *Der totale Hüftgelenkersatz.* Stuttgart: Georg Thieme Verlag, 1973:199–210.
44. Willert H-G, Semlitsch M. Reactions of the articular capsule to artificial joint prostheses. In: Williams D, ed. *Biocompatibility of implant materials.* London: Sector, 1976:40–48.
45. Willert H-G, Semlitsch M. Tissue reactions to plastic and metallic wear products of joint endo-prostheses. In: Gschwend N, Debrunner U, eds. *Total hip prostheses.* Bern: Hans Huber, 1976:205–239.
46. Willert H-G, Semlitsch M. Reactions of the articular capsule to wear products of artificial joint prostheses. *J Biomed Mater Res* 1977;11:157–164.
47. Willert H-G, Semlitsch M, Buchhorn G, Kriete U. Materialverschleiss und Gewebereaktion bei künstlichen Gelenken. *Orthopade* 1978;7;62–83.
48. Zichner L, Willert H-G. Comparison of alumina-polyethylene and metal-polyethylene in clinical trials. *Clin Orthop* 1992;282:86–94.

Biological, Material, and Mechanical Considerations of Joint Replacement, edited by B. F. Morrey. Raven Press, Ltd., New York © 1993.

9

Wear of Polyethylene in Total Joint Arthroplasty

Experimental Studies

*Murali Jasty, *Charles Bragdon, *Kyla Lee, *Amy Hanson, and †William H. Harris

*Orthopaedic Biomechanics Laboratory, †Hip and Implant Unit, Massachusetts General Hospital, †Department of Orthopaedics, Harvard Medical School, Boston, Massachusetts 02114

Largely through the pioneering advances made by Sir John Charnley (7), total replacement of arthritic joints with man-made metal, plastic, and acrylic materials has provided dramatic relief of pain and improvement in function for millions of patients with end-stage arthritis over the past three decades. Approximately one-half million total joint arthroplasties are done each year worldwide, with economic impacts of these procedures in the billions of dollars each year.

Despite the enormous success of these procedures, loosening and periprosthetic osteolysis, frequently necessitating revision surgery, remain major problems. Advances in the materials, designs of the prosthetic components, and surgical techniques have greatly improved the long-term mechanical fixation of components to the skeleton, and femoral component loosening rates now range from 1% to 3% at 10 years with current techniques. However, wear of the polyethylene articulating surfaces and the associated biological reactions to the wear debris have now emerged as the major problem in total joint replacements (16).

The difficulties in maintaining long-term success of total joint replacements can be appreciated when one compares total joint replacements to normal joints. Normal articular cartilage provides a smooth gliding surface with a very low coefficient of friction (0.008), over very large arcs of motion (130°), under high pressures (2,000 psi), over millions of cycles (80 million in 80 years). Substitution of such articulations with man-made articulations is indeed a remarkable achievement.

The introduction of polyethylene at the articulating surface with a very low coefficient of friction (0.02) against metal and excellent mechanical properties and wear characteristics have allowed total joint replacements to become a commonplace operation. Other articulation such as Teflon on metal, polyacetyl on metal, and metal on metal have been used in the past but abandoned either because of an unacceptably high degree of wear or high coefficient of friction.

Even though polyethylene has been extremely successful in total joint replacements, it too undergoes wear with time. Accurate wear measurements are difficult to determine, but linear wear rates (penetration of head into the polyethylene cup) of 0.01 to 0.5 mm per year (average 0.1 mm per year) have been reported on the follow-up radiographs of the total hip replacements (6,12,20). Approximate calculations on the wear volume could be made from these measurements assuming a cylindrical pattern of wear, and these show corresponding wear rates of approximately 40 mm^3 per year.

Although it appears that this is a very low amount of wear and thus would be expected to be compatible with long-term mechanical integrity of the components, in reality, however, wear is a problem in applications such as total joint replacements for reasons involving the integrity of the components as well as the tissue reactions to the wear debris. If a significant amount of material is worn away, the geometrical conformity of the mating parts is altered. This can lead to conditions such as impingement of the femoral neck against the acetabular rim, subjecting the implant-bone interface to detrimental shear and tensile stresses and eventually to loosening (43). With excessive removal of material, the articulations themselves can undergo plastic deformation or fracture. Wear of thin acetabular components and fractures of thin tibial components of total knee replacements are examples of such deleterious effects of wear. This problem is particularly relevant to tibial components, which are normally exposed to high contact stresses and undergo a high degree of localized wear (18,19).

Whereas the mechanical consequences of wear can be largely eliminated by design and surgical techniques, the biological consequences of wear debris remain a major problem. Even small amounts of wear can generate large numbers of wear particles in the periprosthetic tissue, which can lead to periprosthetic osteolysis necessitating revision. Many studies have now shown that the liberation of fine wear particles into the tissues leads to a foreign-body macrophage and giant-cell reaction in the periprosthetic tissues and that this tissue reaction leads to periprosthetic osteolysis by complex mechanisms involving phagocytosis of the particles, and production and release of prostaglandin E$_2$, collagenase, and a variety of other cytokines (2,11, 13,15,21,35,38,41). The amount of bone loss in such circumstances can be massive, leading to component loosening or fracture. Unfortunately, revision surgery in such cases is made particularly difficult, often necessitating the use of special components and massive bone grafts. In some cases the extent of bone loss is so massive as to preclude revision surgery altogether.

Recent information from the follow-up studies of cementless components illustrates the importance of wear in total joint replacements and the urgent need to address this issue. It was initially hoped that longevity of fixation of the components to the skeleton can be improved markedly by using components with porous surfaces into which bone can grow and provide secure and long-lasting skeletal fixation. However, recent reports have shown the development of periprosthetic osteolysis even in the cementless components (21,38). In some cases the osteolysis developed around initially well-fixed components and eventually led to component loosening. Ultrafine polyethylene wear debris (submicron in size) has been shown to migrate along the bone-implant interfaces of these components leading to the foreign-body reaction and osteolysis (35).

Thus, wear of the polyethylene at the articulating surface is now one of the major problems of total joint replacement. There is an urgent need to evaluate the mechanisms involved in the production of fine wear debris and address the problem of wear at the articulating surface in total joint replacement.

MECHANISMS OF WEAR AT THE ARTICULATION

Wear may be defined as the progressive loss of substance from the operating surface of a body as a result of relative motion at the surface. There are various ways in which wear can occur, mechanical, chemical, and electrical (28). The main forms of wear discussed by Rabinowicz (27) relevant to total joint replacements are (i) adhesive wear, (ii) abrasive wear (two- or three-body), (iii) fatigue wear (surface and subsurface), and (iv) corrosive wear. Evaluations of the types of wear are important in identifying the predominant wear mechanisms in order to make modifications in the devices to minimize the adverse forms of wear.

Adhesive Wear

Adhesive wear is a form of wear that occurs when two smooth bodies slide over each other and fragments are pulled off from one surface and adhere to the other (27,28). This is due to the fact that macroscopically smooth surfaces are rough on an atomic scale, and when two such surfaces are brought together under load, contact is made at relatively few isolated asparities. As normal force is applied, the pressure at the asperity becomes extremely high, and cold welding or adhesion at the junctions takes place. With sliding, these junctions are sheared off, some of them not at the interface but within the material. As a consequence, wear fragments are transferred from one surface to the other and with further rubbing, the transferred material may detach to form a loose wear particle. This is by far the most common early wear mechanism between smooth surfaces and applies to polyethylene-metal as well as metal-metal articulations. In this process, not only can both surfaces undergo wear but material from each surface can be transferred to the opposite surface. Rabinowicz and Shooter (28), using radioactive tracers, have shown that transfer of metal to the polyethylene also occurs when polyethylene is worn against metal during sliding. Although most of the wear occurs in polyethylene, the small amounts of metal particles thus transferred can then initiate other forms of wear (abrasive wear).

This type of wear may not necessarily be undesirable, since the transfer of material may further modify the surfaces and reduce wear. In general, the adhesive wear rates are low if abrasive wear is not superimposed. Adhesive wear may appear in wear simulators lubricated with saline or water as a polyethylene film transferred onto the metal head. However, such transfer films can also be due to heating and melting and are affected by lubrication. They are not usually seen when the testing is carried out in serum. Adhesive wear can be minimized by using materials with increased hardness or with low molecular interactions (e.g., dissimilar materials).

Abrasive Wear

Abrasive wear is a more severe form of wear that occurs when a rough hard surface or hard particles between two surfaces slide on softer surfaces leading to grooving of the surface. The material from the grooves is released as a wear particle. When only two materials interact, abrasive wear is referred to as two-body abrasive wear (as in sandpaper), but when third particles are involved (as in aluminum grit used in grinding and lapping), it is called three-body abrasive wear. Surface finish may be very important in this type of wear. The presence of hard, opposed to soft, bodies can accelerate the wear. Surfaces that allow the particles to become embedded, such as polyethylene, can lower three-body wear. The wear rates can decrease with time as the abrasive surface is itself worn and blunted with further wear and the wear particles clog the surface asperities of the worn surface.

Wear polishing is a special form of abrasive wear characterized by the presence of very small abrasive particles (in the micron or submicron range). The worn regions in such cases can appear smooth and reflective. The polishing can take place at light loads, whereas in heavy loads or with larger particles (coarse abrasive wear) the surface damage can predominate.

Fatigue Wear

Fatigue wear is produced when repeating rolling or sliding takes place under repetitive loading and unloading cycles. The material can develop surface or subsurface cracks and this can lead to surface break up and wear. This type of wear can occur even when the surfaces are separated by a lubricant film (thus not susceptible to adhesion or abrasion wear) and are due to large shear stresses that can take place underneath or near the surface. Generally this leads to the formation of large pits, craters, or flakes at the surface and the production of large fragment of wear debris. Brittle materials such as glass can undergo an analogous type of wear (brittle fracture wear), developing tensile cracks in the surface perpendicular to the direction of sliding. This type of fatigue wear generally takes place under high loads involving low-contact areas. It is commonly seen in total knee replacements and less commonly in total hip replacements.

Corrosive Wear

Corrosive wear is a form of wear that takes place in corrosive environments, as the name implies. When rubbing takes place in such an environment, surface reactions lead to the production of reaction products (oxidative films). These can be poorly adherent to the surface and further rubbing causes their removal. Wear of titanium heads against polyethylene sockets is such an example. Although polymers are thought to be relatively resistant to corrosion, it has been shown that some degree of corrosion or oxidation takes place even in the polymers, making them susceptible to corrosive wear.

Experimental wear theories have shown that the wear volume can be simplistically shown as:

$$\text{Wear volume} = \frac{K \times \text{normal force} \times \text{sliding distance}}{\text{hardness of the softer material}}$$

Thus high forces and large sliding distances are expected to increase the wear volume. Harder materials generally have lower wear. The wear coefficient K is related to the intrinsic wear properties of the material and the type of wear taking place. In general, severe abrasive wear produces a large coefficient of wear, whereas mild adhesive wear has a low coefficient of wear. With polyethylene on metal articulations, the wear coefficient is on the order of 10^{-6} to 10^{-7}, with wear volumes being 30 to 100 mm^3 per year.

VARIABLES AFFECTING POLYETHYLENE WEAR

Polyethylene is a semicrystalline polymer of ethylene (carbon and hydrogen). Ultrahigh molecular weight polyethylene (>6 million) is used in orthopaedics because of its superior wear resistance, mechanical properties, and low coefficient of friction.

Ultrahigh molecular weight polyethylene is commonly produced by the Ziegler process, which yields a very high degree of polymerization (17). It is utilized in a wide variety of applications, joint replacement surgery being one of them, and produced by different manufacturers (Hercules, Inc., United States [Hyfax], Hoechst, Inc., Germany [Gur], and others). The ultrahigh molecular weight polyethylene components are then machined from large compression-molded blocks or extruded bars. Ruhrchemie (Oberhausen, Germany), and Westlake Plastics (United States) are some of the manufacturers of these bar stocks.

Different resins are used for molding polyethylene and lead to different molecular weights and structures such as branched, linear, and cross linked. They can alter the mechanical and wear properties. Differences in the molding conditions also introduce variabilities in the crystallinity, structure, and completeness of resin fusion. These variables can profoundly influence the wear, creep, and fatigue resistance of polyethylene (8,10,30). In general, polyethylenes of high molecular weight (>6 million), are thought to be important for their wear resistance. Surgical polyethylene has been inappropriately termed high-density polyethylene in the past, but this is a misnomer, because ultrahigh molecular weight polyethylene used in orthopaedics has a low density and a low crystallinity compared to other forms.

The variabilities in the molecular weight and crystallinity can profoundly influence the wear resistance of polyethylene by any of the mechanisms (29–31) (adhesive, abrasive, and fatigue) described above. In addition, degradation of the mechanical properties and wear resistance can occur *in vitro* and *in vivo* by the corrosive mechanism due to oxidation and chain scission (17,31). Heat sterilization and high-dose radiation can damage polyethylene by chain scission. Most orthopaedic plastics, therefore, are sterilized at approximately 2.5 mrads gamma radiation. Degradation of polyethylene due to oxidation tends to make the polyethylene surface more brittle, decreasing its wear resistance. Absorption of the body lipids into the polyethylene can also degrade the polyethylene, decreasing its fatigue and wear resistance.

RETRIEVAL STUDIES

Acetabular Components in Total Hip Replacements

Morphological and chemical studies of components retrieved from patients years after undergoing total joint replacements have provided many insights into the mechanisms of wear *in vivo*. Dowling et al. (9) evaluated 22 cups at 1 to 14 years after surgery using optical and electron microscopy. They found that the femoral head typically migrates superiorly within the socket producing a well-polished, high-wear area superiorly and an inferior low-wear area where the original machining marks are often visible. These two areas are separated by a distinct ridge. The typical depth of migration is approximately 1 to 2 mm at 10 years. In the high-wear area, features of adhesive wear (fans along with thin smears) were seen. In the low-wear area, plowing and scratch marks indicative of coarse and fine abrasive wear were found. Long cracks 10 to 20 μm in length were seen at the junction and were thought to be the result of surface fatigue. Parallel ripples and bald patches were also found in the high-wear areas, but the significance of these findings was not known. They thought that the initial running-in period was due to abrasive wear but that wear polishing was due to adhesive wear. They sought to determine why polyethylene would wear faster in the human body compared to experimental wear testing and speculated that additional mechanisms (either creep, corrosion in the presence of joint fluid, three-body abrasive wear, fretting, or stress corrosion) may be operating *in vivo*.

Weightman et al. (40) evaluated retrieved cups and found areas of wear polishing containing scratches (abrasive wear) and parallel lines perpendicular to the direction of scratches in the scratches, which they interpreted as tensile cracks due to brittle fracture wear. However, they examined replicas of the worn surfaces, as did Dowling et al., and were not able to appreciate the detail of the worn surfaces. They concluded that the wear of the polyethylene was due to adhesive wear initially, but, with time, abrasive and brittle fracture wear (cracking) predominate in some sockets, producing large fragments of polyethylene and high wear rates. Even though it appeared that polyethylene is not a brittle material and thus unlikely to undergo brittle fracture wear, they speculated that the degradation of polyethylene *in vivo* may be responsible for this type of brittle fracture wear.

Rostoker (32) examined 21 polyethylene cups from total hip and total knee replacements and noted the presence of wear polishing, scratching, folding, pitting, and fretting of the polyethylene. Cracking was rare. The most frequent findings were scratching, folds, and wear polishing. He emphasized the importance of abrasive wear from the bone-cement particles entrapped into the articulating surface and thought that in the absence of three bodies wear was mild.

Kurth et al. (17) examined 250 loose cups and found evidence of wear polishing in 50% of Müller cups, whereas the others showed dull surfaces. Complex wear pattens were found comprising abrasion, adhesion, and fatigue wear, each of these later contributing to the abrasive wear and the abrasive wear being the predominant mode of wear after the running in. They also evaluated the density changes at the cup and found that the density increases with time, presumably due to oxidative degradation *in vivo*. Postcrystallization and material fatigue were thought to reduce the ductility of the surface, thereby decreasing the wear resistance.

Our own studies of cemented cups retrieved at revision surgery subjected to volumetric-wear measurements (rather than calculated from linear-wear measurements) showed an average volumetric wear rate of 100 to 200 mm^3 per year. The wear rates are generally higher in the first 2 years (as much as 900 mm^3 per year), presumably due to wearing in or creep, but then reach a steady state. In contrast to the specimens removed for loosening, the specimens retrieved from patients without loosening at autopsy showed extremely low wear rates of 30 mm^3 per year on the average, suggesting that either the failures were due to high wear rates of the components or that failed cups wear at excessively high rates.

Morphological evaluations of the cups show that when the femoral head wears into the polyethylene, it migrates superiorly creating a new contour (highly worn area) separated by the inferior, less worn area by a ridge (Figs. 1 and 2). Wear polishing is the most common feature in the worn area, present in 100% of the cups. Numerous multidirectional scratches ranging in width from 0.1 μm to several microns are found in this wear polished area, presumably due to three-body wear (Fig. 3). Within these scratches, tears in the material perpendicular to the direction of the scratches are seen under high magnification. Cracks in the nonscratched areas are extremely uncommon but may be found in some extensively worn components (Fig. 4). The morphology of the worn area is consistent with mild abrasive-wear polishing and adhesive wear (which is harder to detect by morphological appearance alone but must have taken place initially) patterns. At the ridge that forms between the worn and unworn areas, many features consistent with fatigue wear or plastic deformation can be found. Numerous pits are present along these ridges, as well as cracks within the polyethylene (Fig. 2). Slightly below this ridge, extensive flaking of the polyethylene can be bound in some specimens. The flakes, however, are large (200–2,000 μm), whereas the scratches in the worn region are much smaller (a few microns or less). In the less worn region, areas of incomplete resin fusion can appear as fluffy granules that are denser than the background. Pieces of acrylic can often be found embedded in the less worn regions.

Thus the findings on specimens retrieved at autopsy or surgery provide several important insights into the wear mechanisms that take place *in vivo*. Wear rates of polyethylene generally are in the range of 100 to 200 mm³ per year in the loosened cups and are somewhat higher than what would be expected from the radiographic penetration rates of 0.1 to 0.2 mm per year. In contrast specimens that were retrieved at autopsy from patients with well-functioning prostheses show low wear rates of 30 to 60 mm³ per year. The wear rates appear to be higher in the first year or two after

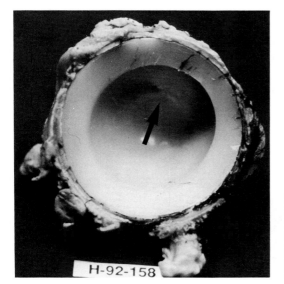

FIG. 1. Cemented polyethylene acetabular component retrieved at revision surgery for loosening at 10 years. *Arrow* indicates the direction of femoral head migration superiorly. The superior highly worn area is highly wear polished and separated by the inferior less worn area by a ridge.

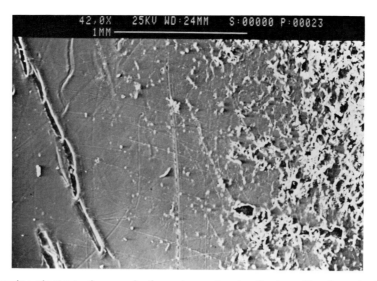

FIG. 2. Scanning electron micrograph of specimen showing the transition from the highly worn to less worn area. The highly worn is polished and smooth at this magnification. Pits are noted in the transitional ridge. Note also the delaminations and flaking inferior to the ridge.

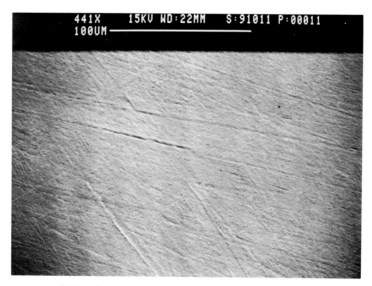

FIG. 3. Numerous multidirectional scratches in the highly worn area of an acetabular component, presumably from three-body wear.

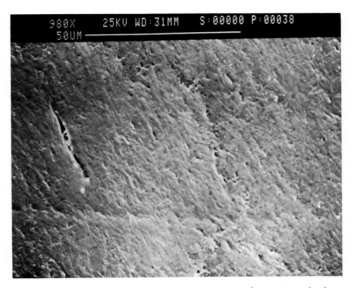

FIG. 4. Cracks in the polyethylene in the highly worn area of an extensively worn cup. These are rare findings.

surgery, either due to initial wearing in or initial plastic deformation of the cup. Extensive fine abrasive wear is commonly present, even though adhesive wear may take place initially. There is far less contribution from fatigue wear and coarse abrasive wear in the hip. The fine two- and three-body abrasive and adhesive wear patterns are consistent with the small wear particle sizes observed in histological studies (35,41). In addition, the retrieved femoral heads also frequently show numerous fine multidirectional scratches providing evidence for three-body abrasive wear (Fig. 5).

Tibial Components in Total Knee Replacements

The mechanisms and patterns of wear of total knee components appear to be somewhat different from those of the hip. The knee joints are generally less conforming than the hip, and complex rolling and sliding motions take place in the knee. The contact stresses are generally greater, as the contact areas are generally lower in the knee compared to the hip. High shear stresses are generated below the surface in the knee as opposed to the hip, where the shear stresses are nearer to the surface (3). For these reasons, polyethylene in the knee is expected to undergo more stress-related fatigue wear. This would lead to the generation of larger wear particles, material failure, and fragmentation of the polyethylene. Coarse abrasive wear with acrylic particles would also be more common in the knee, as the particles are more likely to access the articulation.

Landy and Walker (18) examined 90 retrieved knee components up to 10 years after surgery and found that the wear generally is higher in the knee than the hip. Abrasion from the cement and delaminations are frequent modes of wear. Delaminations consistent with complete break of material into flakes appeared to be initi-

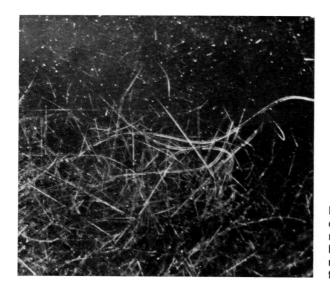

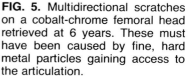
FIG. 5. Multidirectional scratches on a cobalt-chrome femoral head retrieved at 6 years. These must have been caused by fine, hard metal particles gaining access to the articulation.

ated by intergranular material defects and propagated by excessive subsurface stresses beneath the contact zones. Our retrieval studies are also consistent with these features. Figure 6 shows a tibial component retrieved from a patient at 3 years. In this case a portion of the surface had delaminated and exposed the underlying layer. Numerous cracks are noted emanating from this region and reaching the surface. However, this does not mean that other mechanisms in addition to subsurface cracking does not operate in the knee. In the articulating surface different types of wear markings could be seen (Fig. 7). These appear as parallel ripples perpendicular to the axis of sliding (ripples oriented in the medial/lateral directions). The significance of these ripples is not known precisely, but may be due to the cracking and smearing of the polyethylene due to the rolling motion. Figure 7 also illustrates the role of the three-body abrasive-wear polishing of the knee with numerous fine scratches running parallel to the direction of motion.

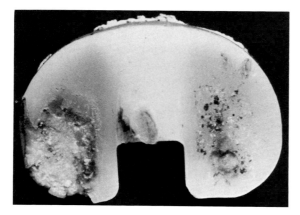

FIG. 6. Uncemented tibial component retrieved at revision surgery for loosening at 3 years. Note coarse pitting, delaminations, and cracking in the polyethylene.

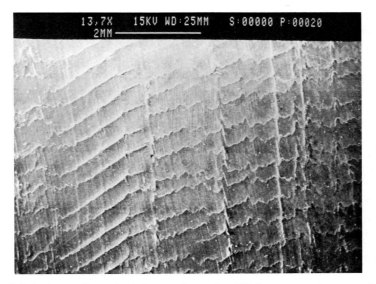

FIG. 7. Parallel ripples at the articulating surface of a tibial component perpendicular to the direction of rolling. Note also the fine abrasive-wear tracks perpendicular to these ripples.

Thus the retrieval studies of polyethylene from total hip and knee replacements not only provide several important insights into the mechanisms of polyethylene wear *in vivo,* but also provide important information pertaining to the design of the experimental wear-testing apparatus and the proper interpretation of the wear-testing results.

EXPERIMENTAL WEAR STUDIES

The difficulties involved in accurately duplicating the *in vivo* wear conditions and the long time that it takes to carry out the wear experiments have limited the widespread use of wear testing of joint replacement components *in vitro.* The types of motions and loads that take place *in vivo,* lubrication, geometrical configuration of the wear specimens to be tested, contaminants introduced into the wear chamber, temperature, and the chemical environments are some of the parameters that affect wear rates and patterns in wear simulators (26). Even if these are adequately controlled, the amount of wear is extremely small and requires sophisticated techniques for measurement (22,26,29). It is also difficult to separate the wear from other processes, such as creep, based on dimensional measurements alone. In spite of these difficulties, however, valuable information has been obtained from experimental studies on wear.

McKellop and Clark (23) provided an excellent review of experimental wear-testing methods and the results. The wear-test machines can be generally grouped into two categories: screening devices and joint simulators. The screening devices are useful in identifying materials of different wear coefficients that may warrant further investigations in the joint simulators. These kinds of testing methodologies include pin-on-disk, cylinder-on-disk, and disk-on-disk type testors. These studies have been enormously valuable in evaluating the material combinations that may produce low wear. For examples, they have shown the low wear rates of ion-implanted titanium against polyethylene and bone compared to nonion-implanted titanium, and the low wear rates of ceramic on polyethylene (23). However, they do not accurately represent the specimen geometry or the loads encountered *in vivo* and thus have limited utility in evaluating the wear in total joint replacement components. As mentioned previously, the mechanisms of wear may be influenced substantially by variables such as the geometrical conformity of the wearing surfaces, the loads imposed, and the presence of third bodies, as noted in the comparison of the wear patterns between the hip and knee components.

Joint simulators, which are more complex than the screening devices, have been used to simulate the *in vivo* wear characteristics. In general, these involve the use of the actual components, simulations of the loading conditions and movements encountered *in vivo*, and lubrication with synovial fluid substitutes. For the hip, most of the studies have used the actual femoral head in the actual type of socket to be tested, simulated flexion extension arcs of the hip (some adding internal and external rotations), simulated loading cycle (39) at low speeds, and used bovine serum instead of distilled water as the lubricant. It is important to note that the speed, temperature, lubrication, and motion can vary the amounts of wear, and these need to be simulated as closely to the *in vivo* condition as possible.

Most testing centers currently weigh the polyethylene cup before and after testing to assess the amount of wear (23,24,26,29). Older studies have used dimensional changes to reflect wear. Rose et al. (29) have shown that at least some of the *in vivo* measurements based on the radiographs may be due to creep. It was their belief that the volume of wear is more accurately measured by recovering the debris worn away. When the wear testing is carried out only for short durations (≤1 million cycles), creep may be a more important contributor to the dimensional change than wear, whereas with longer durations of testing wear may be the predominant mechanism producing the dimensional changes. For these reasons weight methods as used by McKellop and Clark (23) seemed to be the best means to assess true wear rates.

When using the weighing method, however, it is important to control for the water absorption into the polyethylene. For this reason, soaked controls are used and the cups are dried prior to weighing. To control for the creep effects, it may be important to load a cup at the same loading conditions but eliminate the motion.

In spite of the various difficulties with experimental wear testing, valuable information has been obtained when different components are compared in a parametric fashion. Wright and Scales (42) evaluated the wear performance of 25- and 32-mm diameter heads using cobalt chrome against polyethylene and ceramic against polyethylene and found that at 5.2 million cycles, metal on polyethylene wear was approximately twice that of the polyethylene on ceramic. Rose et al. (29) evaluated six Müller polyethylene sockets and found that wear rates varied by as much as 34 times, which in part was related to the variabilities in the molecular weight of the polyethylene. In general, the higher molecular weight polyethylene had better wear resistance. McKellop and Clark (23) found a higher wear rate for 32-mm heads compared to 28-mm heads. The wear of the titanium heads was also greater than the cobalt chrome or stainless steel heads. In follow-up studies, McKellop and Rostlund (26) have shown that the surface treatment of titanium alloy improved the wear resistance of titanium heads but did not significantly improve the polyethylene wear.

As mentioned previously, the role of the three-body abrasive wear has begun to be appreciated (5,14). McKellop and Rostlund (26) introduced two different forms of third bodies, polymethylmethacrylate (PMMA) and commercially pure (CP) titanium, into the wear simulator and found that both of these markedly accelerate the wear of the polyethylene as well as the metal head. Ion implantation offered good protection of the metal surface against third-body wear by PMMA, but the introduction of CP titanium markedly increased the wear, even with ion implantation. With the onset of cementless arthroplasty, which has the capability of producing large amounts of very fine metallic corrosion third-body debris products, the effect of three-body wear may be particularly important.

Alternate materials and improved fabrication techniques have been and are currently being investigated to improve the wear of total joint replacements, based on these retrieval and experimental studies. Femoral heads made out of aluminum or zirconia ceramics have been advocated to improve the surface roughness and abrasion resistance of the counterface and minimize the two- and three-body abrasive wear of the polyethylene, and it appears that ceramics have lower wear rates on polyethylene (36) compared to cobalt chrome alloys. These results were also substantiated in hip wear simulators (42). However, ceramic articulations can be markedly affected by the manufacturing conditions, *in vivo* degradation, surgical positioning, and third-body abrasion. Long-term clinical data are needed to evaluate fully the effect of the ceramics on the wear at the articulation. Other techniques along similar lines that are being investigated involve surface hardening of the metal prosthesis by an ion implantation. Although these techniques appear to be useful on a theoretical basis and have been shown to perform better on wear screening (pin-on-disk machines), adequate wear data from the joint simulators are not yet available.

Fiber reinforcements of the polyethylene with carbon or graphite fiber were initially thought to improve the wear resistance of polyethylene. However, wear studies have shown that graphite-filled polyethylene not only shows a high wear initially, but a late increase in wear rate as well, presumably due to the abrasiveness of the graphite fibers (33). More recently, a highly oriented form of polyethylene (Hylemer, Dupont, Wilmington, Delaware) had been developed to increase the wear resistance of polyethylene. The mechanical properties of the polyethylene, the creep, and fatigue resistance have been substantially improved by this technique (25). However, long-term data with this material are not yet available.

There has also been a resurgence of interest in metal-on-metal articulations in Europe (37). Retrieval studies from selected metal-on-metal implants showed extremely low wear rates (40 times lower than polyethylene on metal). It is hoped that with the contemporary designs in manufacturing techniques, low wear rates could be achieved consistently to allow its use in total joint arthroplasty. However, potential three-body wear from metal particles and the increased coefficient of friction are concerns with these articulations but may be dealt with using good fabrication and techniques.

It is difficult to eliminate the wear completely. Although improvements on wear by improving the material may take several years to develop, proper surgical techniques and selection of components are currently the best means to minimize wear. It is now well established that titanium-based femoral heads perform poorly at the articulation in terms of wear (1,4,26). It is therefore strongly recommended to avoid using titanium heads under the bearing surface and to use cobalt-chrome alloy-based heads or ceramic heads, which seem to perform best in total joint arthroplasty. The use of 32-mm heads against polyethylene in total hip arthroplasty also appears to be suboptimal, compared to 26- or 28-mm heads in terms of volumetric wear (20). Polyethylene components with thicknesses less than 6 to 8 mm should be avoided since the deformability of the components is greatly increased, subjecting them to increased fatigue-related wear (8). This is particularly important in total knee replacements where the fatigue-wear mechanism predominates. The role of the third-body abrasive wear is now being appreciated, particularly with the advent of highly modular cementless prosthesis. The modular connections on the prosthesis can generate very fine metallic corrosion particles that can gain access to the articulation and cause accelerated wear of the polyethylene as well as the metal counterface.

Finally, secure implantation fixation to the skeleton is essential in minimizing the production of third bodies of acrylic or metal generated from loosening and movements at the implant-bone interface.

REFERENCES

1. Agins HJ, Alcok NW, Bansal M, Salvati EA, et al. Metallic wear in failed titanium-alloy total hip replacements. *J Bone Joint Surg* 1988;70:347–356.
2. Anthony PP, Gie GA, Howie CR, Ling RSM. Localised endosteal bone lysis in relation to the femoral components of cemented total hip arthroplasties. *J Bone Joint Surg [Br]* 1990;72:971–979.
3. Bartel DL, Bicknell VL, Wright TM. The effect of conformity, thickness, and material on stresses in ultra-high molecular weight components for total joint replacements. *J Bone Joint Surg [Am]* 1986;72:126–130.
4. Black J, Shefk H, Bonini J, Rostoker WR, Schajowicz F, Galante JO. Metallosis associated with a stable titanium-alloy femoral component in total hip replacement. *J Bone Joint Surg [Am]* 1990;72:126–130.
5. Caravia L, Dowson D, Fisher J, Jobbins B. The influence of bone and bone cement debris on counterface roughness in sliding wear tests of ultra-high molecular weight polyethylene on stainless steel. *Proc Inst Mech Eng* 1990;204:65–70.
6. Charnley J, Halley DK. Rate of wear in total hip replacement. *Clin Orthop* 1975;112:170–180.
7. Charnley J, Kettlewell J. The elimination of slip between prosthesis and femur. *J Bone Joint Surg [Br]* 1965;47:56–60.
8. Collier JP, Mayor MB, Surprenant VA, Surprenant HP, Dauphinais LA, Jensen RE. The biomechanical problems of polyethylene as a bearing surface. *Clin Orthop* 1990;261:107–113.
9. Dowling JM, Atkinson JR, Dowson D, Charnley J. The characteristics of acetabular cups worn in the human body. *J Bone Joint Surg [Br]* 1978;60:375–382.
10. Gold B, Walker P. Variables affecting friction and wear of metal and plastic total hip joints. *Clin Orthop* 1974;100:270–278.
11. Goldring SR, Jasty M, Roueke CM, Bringhurst FR, Harris WH. Formation of a synovial-like membrane at the bone-cement interface. Its role in bone resorption and implant loosening after total hip replacement. *Arthritis Rheum* 1986;29:836–842.
12. Griffith M, Seidenstein M, Williams D, Charnley J. Socket wear in Charnley low friction arthroplasty of the hip. *Clin Orthop* 1978;137:37–47.
13. Harris WH, Schiller AL, Scholler JM, Freiberg RA, Scott R. Extensive localized bone resorption in the femur following total hip replacement. *J Bone Joint Surg [Am]* 1976;58:612–618.
14. Isaac GH, Atkinson JR, Dowson D, et al. The role of cement in the long term performance and premature failure of Charnley low friction arthroplasties. *Eng Med* 1986;15:19–22.
15. Jasty M, Floyd WE III, Schiller AL, Goldring SR, Harris WH. Localized osteolysis in stable, non-septic total hip replacement. *J Bone Joint Surg [Am]* 1986;68:912–919.
16. Jasty M, Smith E. Wear particles of total joint replacements and their role in periprosthetic osteolysis. *Curr Opin Rheumatol* 1992;4:204–209.
17. Kurth M, Eyerer P, Ascherl R, Dittel K, Holz U. An evaluation of retrieved UHMWPE hip joint cups. *J Biomater Appl* 1988;3:33–51.
18. Landy MM, Walker PS. Wear of ultra-high-molecular-weight polyethylene components of 90 retrieved knee prostheses. *J Arthroplasty* 1988;3:73–85.
19. Lindstrand A, Rydl Stenstrom A. Polyethylene failure in two total knees. Wear of thin metal-backed PCA tibial components. *Acta Orthop Scand* 1990;61:575–577.
20. Livermore J, Ilstrup D, Morrey B. Effect of femoral head size on wear of the polyethylene acetabular component. *J Bone Joint Surg [Am]* 1990;72:518–528.
21. Maloney WJ, Jasty M, Harris WH, Galante JO, Callaghan JJ: Endosteal erosion in association with stable uncemented femoral components. *J Bone Joint Surg [Am]* 1990;72:1025–1034.

22. McKellop HA, Clark IC. Evolution and evaluation of materials screening machines and joint simulators in predicting in vivo wear phenomena. In: Ducheyne P, Hastings G, eds. *Functional behavior of orthopaedic biomaterials, vol II, applications.* Boca Raton: CRC Press, 1984: chap. 3.

23. McKellop HA, Clark IC. Degradation and wear of ultra-high molecular weight polyethylene. In: Fraker AC, Griffin CD, eds. *Corrosion and degradation of implant materials: Second Symposium, ASTM STP 859.* Philadelphia: American Society for Testing and Materials, 1985;351–368.

24. McKellop HA, Clark IC, Markolf KL, and Amstutz HC. Wear characteristics of UHMW polyethylene: a method for accurately measuring extremely low wear rates. *J Biomed Mater Res* 1978;12:895–927.

25. McKellop HA, Lu B, Li S. Wear of acetabular cups of conventional and modified UHMW polyethylenes compared on a hip joint simulator. Transactions of 38th annual meeting of the Orthopaedic Research Society, 1992:356.

26. McKellop HA, Rostlund TV. The wear behavior of ion-implanted Ti-6AI-4V against UHMW polyethylene. *J Biomed Mater Res* 1990;24:1413–1425.

27. Rabinowicz E. *Friction and wear of materials.* New York: John Wiley, 1966.

28. Rabinowicz E, Shooter KV. The transfer of metal to plastics during sliding. *Proc Phys Soc [B]* 1952;65:671–673.

29. Rose RM, Nusbaum HJ, Schneider H, et al. On the true wear rate of ultra high-molecular-weight polyethylene in the total hip prosthesis. *J Bone Joint Surg [Am]* 1980;62:537–549.

30. Rose RM, Crugnola A, Ries SB, Cimino WR, Paul I, Radin EL. On the origins of high in vivo wear rates in polyethylene components of total joint prostheses. *Clin Orthop* 1979;145:277–286.

31. Rose RM, Goldfarb EV, Ellis E, Crugnola AN. Radiation sterilization and the wear rate of polyethylene. *J Orthop Res* 1984;2:393–400.

32. Rostoker W. The appearances of wear on polyethylene—a comparison of in vivo and in vitro wear surfaces. *J Biomed Mater Res* 1978;12:317–335.

33. Rostoker W, Galante JO. Some new studies of the wear behavior of ultra high molecular weight polyethylene. *J Biomed Mater Res* 1976;10:303–310.

34. Scales JT, Kelly P, Goddard D. Friction torque studies of total joint replacements—the use of a simulator. *Ann Rheum Dis* 1969(suppl. 28):30.

35. Schmalzried TP, Jasty M, Harris WH. Periprosthetic bone loss in total hip arthroplasty: polyethylene wear debris and the concept of the effective joint space. *J Bone Joint Surg [Am] (in press).*

36. Semlich M, Lehmann M, Weber H, Doerre E, Willert H. New prospects for a prolonged functional life-span of artificial hip joints by using the material combination polyethylene/aluminum oxide ceramic/metal. *J Biomed Mater Res* 1977;11:537.

37. Semlich M, Streicher RM, Weber H. The wear behavior of capsules and heads of CoCrMo casts in long-term implanted all-metal hip prostheses. *Orthopade* 1989;18:377–381.

38. Tanzer M, Maloney WJ, Jasty M, Harris WH. The progression of femoral cortical osteolysis in association with total hip arthroplasty without cement. *J Bone Joint Surg [Am]* 1992;74:404–410.

39. Weightman BO, Paul IL, Rose RM, Simon SR, Radin EL. A comparative study of total hip replacement prostheses. *J Biomech* 1973;6:299–311.

40. Weightman B, Swanson SAV, Isaac GH, Wroblewski BM. Polyethylene wear from retrieved acetabular cups. *J Bone Joint Surg [Br]* 1991;73:806–810.

41. Willert HG, Bertram H, Buchhorn GH. Osteolysis in alloarthroplasty of the hip. The role of ultra-high molecular weight polyethylene wear particles. *Clin Orthop* 1990;258:95–107.

42. Wright K, Scales J. The use of hip joint simulators for the evaluation of wear of total hip prostheses. In: Writer G, Lerey J, deGrousst K, eds. *Evaluation of biomaterials.* New York: John Wiley, 1980:135.

43. Wroblewski BM. Wear and loosening of the socket in the Charnley low-friction arthroplasty. *Orthop Clin North Am* 1988;19:627–630.

*Biological, Material, and Mechanical
Considerations of Joint Replacement,*
edited by B. F. Morrey.
Raven Press, Ltd., New York © 1993.

10

The Role of Particulate Orthopaedic Implant Materials in Peri-implant Osteolysis

Mechanisms of Granuloma Formation and Particle-Induced Osteolysis

*†Jeng-Tzung Wang and *‡Steven R. Goldring

*Department of Medicine, Harvard Medical School, Medical Services (Arthritis Unit),
Massachusetts General Hospital, Boston, Massachusetts 02114; †Harvard School of
Dental Medicine, Boston, Massachusetts 02215; ‡Department of Medicine, New
England Deaconess Hospital, Boston, Massachusetts 02215

BACKGROUND

Periprosthetic osteolysis associated with aseptic component loosening after cemented total hip arthroplasty was first recognized and described by Charnley (3), who noted the presence of a macrophage foreign-body reaction associated with fragmented methacrylate cement. Subsequently, Willert and co-workers (17,18) firmly established that release of prosthetic materials in particulate form into the bone-implant bed could lead to the development of a so-called foreign-body granulomatous reaction that was accompanied by extensive localized bone resorption adjacent to the implant. These authors recognized that this reaction could occur in the absence of local sepsis and speculated that the inflammatory reaction was induced by the particulate prosthetic implant debris. Numerous additional articles have now firmly established that orthopaedic implant materials in particulate form are capable of inducing a granulomatous response at the interface between the implant and adjacent bone. Although these studies have provided important insights into the natural history and the role of biological and mechanical factors in the development of this tissue reaction, the specific cellular and biochemical processes involved in the pathogenesis of the peri-implant osteolysis have not been fully defined. This chapter will provide background into the nature of foreign-body granuloma and discuss the potential role of particle-cell interactions and cytokines in the pathogenesis of this process.

GRANULOMATOUS INFLAMMATORY RESPONSES

Granulomatous tissue reactions have been defined as local cellular responses to materials or substances that have resisted destruction by processes involving components of the acute inflammatory response (16). Although these reactions are classically directed against so-called "foreign" materials, they may also occur in response to endogenous substrates such as sodium urate, which results in the characteristic lesions of gout. In general, these foreign materials share the property of resistance to degradation by host tissues or cells, and the reaction often is accompanied by continuous or repeated exposure to the offending agent. The granulomatous response should not necessarily be regarded as a pathological reaction since it represents, in a sense, an appropriate biological reaction to foreign materials, and this reaction can lead to almost complete resolution with minimal disruption of target-tissue function. Unfortunately, this is not always the case, and in many instances the reaction results in irreversible damage to tissues with severe impairment in function.

Investigators have characterized granulomatous reactions into two major categories based primarily on the cellular features of the tissue reaction. *Nonimmune granuloma* include responses to nondigestible particles, which include the particulate materials derived from orthopaedic implant devices, such as methylmethacrylate, high-density polyethylene, and silicone. The predominant cell types in these lesions are monocyte/macrophages and fibroblasts. *Immune granuloma* are associated with antigenic materials derived from various bacterial, fungal, or viral infectious agents. These tissue reactions demonstrate evidence of involvement of additional components of the immune system including T and B lymphocytes as well as plasma cells, cell types characteristically associated with hypersensitivity responses.

Based on the phenotypic features of the elicited cells, it is therefore possible to determine whether an inflammatory reaction demonstrates features of a hypersensitivity reaction to a foreign agent. In our previously reported series of patients with aseptic loosening after total hip replacement (8), the peri-implant tissue exhibited minimal evidence of lymphocytic infiltration, consistent with a nonimmune granulomatous reaction. Clinical and laboratory assessment of these patients was consistent with the diagnosis of osteoarthritis. Others have reported similar results in patients with osteoarthritis. In contrast, Jiranek, Jasty, and Harris (unpublished) recently evaluated tissues from the regions of focal osteolysis from a series of patients with uncemented prostheses and noted that in half of the patients there were cells expressing T-cell antigenic markers. None of the tissues contained B cells, and clinically it was not possible to distinguish individuals with evidence of T-lymphocyte infiltration from those without evidence of cellular hypersensitivity. Santavirta et al. (15) also noted T-lymphocyte infiltration in tissues from patients with osteolysis associated with uncemented prosthesis. The lymphocytes, however, did not demonstrate evidence of activation, leading the authors to conclude that the tissue response was nonimmunogenic.

Nevertheless, it is likely that in some patients hypersensitivity to the implant materials may modulate the nature of the tissue reaction. For example, Lalor et al. (10) recently demonstrated significant lymphocytic infiltration around titanium-based implants in several patients. Based on the reactivity to metal skin testing of two of the patients, the authors speculated that hypersensitivity to titanium could contribute to the cellular and biological activity of the tissue reaction.

The possible existence of hypersensitivity reactions to implant materials is of significance for several reasons. First, development of hypersensitivity could induce local pain, secondary to the peri-implant immune reaction. These symptoms could

potentially lead to the need for early revision, even in the absence of significant osteolysis. In addition, involvement of T lymphocytes could contribute to am-
plification of the inflammatory reaction, related to the release of soluble inflammatory mediators. In fact, in individuals with silicosis, activated T and B lymphocytes
are often present in the pulmonary nodules and are believed to contribute to the
pathogenic events associated with the destructive capacity and perpetuation of the
tissue reaction. Silicosis thus serves as a disease model in which a presumably "inert" material can evoke a tissue response with features of a hypersensitivity reaction.

We have identified a subgroup of patients with aseptic peri-implant osteolysis
who do exhibit features of an intense immune granulomatous reaction to implant
materials (9). These individuals all had evidence of underlying rheumatoid arthritis. Our findings indicate that in patients with rheumatoid arthritis reactions to so-
called nonimmune, inert particulates could result in concomitant induction of
delayed hypersensitivity. It is of interest that the coexistence of rheumatoid arthritis and silicosis modulates the cellular features of the pulmonary nodules in a similar fashion.

FACTORS AFFECTING CELL-PARTICLE INTERACTIONS

Nonimmune cells such as fibroblasts can bind and even ingest particulate materials with resultant modulation of their functional activities. In this manner they can
function as "facultative phagocytes." However, in nonimmune granuloma, macrophages are likely the principal cell type responsible for mediating the tissue reaction
to these materials. In this paradigm, the macrophages function as the primary "transducers" of the responses to the particulate material. These cells ultimately control
the features of the tissue reaction by the release of soluble mediators such as proteinases and cytokines, which affect remodeling of connective matrices, directly or indirectly, by modulating the activities of other cell types such as resident fibroblasts
(Fig. 1).

It is possible to separate the interaction between the macrophage and particulate
materials into several independent stages (19). The outcome of each of these individual steps ultimately determines the nature of the tissue response. Several studies
have established that the size, shape, relative hydrophobicity or hydrophilicity, composition, and quantity of material are critical factors in defining the consequences of
the particle-cell interaction. In addition, the stage of macrophage activation, as well
as the presence of potential modulating influences, such as lymphocytes or their
products, can profoundly influence the tissue response (16).

The first step in the particle-cell interaction involves *recognition* by the cell of the
particle surface. In this sense the particle surface or its individual components function as surface ligands for putative ligand receptors located on the surface of the cell
membrane. It is possible to classify this ligand-receptor interaction into two major
categories that are defined by the presence or absence of particle opsonization (1).
Opsonins can be defined as any serum protein that can bind to the surface of a
particle to enhance its recognition and facilitate its phagocytosis. This can be accomplished by binding the particle and cell together or binding to the particle alone and
thereby altering its surface properties to enhance its interaction with the cell surface.
The most well-characterized and studied opsonins are immunoglobulins, particularly

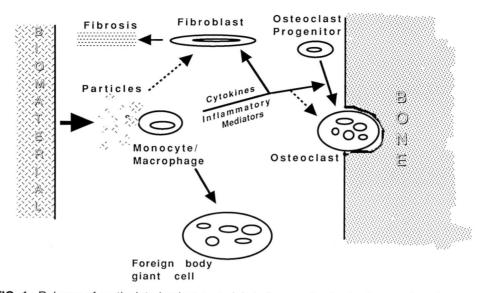

FIG. 1. Release of particulate implant materials induces a foreign-body granulomatous reaction. Interaction of monocyte/macrophages with particles stimulates the release of cytokines and other inflammatory products with the capacity to induce the differentiation and activation of osteoclast-type giant cells, which then mediate the peri-implant osteolysis. The monocyte/macrophage products also induce fibroblasts to produce collagen, leading to formation of fibrous tissue.

of the IgG class, and components of the complement system, but additional serum factors including fibronectin, vitronectin, and a variety of other glycoproteins and peptides can modulate the interaction between cells and particulate matter. Although classically defined as enhancers of phagocytosis, in some instances these serum factors may function to actually inhibit the cell-particle interaction.

Recent studies have stressed the importance of the surface properties of the foreign material in determining properties of the opsonized serum component. For example, Lin et al. (12) showed that increasing the hydrophobicity of silica surfaces alters the binding characteristics for the third component of complement, making it less susceptible to activation and reducing its potential capacity to activate cells through the complement receptor. Similar effects of substrate surface charge on the activity of the adsorbed opsonins have been reported in studies with fibronectin and vitronectin (11).

There have been significant advances in the understanding and characterization of the cell-surface receptors for many of these opsonic ligands and the mechanisms by which binding of these ligands to their specific receptor results in modulation of cell function through specific signal transduction pathways. As stressed by Yin and Stossel (19), the initial binding and recognition of the adsorbed opsonin through these cell surface receptors can result in modulation of cell function through a classical receptor-coupled event independent of the process of internalization.

In addition to particle-cell interactions involving opsonization, it is well established that particle recognition and phagocytosis can occur in the absence of serum factors. Studies have established that particle surface hydrophobicity and charge can markedly affect this system (1), but the nature of the "receptor" involved in this type of interaction and the specific signal transduction mechanisms responsible for modulation of cell function are poorly understood.

An additional factor that influences the biological activity and clinical consequences of granulomatous reactions induced by particulate orthopaedic implant materials is that they are associated with, in most instances, heterogeneous populations of particles. This heterogeneity exists both in terms of the composition of the materials (e.g., high-density polyethylene and methylmethacrylate with cemented implants) as well as particle size and shape. Each subgroup of particles likely exhibits differential capacities to modulate specific cell functions. For example, certain types of particles may be very effective in recruiting cells to the granulomatous reaction. These particles may, because of their size, be resistant to phagocytosis and thus have minimal capacity to induce additional cell responses. These cells, however, become targets for other smaller, readily phagocytosed particles that are present within the granuloma. Interaction with these smaller particles may then result in significant "activation" or modulation of cell function. Similarly, although metal corrosion products or metal wear debris may have relatively limited capacity to induce granuloma formation, they may have significant effects in terms of modulating cell function in tissue reactions initiated by other types of particulates (e.g., high-density polyethylene). Thus, the existence of diverse populations of particulate materials at the bone-implant bed provides the potential for multiple stimuli, each of which may function to modulate and control the tissue and cell reactions in different and specific fashions to augment inflammatory responses. This principle, which we characterize as the "double-hit theory of cell activation," is schematically illustrated in Fig. 2. The existence of multiple stimuli related to the presence of diverse types of particulate materials at the bone-implant bed provides a mechanism for potentiating and modulating the cell responses and likely contributes to the unique pathogenicity of the tissue reaction in terms of peri-implant osteolysis.

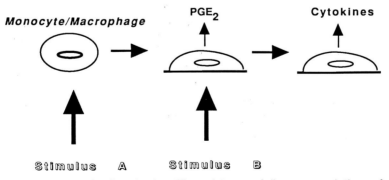

FIG. 2. Double-hit theory of cell activation. The existence of diverse populations of particulate materials at the bone-implant bed provides the potential for multiple stimuli. Each stimulus may function to modulate and control the tissue and cell reaction in different and specific fashions to augment the inflammatory responses by stimulating the release of inflammatory mediators, e.g., PGE_2 and cytokines.

ROLE OF PARTICULATE POLYETHYLENE IN PERI-IMPLANT OSTEOLYSIS

It is now established that the release of polyethylene particulate wear debris into the bone-implant bed after total joint arthroplasty is associated with an intense foreign-body reaction. The presence of this inflammatory tissue reaction in areas of focal osteolysis provides further evidence for an important role for this particulate material in the pathogenesis of peri-implant osteolysis (18).

Examination of the tissue reaction to polyethylene particles from retrieved surgical specimens as well as from animal studies demonstrates that the inflammatory reaction to this material has the histological features of a nonimmune foreign-body granuloma. Thus, there is little evidence that hypersensitivity to polyethylene plays an important pathogenetic role. It is not clear, however, how polyethylene induces focal enhancement of bone resorption.

In order to define the potential mechanism by which polyethylene induces bone resorption Murray and Rushton (14) incubated mouse peritoneal macrophages with particles of high-density polyethylene. They showed that treatment resulted in stimulation of release of PGE_2, as well as soluble products with the capacity to induce bone resorption in an *in vitro* bone-resorption assay. In another study (13) they evaluated the effect of culturing macrophages on bulk surfaces of high-density polyethylene and noted that this surface was considerably less "active" than, for example, tissue culture plastic in stimulating cells to release products with resorbing activity. Bonfield et al. (2) performed similar studies with polyethylene and noted that polyethylene in bulk form demonstrated less capacity to "activate" cells to release cytokines compared to tissue culture plastic. These studies confirm that the transformation of polyethylene from a "bulk" material to particles markedly enhances its capacity to modulate cell function by phagocytic or cell-surface contact.

CELLULAR MECHANISMS INVOLVED IN PERI-IMPLANT OSTEOLYSIS

To study the mechanisms responsible for peri-implant osteolysis we cultured tissue fragments from the bone-implant bed from patients with aseptic peri-implant osteolysis and demonstrated the release of soluble factors that exhibit significant bone-resorbing activity (6,8). PGE_2, interleukin-1, interleukin-6, and tumor necrosis factor-α are among the products implicated in this resorptive process, and these findings have led us to propose the model in Fig. 1. According to this model, released implant particulate materials induce a focal foreign-body granulomatous reaction in the bone-implant bed. The interaction between the elicited cells (macrophages, foreign-body giant cells, and fibroblasts) and the particles induces cell activation, particularly in the cells of monocyte/macrophage lineage. This "activation" results in the release of a variety of inflammatory mediators and cytokines that have the capacity to induce osteoclast recruitment and activation on the adjacent bone surfaces leading to focal induction of bone resorption.

Recently Athanasou et al. (5) proposed an additional mechanism by which particulate orthopaedic implant materials could stimulate focal bone resorption. They cultured inflammatory cells from the joint capsules from patients with granulomatous reactions to particulate implant material. Their results demonstrated that both monocyte/macrophages and cells expressing phenotypic features of foreign-body giant cells could produce bone "resorption pits" in bone slices, although the level of resorption was considerably less than that observed with so-called osteoclast-type giant cells.

Our own studies (5,7) indicate that particulate polymeric orthopaedic implant materials have minimal capacity to induce osteoclast-type giant cells directly and that the bone resoption is mediated by the release from the inflammatory tissue of factors that activate bone-derived cells to resorb the mineralized matrix. In these studies we implanted particles of high-density polyethylene and methylmethacrylate into° soft tissues of rats and analyzed the characteristics of the elicited cells. Based on the absence of several features associated with the osteoclast phenotype, including tartrate-resistant acid phosphatase activity and calcitonin receptors, we concluded that the polykaryons elicited by either polymer did not demonstrate features of osteoclast-type giant cells.

CONCLUSIONS

Analysis of retrieved tissues from patients with aseptic peri-implant osteolysis has established the critical role of particle-induced granulomatous reactions in the pathogenesis of the bone resorption that characterizes this condition. Recent *in vitro* studies have begun to define the cellular, biochemical, and molecular basis for these events. An understanding of these processes is critical for developing more effective therapeutic strategies and improved orthopaedic techniques and materials to eliminate this complication after total joint arthroplasty.

REFERENCES

1. Bodmer JL. Membrane receptors for particles and opsonins. In: Dean, Jessup, eds. *Mononuclear phagocytes: physiology and pathology.* Amsterdam: Elsevier, 1985:55–78.
2. Bonfield TL, Colton E, Marchant RE, Anderson JM. Cytokine and growth factor production by monocytes/macrophages on protein preabsorbed polymers. *J Biomed Mater Res* 1992;26:837–850.
3. Charnley J. The histology of loosening between acrylic cement and bone. *J Bone Joint Surg [Br]* 1975;57:245.
4. Davis GS. The pathogenesis of silicosis. *Chest* 1986;89:166S–169S.
5. Glowacki J, Jasty M, Goldring S. Comparison of multinucleated cells elicited in rats by particulate bone, polyethylene, or polymethylmethacrylate. *J Bone Miner Res* 1986;1:327–331.
6. Goldring SR, Jasty M, Roelke CM, Bringhurst FR, Harris WH. Formation of a synovial-like membrane at the bone-cement interface; its role in bone resorption and implant loosening after total hip replacement. *Arthritis Rheum* 1986;29:836–842.
7. Goldring SR, Roelke M, Glowacki J. Multinucleated cells elicited in response to implants of devitalized bone particles possess receptors for calcitonin. *J Bone Miner Res* 1988;3:117–120.
8. Goldring SR, Schiller AL, Roelke MS, Rourke CM, O'Neill DA, Harris WH. The synovial-like membrane at the bone-cement interface in loose total hip replacements and its proposed role in bone lysis. *J Bone Joint Surg [Am]* 1983;65:575–584.
9. Goldring SR, Wojno WC, Schiller AL, Scott RD. In patients with rheumatoid arthritis the tissue reaction associated with loosened total knee replacements exhibits features of a rheumatoid synovium. *J Orthop Rheumatol* 1988;1:9–21.
10. Lalor PA, Revell PA, Gray AB, Wright S, Railton GT, Freeman MA. Sensitivity to titanium. A cause of implant failure? *J Bone Joint Surg [Br]* 1991;73:25–28.
11. Lewandowska K, Pergament E, Sukenik CN, Culp LA. Cell-type-specific adhesion mechanisms mediated by fibronectin adsorbed to chemically derivatized substrata. *J Biomed Mater Res* 1992;26:1343–1363.
12. Lin Y-S, Hlady V, Janatova J. Adsorption of complement proteins on surfaces with a hydrophobicity gradient. *Biomaterials* 1992;13:497–514.
13. Murray DW, Rae T, Rushton N. The influence of the surface energy and roughness of implants on bone resorption. *J Bone Joint Surg [Br]* 1989;71:632–637.

14. Murray DW, Rushton N. Macrophages stimulate bone resorption when they phagocytose parti-
    cles. *J Bone Joint Surg [Br]* 1990;72:988–992.
15. Santavirta S, Konttinen YT, Hoikka V, Eskola A. Immunopathological response to loose ce-
    mentless acetabular components. *J Bone Joint Surg [Br]* 1991;73:38–42.
16. Wahl SM. Monocytes and granulomatous inflammatory responses. In: Sorg C, ed. *Macrophage-
    derived cell regulatory factors. Cytokines*. Basel: Karger, 1989:173–192.
17. Willert HG, Bertram H, Buchhorn GH. Osteolysis in alloarthroplasty of the hip. The role of bone
    cement fragmentation. *Clin Orthop* 1990;258:108–121.
18. Willert HG, Bertram H, Buchhorn GH. Osteolysis in alloarthroplasty of the hip. The role of ultra-
    high molecular weight polyethylene wear particles. *Clin Orthop* 1989;258:95–107.
19. Yin HL, Stossel TP. The mechanism of phagocytosis. In: *Phagocytosis—past and future*. Orlando,
    FL: Academic Press, 1982:13–27.

Biological, Material, and Mechanical Considerations of Joint Replacement, edited by B. F. Morrey. Raven Press, Ltd., New York © 1993.

Discussion of Ultrahigh Molecular Weight Polyethylene

Timothy M. Wright

Department of Biomechanics, The Hospital for Special Surgery, New York, New York 10021

A panel of 25 surgeons and scientists discussed the current clinical and basic research data relating to the use of ultrahigh molecular weight polyethylene (UHMWPE). The following conclusions are organized according to areas of consensus, areas in which disagreements or differing opinions remain, and areas in which future research and development efforts should be directed.

CONSENSUS

UHMWPE continues to be a standard constituent of the articulation of most prosthetic joints. In general, UHMWPE provides a satisfactory material for articulating surfaces in total joint arthroplasty. The long-term successful performance of total joint replacement is due in large part to the excellent wear of this polymer. Its wear performance can be compromised, however, by many factors, including poor intergranular bonding, porosity, inclusions, oxidation (or degradation), and severe wear conditions (such as third-body abrasion). Efforts to improve the wear resistance of UHMWPE are ongoing and directed toward identifying wear mechanisms and establishing the influence of component design, polymer processing parameters, and clinical factors on these mechanisms.

There is no universal definition of medical grade UHMWPE. A minimal voluntary ASTM standard does exist and is currently under revision. Despite this confusion, it is generally agreed that UHMWPE is biocompatible in bulk form. But large numbers of UHMWPE particles are generated from the component surfaces as a result of wear. For example, even in the best of circumstances, radiographically measured wear rates on the order of 0.1 mm per year in total hip replacements appear unavoidable. This amount of wear relates to the release of billions of small particles (<5 μm in their largest dimension) annually. Particles of this size can be partially phagocytosed. As total joint arthroplasties have been performed in younger, more active patients and as improvements in cemented and uncemented fixation techniques extend the useful life of total joint implants, the problem of osteolysis induced by wear debris has become a more prevalent cause of failure.

This finding suggests that the osteolysis is due to the concentration of particles in the joint tissues. Clinical data reveal that wear particles of hip replacements are quite small, are phagocytosed, and can cause bone lysis. Wear in total knee replacements is dominated by another wear mechanism, delamination, which generates larger particles and less bone lysis. Surface imperfections and subsurface inclusions appear to contribute to the delamination process. It now appears that osteolysis caused by UHMWPE is related to volumetric overload of debris particles in the joint.

CONTROVERSY

Unfortunately, the nature of UHMWPE debris particles is not well characterized in terms of geometry, size, physical and chemical properties, and surface characteristics. Each of these features is thought to have some effect on the cellular response, but little consensus exists on the relative importance of each factor. Similarly, the initial properties of the UHMWPE used to fabricate total joint components are known to vary significantly from batch to batch, but the significance of these differences on clinical performance has not been assessed. Likewise, the wear rate or volume of wear debris required to cause biological reaction is unknown, although clinical evidence exists to suggest a higher incidence of osteolytic lesions in joint replacements with very high rates of wear. The nature of the biological reaction to these particles is also poorly understood, including differences in osseous- versus soft-tissue reactions, the immune response, transport mechanisms, and molecular interactions.

THE FUTURE

Attempts to improve UHMWPE through manufacturing processes aimed at altering the material properties and the use of alternative materials, including ceramics or metals, are under way. No clear choice is seen at this time.

Understanding the characteristics of UHMWPE particles will provide insight into the wear mechanisms responsible for particle generation. Understanding the characteristics of the biological reaction to particles may suggest treatment methods for patients suffering from "particle disease." It may also provide criteria to be met by new designs and materials that may result in different types of wear particles.

A major deficiency restricting research in this area is the lack of means to generate UHMWPE particles comparable in size and shape to those produced *in vivo*. A standardized source of particles would greatly facilitate efforts to study biological reactions in cell culture and in animal models. Such research should be coordinated with expanded experimental and analytical efforts to examine the effects of component design, loading conditions, surface treatments, and degradation on wear mechanisms.

Biological, Material, and Mechanical Considerations of Joint Replacement, edited by B. F. Morrey. Raven Press, Ltd., New York © 1993.

11

Particle Disease Due to Wear of Metal Alloys

Findings from Retrieval Studies

*Hans-Georg Willert, *Gottfried H. Buchhorn, and †Manfred Semlitsch

*Orthopaedic Department, University Hospital of Goettingen,
D-3400 Goettingen, Germany;
†Sulzer Medical Technology, Ltd., CH-8401 Winterthur, Switzerland*

Today several iron- (Fe), cobalt- (Co), and titanium- (Ti) based alloys are used for manufacturing joint endoprostheses. Iron-based alloys are composed chemically of Fe, chromium (Cr), nickel (Ni), molybdenum (Mo), and (additionally) magnesium (Mn), niobium (Nb), and nitrogen (N). Cobalt-based alloys contain Co, Cr, Mo, often Ni, and sometimes also tungsten (W) or Fe. Titanium-based alloys (with the exception of pure titanium) consist of Ti, aluminum (Al), vanadium (V), Fe, or Nb, respectively.

In the compound of the alloy, the specific properties of the pure elements, such as toxicity and allergenicity of cobalt, nickel, and vanadium, become almost entirely insignificant; this fact is responsible for the biocompatibility of these alloys. Moreover, metallic implant materials should be as corrosion resistant as possible.

To use metal alloys to manufacture particular components of an endoprosthesis, their physical and mechanical properties must be adjusted to the requirements for the specific function of that part. Anchoring components (e.g., femoral stems of hip endoprostheses) require high-yield, fatigue, and ultimate tensile strength. If the metal alloy is to be used for gliding surfaces, its wear resistance must be particularly high. Few materials actually qualify for use in bearing surfaces of artificial joints, such as the cast CoCrMo alloys and the wrought iron-based alloys (29,30,34).

ORIGIN OF METAL PARTICLES

Notwithstanding the strength and hardness of the alloys, metal particles may be liberated at different sites and/or levels (Table 1) (Fig. 1). The mechanism of metal particle production is predominantly abrasive or three-body wear. Depending on the mode of origin, material from the counterparts that rub against the metal is also released. We then find, in addition to metal particles, acrylic bone cement and polyethylene within the joint fluid and/or tissue (Fig. 3G–I).

Metal wear from articulating surfaces of the artificial joints (mode I) can be extremely low under ideal conditions. From our experience we can say that cast

TABLE 1. *Modes of metal particle origin*

	Site	
Mode	Cemented hip joints	Noncemented hip joints
I	Articulating surface	Articulating surface
a	Metal/PE/metal	Metal/PE/metal
b	Metal/cartilage and bone	Metal/cartilage and bone
II	Anchoring surface	Anchoring surface
a	Metal/PMMA-bonding	
b	Metal/cartilage and bone-interface (cementing defects)	Metal/cartilage and bone-interface
c	Metal/metal coating	Metal/metal coating
III	Cone	Cone
	Metal/metal/ceramic	Metal/metal/ceramic

CoCrMo and wrought iron-based alloys especially in metal/ultrahigh molecular weight polyethylene (UHMW-PE) bearings produce very little wear debris as long as the joint surface remains smooth and no bone, bone-cement, or other particles are entrapped between the joint surfaces. Under such ideal conditions even cast CoCrMo metal-to-metal bearings showed very low wear over a long period of time (31). In metal/polymer bearings, the softer polymer (like UHMW-PE) is much more prone to wear than the metal and consequently more likely to be found in the surrounding tissue. The situation, however, can change dramatically if particles become entrapped between the joint surfaces. Especially dangerous in this respect are bone-cement fragments (see Color Fig. 1 in color plate following p. 137), since their inclusions of the hard x-ray contrast medium zirconium oxide or barium sulfate may easily abrade the metal. Compared with stainless steel or cast CoCrMo, it has resulted that titanium and its alloys (TiAlV) are much less qualified to be used for bearing surfaces because of the higher vulnerability of their passive layer, for instance, through the friction contact with acrylic cement and its zirconium oxide or barium sulfate inclusions (21,24,29,30,34) or polymerization catalyst particles (titanium/aluminum compound, approximately 20-μm diameter [2]) (4). Kempf and Semlitsch (19) reported on ceramic fragments embedded in a UHMW-PE socket abrading a stainless steel head. Nevertheless in the absence of acrylic or metallic abrasive particles, the wear properties of well-fixed titanium-alloy prostheses are said to be comparable with those of stainless steel or CoCr alloy (24).

Metal wear from the *cone* (mode III) only can develop if fretting between the head and tapered neck occurs. As long as there is an exact taper lock between the head and neck, this should be rather impossible. To our knowledge metal abrasion between head and neck has been observed only in very few exceptional cases (37). Corrosion at the interface of cobalt-alloy heads on titanium-alloy stems has been reported recently (11,12,23). Brown et al. (5) pointed out that fretting-accelerated crevice corrosion might well be caused by a mismatch in hole and cone taper angles resulting in micromovements during weight bearing.

Metal abrasion from the anchoring surfaces of endoprosthetic components is caused by movements either between metal and polyethylmethacrylate (PMMA) in cemented endoprostheses (mode IIa) or between metal and bone in noncemented ones (mode IIb) (Fig. 1A and B). In both instances, the components must be somewhat loose in their cement or bone environment. This can be restricted to a certain area but may also increase in the course of time. In cemented components, again the

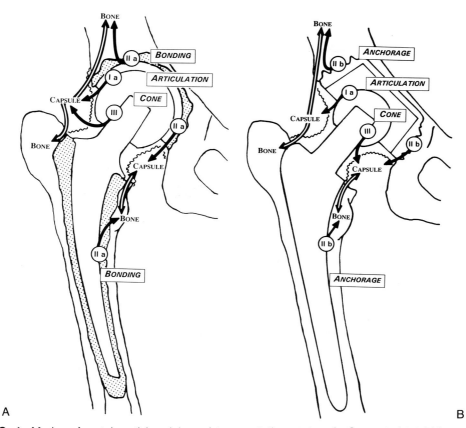

FIG. 1. Modes of metal particle origin and transportation routes. **A:** Cemented total hip endoprosthesis with metal stem, metal head, and metal cup. Mode Ia: Particles originate from the articulating surface, spread first to the joint capsule and from there to bone marrow and implant-bone interface. Mode IIa: Particles originate from the bonding to bone cement, spread, in the case of cement defects, first to the cement-bone interface and from there to the other regions such as bone marrow, the joint capsule, and remote implant-bone interfaces. In the case of intact cement mantle, particle spreading follows mode Ia. Mode III: Particles originate from the cone taper lock and also spread first to the joint capsule and from there to bone marrow and implant-bone interface. **B:** Noncemented total hip endoprosthesis with metal stem, metal head, and metal-backed UHMW-PE cup. Mode Ia: Particles originate from the articulating surface, spread first to the joint capsule and from there to bone marrow and implant-bone interface. Mode IIb: Particles originate from the anchoring surface at the implant-bone interface, spread from there to the bone and joint capsule and then to other regions such as bone marrow and remote implant-bone interfaces. Mode III: Particles originate from the cone taper lock and also spread first to the joint capsule and from there to bone marrow and implant-bone interface.

detrimental properties of the zirconium oxide or barium sulfate inclusions become effective and easily abrade the metal. This mode of origin in our material has produced the greatest amounts of metal particles (Figs. 2 and 3).

If anchoring surfaces of endoprosthetic components are coated, for instance, with wire mesh or beads, abrasion can also occur between metal and metal if the coating becomes loose and rubs against the metal base (mode IIc) (1).

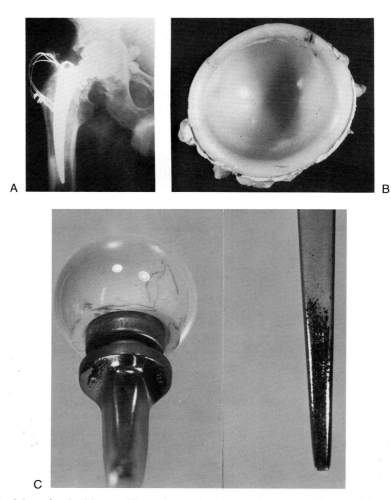

FIG. 2. Revision of a double-cup hip endoprosthesis was done on a 63-year-old man 12 years ago, and a femoral stem with a special large-size ceramic head was cemented while the polyethylene cup was left *in situ*. Recurring pain made another revision necessary. **A:** The x-ray taken prior to the second revision showed endosteal osteolysis of the femoral shaft, especially distal to the tip of the stem. **B:** The retrieved UHMW-PE cup shows wear and oblong deformation in the direction of loading. The joint surface is roughened with embedded bone-cement particles. Fatigue fractures developed at the rim and pole of the cup. **C:** The retrieved Co-NiCrMo stem shows polishing due to metal abrasion. (*Figure continues.*)

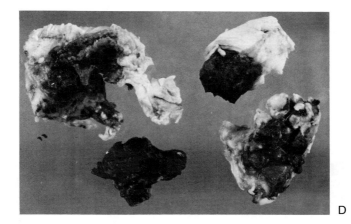

D

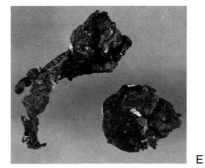

E

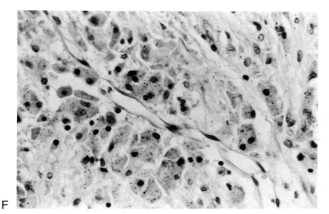

F

FIG. 2. (*Continued.*) **D** and **E:** Tissue samples, taken from the joint capsule (D) and osteolytic area distal to the tip of the stem (E), show an intensive black discoloration. **F:** Tissue from the osteolytic area in the femur. Microscopically the amount of phagocytosed metal particles varied from area to area. Here the phagocytes contain only a few very small ones. Microphotograph, hematoxylin-eosin, ×461.5. (B–E appear on color plate after p. 138.)

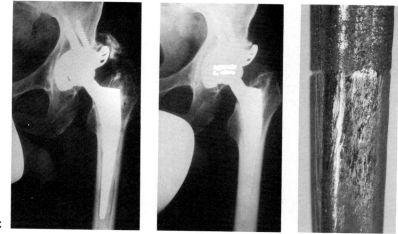

A–C

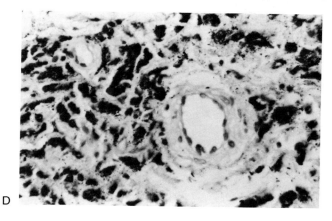

D

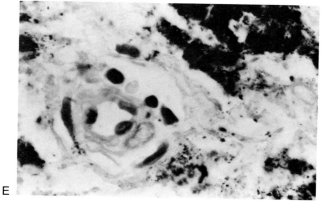

E

FIG. 3. Cemented titanium stem of an artificial hip replacement, implanted 2 years ago in a 49-year-old man, loosened and had to be revised. **A:** Postoperative x-ray: The implantation appears perfect. **B:** X-ray prior to revision: A scalloping osteolytic seam has developed at the cement-bone interface around the distal half of the femoral stem. **C:** Large polished area in the middle of the lateral shoulder of the retrieved TiAlNb stem. (C appears in color plate after p. 138.) **D–I:** Microscopically large amounts of metal particles are seen in the joint capsule (D,E) as well as at the implant-bone interface (F–I). (*Figure continues.*)

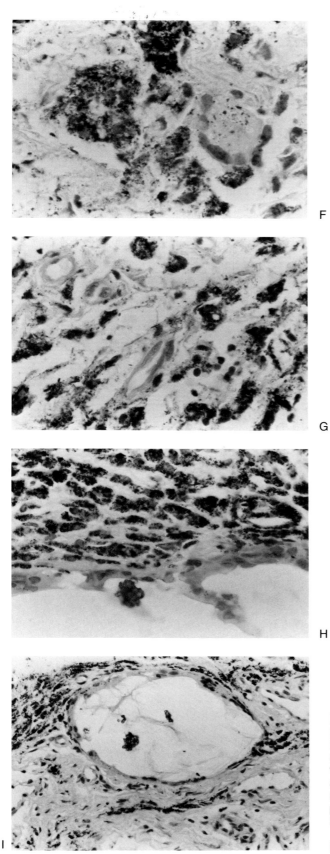

F

G

H

FIG. 3. (*Continued.*) The metal particles were stored mainly in mononuclear macrophages but also in giant cells, sometimes with UHMW-PE. Other giant cells around PMMA fragments were relatively free of metal. Microphotographs, hematoxylin-eosin. Magnifications: D, ×578.5; E, ×1,430; F, ×1,153.75; G, ×871; H, ×721.5; I, ×364.

I

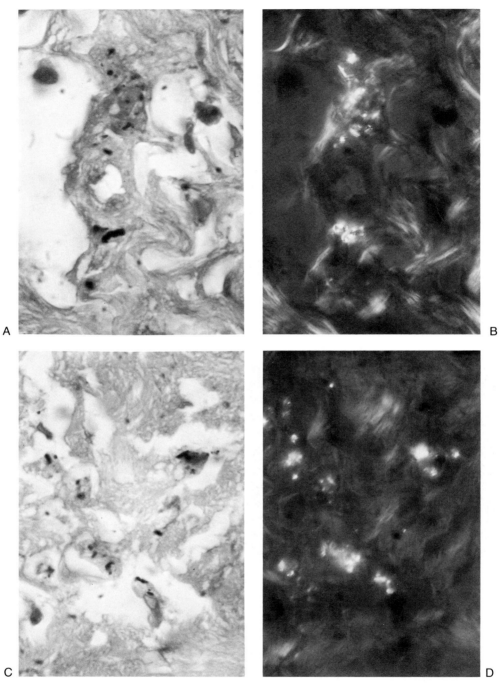

FIG. 4. At revision surgery of a noncemented total hip endoprosthesis with a TiAlV stem and UHMW-PE threaded cup, in a 69-year-old woman 3.5 years after implantation, tissue from the interface with the TiAlV stem was removed. **A–D:** In histological sections very few small black Ti-alloy particles were found after intensive search. Microphotographs, hematoxylin-eosin. A and C: normal, bright transmitted light; B and D: polarized light. Magnification: ×352.5. (A–D appear on color plate after p. 138.) (*Figure continues.*)

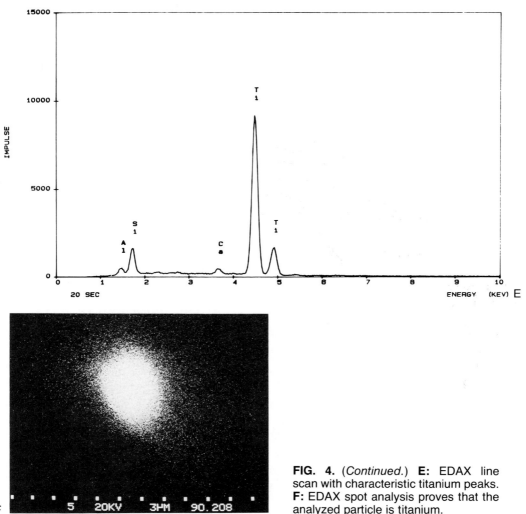

FIG. 4. (*Continued.*) **E:** EDAX line scan with characteristic titanium peaks. **F:** EDAX spot analysis proves that the analyzed particle is titanium.

IDENTIFICATION OF METAL PARTICLES

Several methods are available with which to identify metal particles (41).

Macroscopically, the presence of metal particles in the tissues can be demonstrated by a gray to black discoloration of the areas of deposition (32,33,43,44) (Fig. 2D and E). The intensity of black staining depends on the amount of stored metal.

Analytically, metal inclusions in tissues may be established qualitatively by Debye-Scherrer x-ray diffraction and energy dispersive analysis of x-ray (EDAX). The metal content can be determined semiquantitatively by means of spectral analysis (SpA) and quantitatively by means of atomic absorption spectrometry (AASp), but these methods do not give indications of their localization in specific tissue structures. Scanning electron microscopy, combined with EDAX, allows for local detection and quantitative characterization of wear products (Fig. 4E and F).

Under the *light microscope,* particles from all metal alloys incorporated into the tissues uniformly appear black, if the frozen-, paraffin-, or methacrylate-embedded sections are examined with normal, bright, transmitted light. The metal particles cannot be stained. However, in polarized light, with crossed polarization filters, the light scattering effect on the edges of the particles causes bright yellow-orange shining points, bands, or circumferences. This effect helps to detect metal inclusions in histological sections.

Metal particles in the tissues have to be discriminated from particles of the x-ray contrast medium zirconium oxide or barium sulfate and from formalin pigment. The differentiation by x-ray contrast media is possible by considering the different particle morphology, the birefringency, and the above-mentioned analytical methods. Formalin pigment is a red crystalline material. It can be removed by treating the histological sections with alcoholic ammonium chloride.

SIZE AND SHAPE OF METAL PARTICLES

The dimensions of the metal particles visible with light microscopy range mostly from 0.5 to 5 μm and are only sometimes larger than 20 μm. Particles larger than 20 μm were seldom found. Several authors reported similar size ranges, although the histological material probably differed in origin as well as material and articulation of the joints (10,24,25,27,47) Smaller wear particles were also detected, ranging from 0.1 to 1 μm (sometimes described by means of scanning or transmission electron microscopy) (18,20,26). We have measured size distributions of metallic wear particles in tissues surrounding articulations with different materials by means of television image analysis. Of the visible particles 83% measured less than 1.13 μm^2. The harder the socket material was, the more the size distribution shifted to larger particle areas: cast CoCrMo alloy with UHMW-PE produced small particles, cast CoCrMo alloy with polyethyleneterephthalate (polyester) resulted in larger particles, and cast CoCrMo alloy with cast CoCrMo alloy liberated the largest particles (38).

The shapes of the metal particles are quite irregular, with sharp edges, corners, and points. Although some are oval and others round, there is no predominant shape. This is confirmed by the above-mentioned authors and several others who did not report on particle sizes.

TISSUE REACTION TO METAL PARTICLES

In principle the features of the tissue reaction to metal particles are the same as the reaction to UHMW-PE or PMMA particles. Released into the area surrounding artificial joints, the metal particles likewise will be phagocytosed by cells of the adjacent tissues, with which they come in contact and there induce a foreign-body reaction. Independent of the amount of metal debris released, its content within the phagocytes varies. Thus, the cells may have incorporated only a few metal particles (Fig. 2F) or, in contrast, the cells can be completely filled with metal particles, giving them a totally black appearance (Fig. 3E).

Since the metal particles are mostly small, they are usually phagocytosed by mononuclear histiocytes. Occasionally metal particles are incorporated in multinuclear giant cells. It seems that these giant cells sometimes do not belong primarily

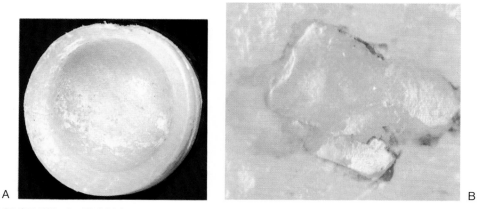

COLOR FIG. 1. PMMA/bone-cement particles have become embedded in the joint surface of polyethylene cup. **A:** UHMW-PE joint surface contains numerous PMMA particles and the superior part of cup shows thinning due to considerable wear. **B:** Enlarged view of a PMMA particle embedded in UHMW-PE.

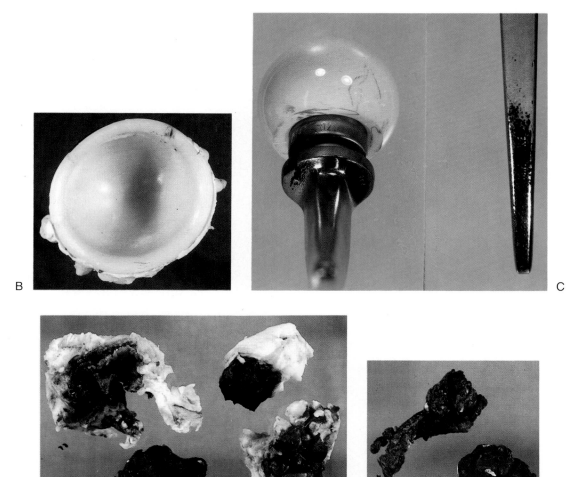

COLOR FIG. 2B–E.

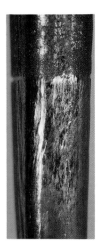

COLOR FIG. 3C.

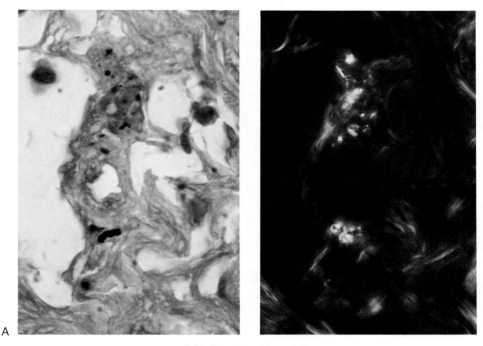

A

B

COLOR FIG. 4A and B.

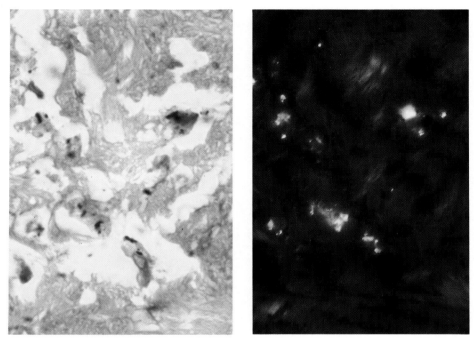

COLOR FIG. 4C and D.

to a cellular reaction against the metal but against UHMW-PE (Fig. 3G) or PMMA. In other cases we see multinucleated giant cells around PMMA inclusions completely free of metal particles (Fig. 3I), although there is extensive phagocytosis of metal debris in the direct neighborhood of these giant cells. This conveys the impression that there would be a kind of division of labor among the phagocytes. On the other hand, the giant cells may contain UHMW-PE or PMMA in addition to small metal particles.

In tissues with prevalent metal storage, mononuclear macrophages are prevalent. Sometimes the metal-containing macrophages appear relatively "meager," but just as often they appear swollen and foamy. These cells usually are densely packed to layers and nodules, forming granulomas, often embedded in strands of fibrous tissue. The extent of granulomatous tissue formation again depends on the amount of particle production. The predominance of mononuclear macrophages and a certain tendency to fibrosis are features that characterize "particle disease" caused by metal wear.

As already described in the findings from retrieval studies with polyethylene in Chapter 8, the proliferation of foreign-body granulomas requires space, and, consequently, we also see the black-stained, particle-storing joint capsules considerably thickened in cases of metallosis (Fig. 2B). Black metal particle-storing cell accumulations are also found in bone marrow and at the implant-bone interface (Fig. 2C). Again the foreign-body granulomas, developing in bone canals and marrow spaces, induce bone resorption resulting in osteolysis (43,44).

Two examples are given for tissue reactions to metal particles:

Case study 1. A 63-year-old man had revision of a double-cup hip endoprosthesis 12 years ago. At that time a femoral stem and special large-size ceramic head were cemented while the polyethylene cup was left *in situ*. Revision again became necessary because of reappearing pain. The radiograph taken prior to the second revision showed extensive, confluent endosteal osteolyses of the femoral shaft, spreading also distally to the tip of the stem, where the bone-cement plug protruded further into the marrow cavity (Fig. 2A).

The retrieved polyethylene cup showed oblong deformation and the bearing was worn out in the direction of the load (Fig. 2B). The bearing surface was roughened, bone-cement particles were embedded, and the unloaded area was discolored. The lack of sufficient mechanical support by bone cement and bone led to fatigue fractures of the rim and pole of the socket. The retrieved CoNiCrMo stem of the endoprosthesis showed marked polishing due to metal abrasion under the collar and over a length of 47 mm at the lateral side of the tip (Fig. 2C).

Tissue samples, taken from the joint capsule and osteolytic area distal to the tip of the stem showed an intensive black discoloration. AASp revealed that the tissue contained 0.34% CoNiCrMo metal.

Microscopically we found pronounced metallosis with a granulomatous tissue reaction (Fig. 2F). The phagocytes contained large amounts of metal particles as well as UHMW-PE and PMMA debris.

Case study 2. A hip joint replacement was done 2 years ago in a 49-year-old man. The femoral component of the endoprosthesis was a straight Müller TiAlNb-alloy stem; the socket was UHMW-PE. Both components were cemented. The head was aluminum oxide. According to the postoperative x-ray the implantation seemed to be perfect (Fig. 3A).

However, because of severe pain, 2 years later revision became necessary. The x-ray prior to revision revealed that a slightly scalloping osteolytic seam had developed at the cement-bone interface around the distal half of the femoral stem (Fig. 3B).

At revision, the femoral component was found to be loose. The retrieved TiAlNb stem showed a large polished area in the middle of the lateral shoulder, indicating massive abrasion of metal (Fig. 3C). The tissue samples, taken from the capsule and cement-implant interface of the proximal femur, showed black surfaces.

Microscopically large amounts of metal particles were seen in the joint capsule and implant-bone interface. The metal particles were stored mainly in mononuclear macrophages as well as giant cells that also contained UHMW-PE. Other giant cells around PMMA fragments were quite free of metal (Fig. 3D–I).

In contrast to some reports in the recent literature (1,4,21,24) and based on our own experience, no risk seems to arise from noncemented, sandblasted titanium endoprostheses that are securely anchored by press fit. For noncemented hip endoprostheses, for more than 10 years we have been using the Zweymüller stem for the femur, which is made of TiAlV resp. TiAlNb alloy. During the first 5 years for the acetabulum, we used an all-polyethylene threaded screw cup. In 1986 a metal backing of pure titanium was added to the polyethylene. The anchoring surfaces of both titanium components are roughened by sandblasting. The primary stability of fixation is achieved by press-fit anchoring, secondary stability by bone ongrowth.

From the first series with the all-polyethylene cup some components became loose because of polyethylene abrasion from the anchoring surface (39). At revision surgery in several cases we gained tissue that had been in contact with the titanium stems. Although we found, using AASp, that in some specimens the metal content was slightly increased above the average, we did not see black staining of the tissue and could detect very few titanium particles in the histological sections (Fig. 4A–D). EDAX also showed titanium particles in very few spots (Fig. 4E and F).

Hence, roughened, noncemented titanium alloy press-fit implants, in our experience, are quite safe, and in regard to possible metallosis as well.

By the techniques available to us, differences in the tissue reaction to particles of the different alloys, which might have been taken as characteristic for the particular metal alloys, could not be established. Furthermore, like Agins and co-workers (1), we did not see changes of the cells and tissues that had to be attributed to toxic effects of the metal particles. Any such changes we would have taken as necrosis of individual cells laden with debris as well as damage to the vessels (40). Necrosis, which goes along with extensive granulomatous reactions, develops quite regularly in the center of large granulomas, probably due to a disturbance of blood supply. The larger the granulomas grow, the more pronounced is their tendency to necrosis. But, as with UHMW-PE wear, and in the cases of metallosis as well, it seems to be the excessive amount of particles, and not a suspected toxicity, that causes the adverse effects to bone and other tissues surrounding an artificial joint. Furthermore, on the basis of our retrieval studies we are not able to classify the alloys used by those that are better and those that are less well tolerated. However, we approached this question experimentally.

Resorption and transport of metal wear particles have been studied in an animal model. We produced metal powders of several metal alloys used for orthopaedic implants (stainless steel, CoCr cast and forged, CoNiCrMo forged, CP-Ti, TiAlV, TiAlNb) (6,8,9,42). These powders showed a size distribution quite similar to the one of metal particles stored in tissues surrounding joint replacements (38). They were suspended in a viscous liquid and injected through a needle into the neck, knee joint, and femoral muscles in rats. The vehicle served as a delivery system, prohibited clot formation, and allowed for a continuous uptake of particles. The tissue reactions were analyzed up to 52 weeks postinjection and graded on a four-point scale (none to + + +). The amounts of erythrocytes, granulocytes, lymphocytes, histiocytes, foreign-body giant cells, fibrocytes, collagen, and blood vessels were recorded. All particles were subjected to transportation, the fibrous membrane around the vehicle and the capsular tissues were free of particles at least 26 weeks after injection. The vessels were frequently surrounded by broad strips of macrophages densely packed with metal powder. Occasionally we were able to find regional lymph nodes; they were densely packed with wear debris. In stainless steel and cobalt-based alloys in particular, scarring and increased vascularization were typical. The titanium-based alloys showed the least tendency to scar formation, many extracellular particles, especially in muscle, were found. No persistent signs of immunologic reaction or necrosis could be found in any of the materials. In general, our study showed that stainless steel evoked the strongest reactions, cobalt-based alloys were tolerated, and titanium alloys were the most compatible (6,8,9).

AMOUNT OF RELEASED METAL PARTICLES

The amount of released metal particles undoubtedly correlates with the mode of origin, the properties of the metal alloy, and the counterpart material against which the metal has rubbed. In some cases very little metal could be found and appeared more as a secondary finding to a prevailing deposition of polyethylene and/or PMMA debris. In other cases, extensive amounts of metal particles were present and dominated the histological picture.

CORROSION OF METALLIC WEAR DEBRIS

The alloys used at present for joint replacements demonstrate passivation of superior quality, which reduces the risk of persistent corrosion and liberation of metal ions. After deterioration of surfaces, the alloys especially manufactured for long-term use rebuilt their passivation layers very quickly, thus reducing the rate of ions released. Repassivation is induced in the articulation, on the surfaces of wear particles, and on anchoring surfaces under mechanical attack in case of loosening.

Elements used as constituents of implant alloys in significant concentrations naturally occur in tissues of the human body. For example, aluminum, chromium, cobalt, molybdenum, nickel, and vanadium are always present, and, except for some uncertainty concerning nickel, have been proven to be essential. Titanium and niobium appear to be indifferent, neither essential nor toxic at physiological levels.

Physiological storage areas for cobalt are known to be in bone, muscle, hair, and soft tissues; for molybdenum in kidneys, liver, spleen, and bone. Chromium, nickel, and niobium are reported to be present in all tissues; values of nickel are elevated in the aorta and skin. As for all essential elements, regulatory mechanisms do exist for excretion and storage of iron, cobalt, chromium, molybdenum, nickel, niobium, and vanadium ions. Further information on metabolism and toxicities of alloys is to be found in refs. 3,22,35,45,46.

SpA and AASp were performed on selected tissue specimens surrounding implants made of cast CoCr alloys. We determined the existence of wear particles and tried to control both their chemical composition and corrosion (7,32,33,36,40).

The chemical treatment of acid digestion applied to the tissue samples dissolves tissues, corrosion products, and wear particles. Thus, the values gained are cumulative and represent the natural content of elements, as well as elements bound as oxides and hydroxides, or, for example, combined with proteins, the passivation layers of the particles as well as the particles stored. For cast CoCr alloys we found higher values of chromium than cobalt. This finding is reported in numerous reports and can be explained by the insolubility of chromium oxide in the pH of the tissues surrounding the joints. Values of the elements nickel and molybdenum did not show a uniform pattern of enrichment or elimination in the tissues. They never were elevated and only seldom were in accordance with the corresponding amount in the alloy. However, both the total number of particles of the alloy stored in a tissue sample and the amount of metallic reaction products are of great interest. A calculation was made to evaluate the theoretical amount of particles in the state of the alloy according to the proportional content of the major elements. This calculation was based on the elements cobalt, chromium, molybdenum, magnesium, and nickel. As a result, in CoCrMo/polyethylene articulations on average 64% and in CoCr/CoCr articulations on average 43% of the ions detected are still bound in the form of the alloy (7). For the rest it can be speculated that the ions must have been liberated. Depending on the character and solubility of the reaction products, these ions are still bound in the tissues, have been transported to distant organs, or have been excreted e.g., through urine, feces, skin, hair, and nails.

Preliminary results of a running study including AASp measurements of tissues surrounding implants made from TiAlV alloys revised at our University Hospital show a wide range of values of the metals titanium and aluminum. For an increase of titanium values above the proportional concentration in the TiAlV alloy, the relative insolubility of the titanium oxide and the excretion of aluminum can serve as an explanation (in preparation).

In combination with the histological specimen examined we feel safe with TiAlV or TiAlNb alloys in those clinical applications in which the design of the implants promises a minimal amount of particle release and minimal deterioration of the passivation layers (39). In 1988 Agins and co-workers (1) studied tissues surrounding eight failed cemented and one failed noncemented TiAlV femoral stems. They analyzed each specimen with AASp for TiAlV wear and corrosion products and stated that the metal ions found were in the same ratio as the implant alloy. In conclusion they warned against "toxic local concentrations of metal debris" that "may contribute to infection and loosening."

In 1991 Jacobs and co-workers (16) published their work on the release and excretion of metal from TiAlV hip components. In this study patients had an increased serum concentration of titanium. "The toxicological importance of this finding is not known." No elevation in serum and urine concentration of aluminum was found by these authors. The latter result is calming fears of possible hazards to the nervous system (e.g., encephalopathy) due to increased aluminum levels.

Our own research extends the method described by Jacobs et al. as we not only collected urine of patients awaiting revision of loosened TiAlV femoral components but also asked the consent of 13 patient to medical treatment with Desferal. This drug released the aluminum bound in the tissues. Therefore, the values measured after application of Desferal represented the long-term accumulated amount of aluminum rather than the actual, and obviously misleading, level of aluminum. We conclude that the results obtained so far give no reason to assume an elevated risk for patients due to levels of aluminum in the body (13,14).

Undoubtedly the elevation of ion concentrations in the tissues surrounding metallic implants leads to an impregnation of neighboring tissues and organs. As there are diffusion of ions and probably transport as well, a possible tissue response decreases with growing distances and decreasing concentrations. It is obvious that tissues in direct contact are most endangered by toxic levels of ion, oxide, and hydroxide accumulations. From our findings thus far, we cannot describe variations in cellular reactions directly attributable to the concentration of ions.

Wear particles are transported away from their site of origin, and the continuing liberation of corrosion products might lead to accumulation at distant places of storage.

Only a few patients are known to be allergic to one or more elements used in implant alloys. The probability that these hypersensitivities result from implant alloys is very low as there is a much greater hazard caused by industrial or jewelry-related exposition (40).

SPREAD OF PARTICLES TO TISSUES REMOTE FROM THEIR SITE OF ORIGIN

If metal particles originate from the articulating surface (mode I) or the head-taper interface (mode III), they are released into the joint cavity. There they initially come into contact with the joint capsule from which they are subsequently phagocytosed. In mode II of origin from an anchoring surface, it is more likely that the released particles at first come in contact with the tissue at the implant-bone interface, which then again starts phagocytosis.

Free particles are found only in the joint fluid and fibrin exudations on the surface of the joint capsule or at the implant-bone interface. Within the tissues the particles usually are incorporated by cells.

In the course of time, the metal particles become distributed over the whole area surrounding of the endoprosthesis, regardless of the site at which they were produced, and can be recognized by the black staining of the affected tissues, like on the inner surface of the joint capsule and at the implant-bone interface.

The transportation routes depend on the site of particle production. If the particles are generated in the joint (mode I) or the head-taper interface (mode III) and phagocytosed by the joint capsule, then further spreading to bone marrow and implant-bone interface proceeds from there. If the particles originate from an anchoring surface (mode II) and are primarily absorbed by the tissue at the implant-bone interface, they spread from there to other regions such as bone marrow, the joint capsule, and remote implant-bone interfaces.

The three mechanisms of spreading, described in Chapter 8, are also applicable to metal particles:

1. Transport via perivascular lymph spaces.
2. Regional spread *per continuitatem*
3. Passive dissemination of free particles via open communicating spaces

Transport of particles by macrophages via the perivascular lymph spaces also occurs in metallosis, since we regularly see accumulations of metal particle-containing phagocytes around the vessels (Fig. 3D and E). This transport is also found quite distant from the site of particle production in the newly formed capsule around the joint, bone marrow, and the tissue at the implant-bone interface as well. In this way metallic wear debris can also be carried away centripetally from the area surrounding the implant and arrive in the regional lymph nodes.

As we stated in Chapter 8, the production and spread of wear debris, tissue reaction, treating the particles as foreign bodies, and even the development of osteolysis due to granuloma formation at the implant-bone interface in principle are not specific for any particulate material. We have been able to show repeatedly that very similar processes, as described here for metallosis (except the intensive black staining of the tissue), can be induced by almost every other material, such as Teflon, polyester, polyacetal, polyethylene, silicone rubber, alumina ceramic, and PMMA. The formation of granulomas and their adverse effects, however, are not so much the result of a suspected behavior or toxicity of the material involved but depend first on the amount, and, second, regarding the cellular characteristics, on the size of the released particles. Terms like "metal disease" (28), "cement disease" (17), or "polyethylene disease" (15) seem inappropriate for the principle in general. We therefore propose that the clinical sequelae of metallosis be called particle disease.

ACKNOWLEDGMENTS

No benefits in any form have been received from a commercial party directly or indirectly to the authors of this chapter. Parts of this work were funded by the Deutsche Forschungsgemeinschaft (grant no. Wi 346). The assistance of Dr. Ingeborg Lang is gratefully acknowledged.

REFERENCES

1. Agins HJ, Alcock NW, Bansla M, et al. Metallic wear in failed titanium-alloy total hip replacements. *J Bone Joint Surg [Am]* 1988;70:347–356.
2. Birnkraut HW. Synthesis of UHMW-PE. In: Willert H-G, Buchhorn GH, Eyerer P, eds. *Ultrahigh molecular weight polyethylene as biomaterial in orthopaedic surgery*. Toronto, Lewiston, Bern, Goettingen, Stuttgart: Hogrefe & Huber, 1991:3–5.
3. Black J. *Biological performance of materials—fundamentals of biocompatibility*. New York/Basel: Marcel Dekker, 1981.
4. Black J, Sherk H, Bonini J, Rostocker WR, Schajowitz F, Galante J. Metallosis associated with a stable titanium-alloy femoral component in total hip replacement. *J Bone Joint Surg [Am]* 1990;72:126–130.
5. Brown SA, Flemming CAC, Kawalec JS, et al. Fretting accelerated crevice corrosion of modular hips. Transactions: Implant Retrieval Symposium 1992, Society of Biomaterials, Minneapolis, 1992:59.
6. Buchhorn GH, Bertram H, Willert H-G. Biokompatibilität feinster Metallpulver von Eisen- und Kobalt-Basislegierung. *Mitteilungsblatt der DGOT* 1986;3:78.

7. Buchhorn GH, Willert H-G, Semlitsch M. Distribution of elements in tissues surrounding total joint endoprostheses with metal components. Transactions 7th Annual Meeting Society for Biomaterials, May 28–31, 1981, Troy, NY, p. 13.

8. Buchhorn GH, Willert H-G, Semlitsch M, Schoen R, Steinemann S, Schmidt M. Preparation, characterization, and animal testing for biocompatibility of metal particles of iron-, cobalt, and titanium-based implant alloys. In: John KRS, ed. *ASTM STP 1144—Particulate debris from medical implants: mechanisms of formation and biological consequences*. Philadelphia: ASTM, 1992:177–188.

9. Buchhorn GH, Willert H-G, Semlitsch M, Thoma E. Biocompatibility of TiAlNb-alloy compared to titanium and TiAlV-Alloy; an animal experiment with implant alloys implanted in powdered form. Abstracts on European Congress on Biomaterials, September 14–17, 1986, Bologna, Italy, p. 250.

10. Charosky CB, Bullough PG, Wilson PD. Total hip replacement failures—a histological evaluation. *J Bone Joint Surg [Am]* 1973;55:49–58.

11. Collier JP, Surprenant VA, Jensen RE, Mayor MB. Corrosion at the interface of cobalt-alloy heads on titanium-alloy stems. *Clin Orthop* 1991;271:305–312.

12. Collier JP, Surprenent VA, Jensen RE, Mayor MB, Surprenent HP. Corrosion between the components of modular femoral hip prostheses. *J Bone Joint Surg [Br]* 1992;74:511–517.

13. Dittert D-D, Warnecke G, Willert H-G. Aluminiumserumspiegel bei Ti-Al-V- und Ti-Al-Nb-Hüftendprothesenträgern. In: Hipp E, Gradinger R, Ascherl R, eds. *Die zementlose Hüftprothese*. Gräfelfing: Demeter Verlag, 1992:49–53.

14. Dittert D-D, Willert H-G, Warneke G. Aluminum excretion and levels in serum in patients with Ti-Al-V and Ti-Al-Nb total hip replacements *(submitted)*.

15. Guttmann D, Schmalzried TP, Jasty M, Harris WH. Light microscopic identification of submicron polyethylene wear debris: specificity of "Willert's phenomenon." Implant retrieval symposium of the Society for Biomaterials. Transactions, Society for Biomaterials, Minneapolis, 1992:84.

16. Jacobs JJ, Skipor AK, Black J, Urban RM, Galante JO. Release and excretion of metal in patients who have a total hip-replacement component made of titanium-base alloy. *J Bone Joint Surg [Am]* 1991;73:1475–1486.

17. Jones LC, Hungerford DS. Cement disease. *Clin Orthop* 1987;225:192–206.

18. Jones SMG, Pinder IM, Morran CG, Malcolm AJ. Polyethylene wear in uncemented knee replacements. *J Bone Joint Surg [Br]* 1992;74:18–22.

19. Kempf I, Semlitsch M. Massive wear of a steel ball head by ceramic fragments in the polyethylene acetabular cup after revision of a total hip prosthesis with fractured ceramic ball. *Arch Orthop Trauma Surg* 1990:109:284–287.

20. Lee J-M, Salvati EA, Bets F, DiCarlo EF, Doty SB, Bullough PG. Size of metallic and polyethylene debris particles in failed cemented total hip replacements. *J Bone Joint Surg [Br]* 1992;74:380–384.

21. Lombardi AV, Mallory TH, Vaughn BK, Drouliiard P. Aseptic loosening in total hip arthroplasty secondary to osteolysis induced by wear debris from titanium-alloy modular femoral heads. *J Bone Joint Surg [Am]* 1989;71:1337–1342.

22. Luckey HA, Kubli F, eds. *Titanium alloys in surgical implants*. ASTM STP 796. Philadelphia: ASTM, 1983.

23. Mathiesen EB, Lindgren JU, Blomgren GGA, Reinholdt FP. Corrosion of modular hip prostheses. *J Bone Joint Surg [Br]* 1991;73:569–575.

24. McKellop HA, Sarmiento A, Schwinn CP, Ebramzadeh E. In vivo wear of titanium-alloy hip prostheses. *J Bone Joint Surg [Am]* 1990;72:512–517.

25. Mirra JM, Amstutz HC, Matos M, Gold R. The pathology of the joint tissues and its clinical relevance in prosthesis failure. *Clin Orthop* 1976;117:211–240.

26. Nasser S, Campbell PA, Kilgus D, Kossovsky N, Amstutz HC. Cementless total joint arthroplasty prostheses with titanium-alloy articular surfaces—a human retrieval analysis. *Clin Orthop* 1990;261:171–185.

27. Peters PC, Engh GA, Dwyer KA, Vinh TN. Osteolysis after total knee arthroplasty without cement. *J Bone Joint Surg [Am]* 1992:74:864–876.

28. Santavirta S, Hoikka V, Eskola A, Konttinen YT, Paavilainen T, Tallroth K. Aggressive granulomatous lesions in cementless total hip arthroplasty. *J Bone Joint Surg [Br]* 1990;72:980–984.

29. Semlitsch M. Titanium alloys for hip joint replacements. *Clin Mater* 1987;2:1–13.

30. Semlitsch M. Twenty years of Sulzer experience with artificial hip joint materials. *Proc Inst Mech Eng* 1989;20:159–165.

31. Semlitsch M, Streicher RM, Weber H. Verschleissverhalten von Pfannen und Kugeln aus CoCrMo-Gusslegierung bei langzeitig implantierten Ganzmetall-Hüftprothesen. *Orthopäde* 1989; 18:377–381.

32. Semlitsch M, Vogel A, Willert H-G. Kombination moderner Mikroanalysemethoden zur Untersuchung von Gelenkendoprothesen-Abrieb im Bindegewebe der Gelenkkapsel. *Medizinalmarkt/Medicotechnica* 1971;19:38–41.

33. Semlitsch M, Willert H-G. Gewebsveränderungen im Bereiche metallischer Hüftgelenke; mikroanalytische Untersuchungen mittels Spektralphotometrie, Elektronenmikroskopie und der Elektronenstrahl-Mikrosonde. *Mikrochimica Acta* 1971;1:21–37.
34. Semlitsch M, Willert H-G. Metallic materials for artificial hip joints. In: Webster JG, ed. *Encyclopedia of medical devices and instrumentation.* New York: John Wiley, 1988:137–149.
35. Venugopal B, Lukey TD. *Metal toxicity in mammals,* vols 1 and 2. New York: Plenum Press, 1978.
36. Willert H-G. Tissue reactions around joint implants and bone cement. In: Chapchal G, ed. *Arthroplasty of the hip.* Stuttgart: Georg Thieme Verlag, 1973:11–21.
37. Willert H-G, Buchhorn GH. Biocompatibility of endoprosthetic materials. In: Morscher E, ed. *The cementless fixation of hip endoprostheses.* Berlin, Heidelberg, New York, Toronto, Springer-Verlag, 1984:29–38.
38. Willert H-G, Buchhorn G, Buchhorn U, Semlitsch M. Tissue response to wear debris in artificial joints. In: Weinstein A, Gibbons D, Brown S, Ruff W, eds. *Implant retrieval: material and biological analysis,* NBS, SP 601. Gaithersburg, MD: U.S. Department of Commerce, National Bureau of Standards, 1981:239–267.
39. Willert H-G, Buchhorn GH, Hess T. No risk with non-cemented TiAlV-femoral stems—results from retrieval analyses. Transactions: Implant Retrieval Symposium 1992, Society of Biomaterials, Minneapolis, 1992:47.
40. Willert HG, Buchhorn GH, Semlitsch M. Die Reaktion des Gewebes auf Verschleissprodukte von Gelenkendoprothesen der oberen Extremitäten. *Orthopade* 1980;9:94–107.
41. Willert H-G, Buchhorn GH, Semlitsch M. Recognition and identification of wear products in the surrounding tissue of artificial joint prostheses. In: Dumbleton JH, ed. *Tribology of natural and artificial joints.* Amsterdam: Elsevier, 1981:381–419.
42. Willert H-G, Buchhorn GH, Semlitsch M, Arnemann H-J. Recommended practice for the preparation of metal wear products for biocompatibility testing. In: Tsuruta T, ed. *Transactions 4th World Biomaterials Congress, April 21–25, 1988,* Kyoto, Japan, 344.
43. Willert H-G, Semlitsch M. Tissue reactions to plastic and metallic wear products of joint endoprostheses. In: Gschwend N, Debrunner U, eds. *Total hip prostheses.* Bern: Hans Huber, 1976: 205–239.
44. Willert H-G, Semlitsch M, Buchhorn G, Kriete U. Materialverschleiss und Gewebereaktion bei künstlichen Gelenken. *Orthopade* 1978;7:62–83.
45. Williams DF, ed. *Systemic aspects of biocompatibility,* vol 1. Boca Raton, FL: CRC Press, 1981.
46. Williams DF, ed. *Biocompatibility of orthopaedic implants,* vol 1. Boca Raton, FL: CRC Press, 1982.
47. Winter GD. Identification of wear and corrosion products in tissues and the reactions they provoke. In: Williams D, ed. *Biocompatibility of implant materials.* London: Sector, 1976.

Biological, Material, and Mechanical Considerations of Joint Replacement, edited by B. F. Morrey. Raven Press, Ltd., New York © 1993.

12

Particulate Metals

Experimental Studies

Katharine Merritt and Stanley A. Brown

Department of Biomedical Engineering, Case Western Reserve University, Cleveland, Ohio 44106-7207

The importance of generation of particulate debris as a potentiator of failure of total hip arthroplasties was evident in the early investigations by Sir John Charnley with the use of Teflon as a bearing surface (15,16). This was further amplified by Willert and Semlitsch (62) with the diagram of the generation of polyethylene (PE) wear debris contributing to tissue responses associated with loosening of the device. Analysis of tissue obtained at revision surgery for failed total joint replacements (TJR) reveals PE debris, bone cement (polymethylmethacrylate [PMMA]) debris, and metal debris. The histologic results from our retrieval study show high levels of PE, PMMA, and metal debris in some patients. The question to be answered for the TJR patient is what role does each of the materials (PE, PMMA, and metal) play in the tissue response leading to failure. The importance of PE and PMMA has been discussed earlier in this volume. The delineation of the role of metal debris in the TJR patient remains a problem to solve since all devices in current use have PE as a bearing surface and PE debris may be produced concurrently. The metal articulating with metal devices used previously had a high level of metal debris, an association of metal allergy responses (20,21), and their implantation was discontinued. The patient reactions were assumed to be associated with metal debris; however, these devices were all used with PMMA. The return to metal articulating with metal devices for use without the PMMA has been proposed and prototypes are available; however, a PE ring is present that could generate PE debris in a dislocation or loose prosthesis. Thus, experimental studies *in vitro* and in animal models have been undertaken to investigate the role of metal debris in the absence of polymer debris in the development of untoward biological responses. Various approaches have been taken over the past 20 to 25 years, and an attempt will be made here to address the important issues and findings. Literature citations are mostly review articles and our own work from which the reader can obtain the original references. The literature citations will commonly occur at the end of the section without specific reference to each item.

A major problem in putting together this analysis is terminology. There are many terms being used that to each of us involved in these experiments has a particular meaning, and it is not necessarily in agreement with other investigators. Some of the differences in results may be muted when the terminology is clarified. When one looks at the dictionary (Webster) definition of the following terms commonly used in the reports on experimental results, problems become evident.

—particle: a small bit
—debris: the remains of something destroyed
—an ion: an electrically charged particle
—a salt: a substance formed from an acid and a metal
—a complex: has many parts
—a metal: any of a number of substances with the following characteristics: good conductor of heat and electricity, malleable and ductile, crystalline solid at or near room temperature, lustrous, capable of losing electrons to form a cation, capable of forming metallic bonds
—an alloy: a mixture of metals

These authors are therefore going to define the task of addressing the issue of biological responses to particulate metals to include all of the above and attempt to determine what is known and what is needed. Thus, accepting the definition of an ion as a charged particle, studies with salts (ions) that become undefined organometallic complexes when used *in vivo,* metals mixed with specific proteins *in vitro* forming preformed organometallic complexes of known composition, microscopic particles of metals and alloys, and debris that may be micro- or macroscopic will be considered all to be part of understanding the response to particulate metals.

It is well-known in the medical literature that humans exhibit various biological responses to particulate metals. Sensitivity reactions to nickel from the wearing of jewelry and the metal industry, to chromium from working in the cement and concrete industry, and cobalt primarily from the leather industry are well documented (18,38,40,41). Inhalation of metal particles in the workplace was known to cause immune complex diseases or sensitivity reactions (18,38,40,41). Carcinogenicity was documented to occur from repeated contact with some metal compounds (18,31,33,58,59). In addition, some metals were toxic and caused cell death without the intervention of the host immune or genetic responses. The question of whether there was any relevance of this for recipients of TJRs became an issue.

It was thought by some that since the alloys used for these devices were corrosion resistant, metal particles would not be released, and therefore there could be no adverse host responses. Considerable effort was put forth in the 1970s to determine this. It became evident from the work of many individuals that the alloys had various corrosion tendencies, but none completely resisted corrosion. All of the alloys when subjected to wear against other components had generation of ions, particles, or debris. This was shown in laboratory studies on corrosion, fretting-initiated corrosion, tribological properties are confirmed with laboratory studies on body fluids and tissues retrieved from experimental animals and from patients (3,4,9,17,22,63,64). The work of the 1980s and 1990s has demonstrated that even titanium and its alloys (61) and the ceramics (30) are not immune to the generation of particles under conditions of wear. It is now well accepted that metal is released in some form from all of the metal devices. The question remains as to what biological responses are stimulated.

It thus became important to understand which metals and which particles were involved in or initiated these responses, and in what forms they were active or inactive. Therefore, studies on corrosion of the devices were done in acid, saline, and serum. Similarly corrosion rates of particles of the alloys were studied under these same various conditions. Studies on protein and cell binding were undertaken in the presence of serum proteins and in the presence of the complex components of cell culture. Toxicity studies were also undertaken using various cell culture systems.

The *in vitro* studies were important and led to much information; however, a cell culture is a closed system that does not allow for metabolism or transport of the components by the host and thus underpredicts toxicity of some complexes that would be formed *in vivo* with components not represented *in vivo,* and overpredicts toxicity of the particles. Therefore, the *in vivo* studies, although a more complex system, were also important in evaluating the biological responses.

The biological responses to foreign material, including metal particles, are to eliminate it; ignore it; mount an inflammatory response to clean it up, detoxify it, and neutralize it; to mount an immune response against it that will detoxify and eliminate it but might result in an allergic response; and finally to undergo genetic aberrations. The ideal situation for patients with TJRs would be for the particles to be ignored or promptly eliminated. This, however, is not usually the situation.

This chapter will look at the various ways that the biological role of metals has been studied. The format will be to look at the use of metal salts *in vitro* and *in vivo,* micro- and macroscopic particles *in vitro* and *in vivo,* metals *in vitro* and *in vivo,* alloys *in vitro* and *in vivo,* and ceramics *in vitro* and *in vivo.* The field of orthopaedic surgery shares with implant dentistry many of the same materials and problems. Thus, relevant studies from the dental literature may be cited.

STUDIES ON THE EFFECTS OF METAL SALTS

In Vitro—in Solutions

The use of metal salts allows the investigator to easily obtain metal ions of known concentration and known valence. The preferential salt to use is a metal chloride since most solutions are sodium chloride (saline) based and thus the effect of the anion will be minimal. However, not all the elements are available as chloride salts and thus sulfates, phosphates, and other oxygen-based salts (ates) are used. When assessing the role of the metal, the role of the other components and the relevance to biological situations need to be considered. These salts studies have shown that metals bind to proteins and thus form organometallic complexes. The answer to the question of on what they bind to varies from investigator to investigator and the conditions of their experiments. Metal salts added to serum or plasma will all show strong binding to albumin, not because albumin has special binding sites, but because it is there in high concentration. Binding to the other proteins occurs, especially when conditions are adjusted to raise the concentration of one over another. There are also specific metal-binding/transport proteins including transferrin and ceruloplasmin that have specific binding and dissociation properties for the different metals. However, the bulk of the studies on binding and effects have focused on albumin since it is the protein in highest concentration in blood plasma or serum, in tissue fluids, and other serous exudative fluids. The important message here is that metals used as ions do not stay as ions in the presence of proteins and a variety of organometallic complexes are formed. The simplest action of the protein is as a chelator; i.e., it binds positively charged ions. Thus, the use of other chelators, such as EDTA and citrate commonly used in obtaining serum, with strong binding affinities for cations, will result in those metal complexes and alter formation of organometallic complexes. There is no indisputable evidence that one protein-metal complex behaves differently from another. (See refs. 31,39–40,43.)

In Vitro—in Cell and Organ Culture

Cell and organ culture studies have provided much information on the role of the individual ions and the protein-cell interactions. Some of these studies have been short term and have looked at effects on cell function and morphology for a few hours, and some have had extended culture times from a few days to a few weeks. The cells/organs examined have included white blood cells, various sources of fibroblasts, synovial tissue, and fetal bone cultures. From these studies it became evident that the toxic elements were nickel and vanadium. Cobalt had some toxicity. Chromium-3^+ was nontoxic and had little cellular uptake. Chromium-6^+ had cellular uptake and genetic aberrations were a concern. Molybdenum has not been extensively studied, but it is apparently nontoxic. Titanium was difficult to maintain as a salt, and thus questions have continued to be raised about the form in which it is used. However, titanium appears to be nontoxic but does have some cellular uptake and attachment. (See refs. 1,3,42.)

In Vivo

Results from the use of metal salts *in vivo* have not entirely agreed with the results from *in vitro* studies. The *in vitro* studies were in a confined system, whereas *in vivo*, there are distribution and metabolic events to consider. However, the route of administration must be considered.

Metal salts have been used commonly in the practice of dermatology and allergy to detect metal sensitivities. Nickel, chromium, and cobalt are known to be causes of contact dermatitis. Application of the metal salts onto or just under the skin will evoke a response in sensitive people, and this has been confirmed in laboratory animals. Application of metal salts in other sites gives variable results with one of the more interesting ones being a reaction at any site of previous cutaneous contact. The issue of oral contact is still of concern. Indications are that ingestion in low quantities rarely causes problems, but oral mucosa contact can result in hypersensitivity reactions. (See refs. 38–40,42,43,45,46.)

Our own data would indicate that deep-tissue administration of metal salts by injection intraperitoneally or intramuscularly into rodents results in rapid elimination of nickel, molybdenum, vanadium, and cobalt. Chromium and titanium are not rapidly eliminated in the urine with chromium being transported to the blood and chromium-6^+ being taken up in red cells. Titanium had limited transport to the blood with most of it remaining at the site of injection. A few studies were done with injection of salts into the medullary canal, and the elimination of the salts followed the deep-tissue pattern.

The issue of nickel sensitivity and nickel processing has led us to try dermal application of nickel. It is apparent that nickel applied to the skin is not transported and not eliminated as rapidly as that following intramuscular injection. These data do not conflict with other data in the literature and have important implications for patients with total joint arthroplasties since that is a deep-tissue not dermal contact.

Thus, although vanadium and nickel are toxic, they are rapidly eliminated from deep tissues and are unlikely to cause toxicity. On the other hand, chromium and titanium, although less toxic or nontoxic in cell culture, are not eliminated, accumulate, and may cause more of a biological response than expected.

MICROSCOPIC AND MACROSCOPIC PARTICLES

There have basically been three types of approaches to studying the biological effects of these particles. One approach has been to use microspheres and mesh, the second has been to use scraping and wear debris, and the third has been to generate corrosion products from implant materials by electrolytic or fretting corrosion. Comparison of the results of the studies has been difficult because of the tremendous variation in size and properties of the components, but there are some underlying similarities.

In Vitro—in Solutions

Microspheres, mesh, and particles have been placed in saline and serum solutions for periods of time from hours to months. Analysis has revealed that metal species are dissociated with binding to proteins. Whether the elements come off in the ratio of implant composition, the actual quantities coming off and the role of individual proteins remain controversial. Some elements such as nickel may dissolute in disproportionately high values. All of the elements including nickel, cobalt, chromium, and titanium can be detected in solution. The presence of proteins and chelating agents have been shown to affect and mostly enhance metal release. (See refs. 2,3,28,61,69.)

Particles in Cell and Organ Culture

Cell culture studies have demonstrated that many of the particles are toxic to cells or fetal bone. The toxicity seems to be related to the dissolution of metals from the particles. The bulk of these studies have used particles from alloys, and this information will be discussed in the section on alloys. However, one of the purposes of using metal particles has been to look at the effect of particle size. Particles that are small will be phagocytosed and cell function may be altered by internalization. Particles of the same weight but different size (i.e., changes in surface area) show that increased surface area (increased metal dissolution) results in increased cell damage or increased cell uptake. (See refs. 3,30,54–56,61.)

In Vivo

The implantation of particles *in vivo* into different sites has been done to examine (a) the effects of site (bone, intramuscular, subcutaneous, intra-articular), (b) the role of particle size, (c) the role of the alloy (discussed in later section). The results of the studies addressing the site are basically in agreement with the salts studies showing that the site of application does not alter the toxicity rating of the particles. However, intra-articular particles cause more damage from three-body wear than do particles in the other locations. The issue of particle size remains a very important topic of extreme controversy. The issue of particle size has yet to be distinguished from particle shape and particle composition. Particles of exactly the same shape and composition are not available in the same sizes.

What are the appropriate sizes? Particles less than 5 μm can be phagocytosed or pinocytosed, particles larger than 50 μm cannot. The issue becomes the fate of the particles between 5 and 50 μm, which are the commonly observed sizes in the histopathology sections from tissues surrounding a failed TJR. Why are these the commonly seen ones? The supposition (dataless conclusions) of the authors are that particles less than 5 μm are phagocytosed, "digested," and are in a nonvisible form. In addition, the resolution of most optical microscopes would require an oil immersion lens to detect particles less than 5 μm, and oil immersion lenses are rarely used in routine histopathologic diagnoses, and if we see the 5 to 50 μm particles so easily, do we really need to see the smaller ones? The large metal chunks greater than 50 μm are difficult to section with the routine paraffin-embedding procedures, and many of these are probably lost to "pluck out" in sectioning. Again, their loss may not be significant in the overall evaluation. However, this still does not address the issue of which particle sizes should be evaluated: less than 5, 5 to 10, and 10 to 50, and greater than 50 μm? (See refs. 3,14,19,26,27,29,30,36,57,61,65,67.)

METALS

In Vitro

The studies of protein absorption to, and metal dissolution from, pure metals have provided some important information on toxicity. Thus, metals in pure form, predominantly those used for dentistry, have been studied. The pure metals studied that are of interest to orthopaedic applications are primarily nickel and titanium, with some on cobalt and chromium. As would be expected from the results with salts and particles, the nickel shows little protein attachment and dissolution is rapid. Titanium shows strong protein attachment and little dissolution. (See refs. 2–4,63,64.)

In Cell and Organ Culture

Again the relevant pure metals studied most have been nickel and titanium. The results are consistent with the others showing that nickel is toxic to cell and fetal bone and titanium is nontoxic. Cell attachment to titanium has been observed. (See refs. 23,63,64.)

In Vivo

Nickel has been implanted only seldom, with the predictable massive toxicity. The implantation of titanium for dental, soft tissue, and orthopaedic evaluations has a literature that is too massive to even approach. The results have indicated that there are cell attachment to titanium and excellent biocompatibility. (See refs. 37,63–65.)

ALLOYS

In Vitro

The use of cobalt-chromium alloy (F75) microspheres and of metal scrapings in saline and in serum has shown dissolution of metal species into solution with protein binding. The rate of dissolution depends on (a) the type of solution: acids highest, saline low, and the presence of proteins and other chelators often hastening dissolution to be between that in acids and that in saline, (b) the surface area of the material: increases in surface area result in increased metal dissolution, (c) agitation of the particles: with increased release with motion. The release of metals from implant-quality alloys 316L stainless steel, F75, or F90 cobalt-chromium alloys by enhanced corrosion mechanisms demonstrated a marked effect of the presence of protein solutions. The effects on electrolytic corrosion varied with proteins protecting against corrosion when the applied potential was below the breakdown potential in serum or acid, but markedly accelerating corrosion when the applied potential was above the breakdown potential. The use of fretting corrosion demonstrated protection afforded by proteins. (See refs. 2,5–7,10–12,44,61,63–66,69.)

In Cell and Organ Culture

There have been numerous studies on the effect of alloys on cells in culture. Having progressed from the salts to the particles to the metals to the alloys, the results are predictable. However, this is not how the research progression went. The research progression went in the opposite direction for the most part starting with the alloys, then the metals, then the salts, and now the particles. In short, stainless steel is the most toxic of the alloys and titanium alloys are the least toxic. The reasons are now explainable due to the results with salts, particles, and pure metals. (See refs. 23,34,35,61.)

In Vivo

Again, this literature is too vast to consider approaching. It is also difficult to separate alloy from device in some of the studies. An oversimplified summary of the data would indicate that all the currently used alloys (316L, Co-Cr-Mo, Co-Cr-W, Ti64), used in passive applications, are biocompatible, although there may be dissolution of metal species. Cell attachment has been reported with titanium and its alloys, and fibrous capsules of various thicknesses have been associated with stainless steel and cobalt-chromium alloys.

However, when the alloys are used in situations of active wear against themselves or bone, or subjected to corrosion, a different situation is encountered. Under these conditions of wear and corrosion, there is massive release of metal species with various degrees of transport and accumulation. The summary of the numerous reports would indicate that nickel is excreted, cobalt is excreted slowly, chromium is largely cell bound with organ accumulation, the titanium shows minimal transport and large accumulation at the site where the metal particles are generated. Levels of vanadium and molybdenum are low in these alloys and not detectable *in vivo*. The rapid elimination of vanadium and molybdenum, when given as salts, would indicate that rapid elimination when released from the alloy also is a factor in lack of detectability at implant-site evaluation.

When the alloys are injected or implanted as particles, toxicity is seen and is related to particle composition, size, shape, and location of implantation. The role of these different variables has not been sorted out, as described previously. (See refs. 5,7,8,13,37.61,63–65,67–69.)

CERAMICS

In Vitro

The ceramics alumina, zirconia, and hydroxyapatite (HA) have been studied under conditions similar to those of the metals. The *in vitro* studies have demonstrated some protein attachment to the materials and general biocompatibility in cell and organ culture. Release of aluminum from alumina is small and slow, zirconia has been studied minimally, and HA behaves basically as a bone culture with some release of calcium and phosphate.

Studies on cellular reactions to particles demonstrate that particles are particles. Small particles are phagocytosed and large particles are not. HA particles are resorbed, remodeled, incorporated. Alumina and zirconia particles are more difficult for the cells to metabolize and can cause cell death. (See refs. 30,52,53.)

In Vivo

Particles of alumina have been injected into animals (usually mice) and large macrophages with particles, giant cells, and granulomas have been observed. In the absence of particle generation, alumina and zirconia have been biocompatible with at most a thin fibrous capsule.

HA has been studied extensively. HA particles in the vicinity of bone seem to be rapidly incorporated or eliminated with no long-lasting biological consequences. The application of HA into soft-tissue sites has been associated with a variety of results from rare fibrous encapsulation, to the more common slow resorption, to heterotopic bone formation. These soft-tissue studies have been done to evaluate various features of drug-delivery systems and bone formation/stimulation studies and are not pertinent to aspects of biological responses discussed here. (See ref. 30.)

CONCLUSION OF BIOLOGICAL CONSEQUENCES OF PARTICULATE METALS BASED ON EXPERIMENTAL STUDIES

The possible biological consequences listed previously are eliminate, ignore, mount inflammatory responses, form immune responses, and undergo genetic aberrations. The issue will now be addressed from a different material perspective by reclassifying the materials from the viewpoint of biological function.

Biological Consequences of Metal Particles of Known Trace Elements

Nickel, cobalt, chromium, molybdenum, aluminum, and vanadium are all trace elements in the animal body. All except vanadium are known to be essential for animals and humans, and vanadium is essential for some animals and perhaps humans. Thus, mechanisms are available to rapidly control their concentration. All are toxic in elevated levels, but toxicity is repaired as the element is eliminated. Aluminum has perhaps the most severe consequences, not fully proven, as a bone-formation inhibitor and from accumulation in the brain. Orthopaedic sources of aluminum are minor compared to activities of daily living (ADL) including drinking water in animal studies and water and tissue culture media in *in vitro* studies. Direct deep-tissue application of aluminum does not mimic ADL; however, the data indicate that most of this aluminum is excreted. Therefore, although these elements are toxic in the closed system of cell culture, they are not toxic in doses that would be released from implants under normal situations in animals with normal metabolism. The issue of chromium carcinogenicity from cell uptake of chromium-6$^+$ can never be excluded, but evidence to date does not indicate major consequences.

The mechanism of acquisition of the substance will affect the elimination. Salts will be rapidly handled, particles will be slowly corroded and eliminated with some cellular reaction while this is occurring. Those materials in a passive state with no release of the metals as salts of organometallic complexes will be walled off and ignored/accepted by the host.

Substances such as HA, which are similar to host tissue, will also be easily accepted or eliminated by the body. Only minor transient cell function perturbations will occur from release of substances such as calcium and phosphate.

The exception to the above statements is the remaining, underevaluated problem of the immune response, which is a memory response evoking faster and stronger responses with each stimulus. Some of these immune responses cause harm to the host body as hypersensitivity reactions, which will be discussed elsewhere in this volume. (See refs. 18,20,21,30,33,34,39,40,49,58,59.)

Biological Consequences of Particles of Metal That Are Not Trace Elements

Elements that are not trace elements and utilized may not be readily eliminated by the body. Thus, a different tissue response may be seen. The two elements of interest in this section are zirconia and titanium, which appear to be ignored by the body. The data on zirconia are scanty and will not be discussed further, and further study is encouraged.

The response to titanium is of major concern and interest. Our daily contact with titanium dioxide is more extensive than previously thought with toothpaste being a prime example of an ignored titanium source. However, there is still no evidence that titanium is an essential or unessential trace element utilized or metabolized by the host. The nonmetabolizable particles of PMMA and PE discussed in other chapters in this volume result in the stimulation of chronic inflammation and giant cells in the tissue. This does not seem to be the case with titanium. Retrieval studies in animals and humans show deposition of large amounts of titanium debris with no cellular response at all. It is unusual for the body to ignore a foreign material: no evident cytotoxicity, no evidence of inflammation or immune responses, and no evidence of a fibrous capsule. How long this will remain inert without evoking a response is a major question. Of concern in these studies is that we have focused on cytotoxicity studies and not on cell proliferation, with the exception of immune responses and carcinogenicity. Some of these materials may stimulate effects on distant cells and tissues through the elaboration of soluble mediators such as cytokines and hormones not routinely detected. (See refs. 30,61,63,64.)

WHAT HAVE WE LEARNED AND WHAT DO WE NEED TO KNOW?

In general the experimental studies have provided much information on the biological effects of these materials and particles. Protocols are in place for studying effects of salts and corrosion products *in vitro* in various solutions and in cell culture. These initial studies can provide much information on how to evaluate the *in vivo* performance; i.e., these studies can indicate cell and protein binding, and thus non-cell binding materials should be assessed in the urine and cell-binding substances should be assessed in red blood cells and tissue. However, *in vitro* studies, an important first step, do not mimic the *in vivo* performance—especially when a material, and not a device, is studied. Careful *in vivo* studies, under some extremes of wear and corrosion, are required.

The scientific community continues to make advances in our understanding of complex cellular interactions. Many of these will provide us with ways of predicting *in vivo* performance without resorting to use of experimental animals. Interaction among molecular biologists, bone and cartilage biologists, and biomechanical and material scientists is essential to fully understand the biological responses to particulate metals from TJR devices. (See refs. 24,25,32,50,51,60.)

Metals as ions forming organometallic complexes and particles that will also slowly form organometallic complexes are released *in vitro* and *in vivo* from materials used in joint replacement devices. Although dose-response relationships are not known and the subject of much controversy, everyone agrees that it is important to minimize the release. The quantity, nature, and function(s) of the various organometallic complexes formed are also a subject of much controversy among investigators. It is important to continue to explore the formation and function of these complexes using salts, particles, metals, and alloys. These complexes are the stimulators of the biological responses of concern in the orthopaedic patient. Finally, these biological responses may be stimulated by a complex acting on one cell resulting in a cascade of release of stimulators acting at some distance from the original metal complex formation. The end cell responding may have no interaction with the original metal released. The tools and findings of the molecular biologist are important in evaluating the end stages of the response to the presence of a metal (or polymer) device.

REFERENCES

1. Bearden LJ, Cooke FW. Growth inhibition of cultured fibroblasts by cobalt and nickel. *J Biomed Mater Res* 1980;14:289–309.
2. Bence JL, Black J, Mitchell SN. Role of plasma proteins in corrosion of 316L stainless steel in vitro. In: Williams JM, Nichols MF, Zingg W, eds. *Biomedical materials,* vol 55. Pittsburgh, PA: MRS, 1986:387–393.

3. Black J. Systemic effects of biomaterials. *Biomaterials* 1984;5:11–18.
4. Black J. Does corrosion matter? *J Bone Joint Surg [Br]* 1988;70:517–520.
5. Brown SA, Farnsworth LJ, Merritt K, Crowe TD. In vitro and in vivo metal ion release. *J Biomed Mater Res* 1988;22:321–338.
6. Brown SA, Hughes PJ, Merritt K. In vitro studies of fretting corrosion of orthopaedic materials. *J Orthop Res* 1988;6:572–579.
7. Brown SA, Margevecius RW, Merritt K. Fretting and accelerated fretting corrosion of titanium in vitro and in vivo. In: Heimke G, Sultesz U, Lee AJC, eds, *Clinical implant materials*. Amsterdam: Elsevier, 1990:37–42.
8. Brown SA, Merritt K, Farnsworth LJ, Crowe TD. An in vivo model for quantification of metal ion release and transport. In: Pizzoferrato et al, eds. *Biomaterials and clinical applications*. Amsterdam: Elsevier, 1987:717–722.
9. Brown SA, Merritt K, Farnsworth LJ, Crowe TD. Biological significance of metal ion release. In: Lemons J, ed. *Quantitative characteristics and performance of porous implants*. STP 953. Philadelphia: ASTM, 1987:163–181.
10. Brown SA, Merritt K. Fretting corrosion in saline and serum. *J Biomed Mater Res* 1981;15:479–488.
11. Brown SA, Merritt K. Electrochemical corrosion in saline and serum. *J Biomed Mater Res* 1980;14:173–175.
12. Brown SA, Merritt K. Fretting corrosion of plates and screws: an in vitro test method. In: Fraker AC, Griffin CD, eds. *Corrosion and degradation of implant materials*. STP 859. Philadelphia: ASTM, 1985:105–116.
13. Brown SA, Zhang K, Merritt K, Payer JH. Quantification of in vivo release and transport of Ni Co Cr and Mo from accelerated anodic corrosion (AAC) of porous coated CoCrMo. *Adv Biomater (in press).*
14. Buchhorn GH, Willert HG, Semlitsch M, Schoen R, Steinemann S, Schmidt M. Preparation, characterization and animal testing for biocompatibility of metallic particles of iron-, cobalt-, and titanium-based implant alloys. In: St. John KR, ed. *Particulate debris from medical implants*. STP 1144. Philadelphia: ASTM, 1992:177–189.
15. Charnley J, Kamangar A, Longfield MD. The optimum size of prosthetic heads in relation to the wear of plastic sockets in total replacement of the hip. *Med Biol Eng* 1969;7:31–39.
16. Charnley J. Tissue reactions to implanted plastics. In: *Acrylic cement in orthopedic surgery*. Baltimore: Williams & Wilkins, 1970:1–9.
17. Coleman RF, Herrington J, Scales JT. Concentration of wear products in hair, blood, and urine after total hip replacement. *BMJ* 1973;1:527–529.
18. Collery P, Poirier LA, Manfait M, Etienne JC. *Metal ions in biology and medicine*. Paris: John Libbey Eurotest, 1990.
19. Cuckler JM, Mitchell J, Baker D, Ducheyne P, Imonitie V, Schumacher HR. A comparison of the biocompatibility of polymethyl methacrylate debris with and without titanium debris: comparison of two in vivo models. In: St. John KR, ed. *Particulate debris from medical implants*. STP 1144. Philadelphia: ASTM, 1992:118–126.
20. Elves MW, Wilson JN, Scales JT, Kemp HBS. Incidence of metal sensitivity in patients with total joint replacements. *BMJ* 1975;4:376–378.
21. Evans EM, Freeman MAR, Miller AJ, Vernon-Roberts B. Metal sensitivity as a cause of bone necrosis and loosening of prostheses in total joint replacements. *J Bone Joint Surg [Br]* 1974;56:626–642.
22. Ferguson Jr AB, Laing PG, Hodge ES. The ionization of metal implants in living tissues. *J Bone Joint Surg [Am]* 1960;42:77–90.
23. Gerber H, Perren SM. Evaluation of tissue compatibility of in vitro cultures of embryonic bone. In: Winter G, Leray J, deGroot K, eds. *Evaluation of biomaterials*. Chichester: Wiley, 1980:307–314.
24. Goldring MB, Goldring SR. Skeletal tissue response to cytokines. *Clin Orthop* 1990;258:245–278.
25. Goldring SR, Bennett NE, Jasty MJ. In vitro activation of monocyte/macrophages and fibroblasts by metal particles. In: St. John KR, ed. *Particulate debris from medical implants*. STP 1144. Philadelphia: ASTM, 1992:236–242.
26. Goodman SB, Davidson J, Fornasier VL. The histological reaction to titanium alloy and hydroxyapatite particles implanted in the rabbit tibia. *Transactions of the 4th World Biomaterials Congress*, 1992, 317.
27. Goodman SB, Fornasier VL, Lee J, Kei J. The effects of bulk versus particulate titanium and cobalt chrome alloy implanted into the tibia. *J Biomed Mater Res* 1990;24:1539–1549.
28. Healy KE, Ducheyne P. The mechanisms of passive dissolution of titanium in a model physiological environment. *J Biomed Mater Res* 1992;36:319–338.
29. Howie DW, Vernon-Roberts B. The synovial response to intraarticular cobalt-chromium wear particles. *Clin Orthop* 1988;232:244–254.
30. Hulbert SF, ed. *Bioceramics*, vol 3, Terre Haute: Rose Hulman Institute of Technology, 1992.

31. Langard S, Hensten-Pettersen A. Chromium toxicology. In: Williams DF, ed. *Systemic aspects of biocompatibility,* vol 1. Boca Raton: CRC Press, 1981:143–161.
32. Lorenzo JA. The role of cytokines in the regulation of local bone resorption. *Crit Rev Immunol* 1991;11:195–213
33. Marnett LJ. The role of oxidative damage in metal carcinogenicity. *Chem Res Toxicol* 1992;4:i.
34. Maurer AM, Merritt K, Brown SA. Biocompatibility of titanium wear products with blood components and fibroblast cell cultures. *Trans Soc Biomater* 1991;14:37.
35. Maurer AM, Merritt K, Brown SA. Cellular uptake of titanium and vanadium from addition of salts or fretting corrosion in vitro. *J Biomed Mater Res (submitted).*
36. Meachim G, Brooke G. The synovial response to intra-articular Co-Cr-Mo particles in guinea pigs. *Biomaterials* 1983;4:153–159.
37. Meachim G, Williams DF. Changes in nonosseous tissue adjacent to titanium implants. *J Biomed Mater Res* 1973;7:555–572.
38. Merritt K. Role of medical materials, both in implant and surface applications, in immune response and in resistance to infection. *Biomaterials* 1984;5:47–53.
39. Merritt K. Biochemistry/hypersensitivity/clinical reactions. In: Lang B, Morris J, Rassoog J, eds. *International workshop on biocompatibility, toxicity, and hypersensitivity to alloy systems used in dentistry.* Ann Arbor: University of Michigan Press, 1986:195–223.
40. Merritt K. Allergic reactions to materials used in prosthetic surgery. In: Pizzoferrato A, Marchetti P, Ravaglioli U, Lee ACL, eds. *Biomaterials and clinical applications.* Amsterdam: Elsevier, 1987:711–716.
41. Merritt K, Brown SA. Metal sensitivity reactions to orthopedic implants. *Int J Dermatol* 1981;20:89–94.
42. Merritt K, Brown SA, Sharkey NA. Blood distribution of nickel, cobalt, and chromium following intramuscular injection into hamsters. *J Biomed Mater Res* 1984;18:991–1004.
43. Merritt K, Brown SA, Sharkey NA. The binding of metal salts and corrosion products to cells and proteins in vitro. *J Biomed Mater Res* 1984;18:1005–1015.
44. Merritt K, Brown SA. Effect of proteins and pH on fretting corrosion and metal ion release. *J Biomed Mater Res* 1988;22:111–120.
45. Merritt K, Crowe TD, Brown SA. Elimination of nickel, cobalt and chromium following repeated injections of high dose metal salts. *J Biomed Mater Res* 1989;23:845–863.
46. Merritt K, Margevicius RM, Brown SA. Storage and elimination of titanium, aluminum, and vanadium salts in vivo. *J Biomed Mater Res* 1992 *(in press).*
47. Merritt K, Wenz LM, Brown SA. Cell association of fretting corrosion products generated in a cell culture. *J Orthop Res* 1991;9:289–296.
48. Mizel SB. The interleukins. *FASEB J* 1989;3:2379–2388.
49. Mjoberg B. Aluminum may cause senile dementia and bone fragility. *Calcif Tissue Int* 1990;47:259–260.
50. Mundy GR. Inflammatory mediators and the destruction of bone. *J Periodont Res* 1991;26:213–217.
51. Murray DW, Rushton N. Macrophages stimulate bone resorption when they phagocytose particles. *J Bone Joint Surg [Br]* 1990;72:988–992.
52. Pizzoferrato A, Vespucci A, Ciapetti G, Stae S. Biocompatibility testing of prosthetic implant materials by cell cultures. *Biomaterials* 1985;6:346–351.
53. Pizzoferrato A, Vespucci A, Ciapetti G, Stae S, Tarabusi C. The effect of injection of powdered biomaterials on mouse peritoneal cell populations. *J Biomed Mater Res* 1987;21:419–428.
54. Rae T. A study of the effects of particulate metals of orthopaedic interest on murine macrophages in vitro. *J Bone Joint Surg [Br]* 1975;57:444–450.
55. Rae T. The toxicity of metals used in orthopaedic prostheses: an experimental study using cultured human synovial fibroblasts. *J Bone Joint Surg [Br]* 1981;63:435–440.
56. Rae T. The biological response to titanium and titanium-aluminum-vanadium alloy particles. I. Tissue culture studies. *Biomaterials* 1986;7:30–36.
57. Rae T. The biological response to titanium and titanium-aluminum-vanadium alloy particles. II. Long term animal studies. *Biomaterials* 1986;7:37–40.
58. Standeven AM, Wetterhahn KE. Chromium VI toxicity: uptake, reduction, and DNA damage. *J Am Toxicol* 1989;8:1275–1283.
59. Standeven AM, Wetterhahn KE. Is there a role for reactive oxygen species in the mechanism of chromium VI carcinogenesis. *Chem Res Toxicol* 1992;4:616–625.
60. Stashenko P, Obernesser MS, Dewhirst FE. Effect of immune cytokines on bone. *Immunol Invest* 1989;18:239–249.
61. St. John KR, ed. *Particulate debris from medical implants.* STP 1144. Philadelphia: ASTM, 1992.
62. Willert HG, Semlitsch M. Reaction of articular capsule to wear products of artificial joint prostheses. *J Biomed Mater Res* 1977;11:157–164.
63. Williams DF, ed. *Systemic aspects of biocompatibility,* vol 1. Boca Raton: CRC Press, 1981.
64. Williams DF, ed. *Biocompatibility of orthopaedic implants,* vol 1. Boca Raton: CRC Press, 1982.

65. Williams DF. Tissue reaction to metallic corrosion products and wear particles in clinical orthopaedics. In: Williams DF, ed. *Biocompatibility of orthopaedic implants,* vol 1. Boca Raton: CRC Press, 1982:231–248.
66. Williams RL, Brown SA, Merritt K. Electrochemical studies on the influence of proteins on the corrosion of implant materials. *Biomaterials* 1988;9:181–186.
67. Woodman JL, Black J, Jimenez S. Organometallic corrosion products of 316L SS and HS-21 in serum: in vitro and in vivo comparison in an acute rat model. In: Winter G, Gibbons D, Plenk H, eds. *Biomaterials 1980*. Chichester: Wiley, 1982:245–250.
68. Woodman JL, Black J, Nunamaker DM. Release of Co and Ni from a new total finger joint prosthesis made of vitallium. *J Biomed Mater Res* 1983;17:655–668.
69. Zabel DD, Brown SA, Merritt K, Payer JH. AES analysis of stainless steel corroded in saline, serum, and in vivo. *J Biomed Mater Res* 1988;22:31–44.

Biological, Material, and Mechanical Considerations of Joint Replacement, edited by B. F. Morrey. Raven Press, Ltd., New York © 1993.

Discussion of Materials and Ceramics, Including Hydroxylapatite

Jack E. Lemons

Laboratory Research, Division of Orthopaedic Surgery, Departments of Surgery and Biomaterials, University of Alabama at Birmingham, Birmingham, Alabama 35294-3295

The workshop group consisting of 22 surgeons and scientists have categorized opinions for (i) metals, alloys, and polymers and (ii) ceramics (calcium phosphates) according to consensus, areas of contention, and future needs.

METALS, ALLOYS, AND POLYMERS

In an attempt to separate the information into subcategories, opinions on metals, alloys, and polymers have been divided into areas as follows:

1. Particulates and osteolysis,
2. Corrosion and biodegradation,
3. Wear resistance,
4. Models,
5. Definitions and observations,
6. General opinions.

Consensus

Particulates and Osteolysis

Particulates of metals and alloys, ceramics, polymers, and combinations of various sizes, geometries, and distributions can cause significant reactions within biological environments.

Metallic particles are very different from polymeric particles (a mix of ions, small particles, alloy, etc.).

Polymeric wear debris is of more concern than metallic wear debris in terms of device loosening and osteolysis, probably because of the relative volume of particulate generated (in conventional metal/polyethylene hips).

Metallic particulates *in vivo* should not be fully equated with laboratory-prepared particulates.

The process of osteolysis is a complex continuum involving soluble mediators, cells, and mechanical aspects.

Osteolysis can be mediated by particulates, both metallic and polymeric, through macrophage activity, and this is primarily a biological problem.

Very small volumetric changes in a metal implant (through wear, abrasion, or fretting) can release such high quantities of small metallic particulate as to strongly discolor tissues. The inference is that metallic particles are not as inductive to osteolysis as polyethylene particles. This may be a false inference due to differences in volume. Polyethylene debris probably occurs at several orders of magnitude greater than metal debris.

Corrosion and Biodegradation

Metal ion release due to corrosion and wear phenomena is of concern regarding its effect on cell behavior. Wear is a means of creating high surface areas that will amplify the corrosion phenomena.

Wear Resistance

Wear resistance of metals and alloys can be improved through state-of-the-art technology improvements more readily than improvement of polymer wear resistance.

Models

Osteolysis is a complex biological problem that requires an animal model in which metal particles can be generated to test the cellular (including osteoblasts and osteoclasts) reactivity. The chemical composition of metallic particulate debris must be delineated and the volume of material released must be quantified.

Particles used for *in vitro* studies need to be fabricated in protein or other biologically representative solutions of *in vivo* debris.

Definitions and Observations

The term adverse biological response is preferred to toxicity.

Blackening of tissue is not necessarily an accurate measure of volumetric loss or toxicity of metallic debris.

General Comments

It is important to integrate biological/biomaterial/biomechanical considerations, because it is unknown which is the primary etiology resulting in osteolytic phenomena.

Debris from *in vivo* devices usually include several components, thus preventing descriptions of cause-effect relationships.

The process has a cascade effect.

Metal/metal articulation may release higher metal levels than current metal/polyethylene devices (maybe only through corrosive release); this may be a problem systemically (e.g., toxicity, carcinogenicity), but not in terms of osteolysis.

We need to understand how metals regulate cell and tissue biology; the concept of toxicity is inadequate to describe the effects of materials on bone formation and resorption.

Areas of Contention

Particulates and Osteolysis

Metal particles have been shown to be present in tissues with little or no evidence of osteolysis.

Particulates per se can be a stimulus to cells versus corrosion products being released.

Can metallic debris cause osteolysis in the absence of other particulates?

Corrosion and Biodegradation

What is the role of metal ions (corrosion)?

Wear Resistance

What is the role of a metal/metal articulating surface for a total joint replacement prosthesis? Can the quality be adequately controlled? Will it improve or worsen the situation? What is the advisability of metal/metal articulating surfaces?

Models

Relevant *in vitro* and *in vivo* models that emphasize environmental responses to metals and polyethylene must be developed.

General Opinions and Unanswered Questions

Is there actually a consensus that osteolysis around a noncemented implant is primarily caused by particulates, metal or otherwise? What about other etiologies such as the biomechanics of force transfer?

Basic data on synergism of different biomaterial particulates *in vivo* have not been adequately evaluated (cause-effect relationship).

The basic biological responses that cause cytokine release need to be investigated for separate and combined substances using standardized test methodologies. Current data, although of value, have significant limitations.

Future Needs

Particulates and Osteolysis

Standardized methods for study and characterization of both polymeric and metallic particulates need to be emphasized.

Considering polyethylene, polymethylmethacrylate, or metal as the same dimension particles: do they do the same thing *in vivo?* We need dose-response curves for all three.

Wear Resistance

Are there bearing surface materials that we can expect to last the lifetime of the joint? There is a need for the development of highly wear-resistant metals and alloys.

Industrial bearings are available that last for long periods. Is it realistic to expect this for implants?

Models

There is a need to develop realistic *in vitro* models to study *in vivo* environmental influences to assess material responses (biological activities), model systems for particulate generation (*in vitro* system and environment), and standardized *in vitro* cultures and laboratory animal models. We also need *in vivo* generators for the chronic delivery of particulates in laboratory animals.

An *in vitro* model system should be developed that deals with protein absorption.

Definitions and Observations

Has there, in fact, been a change in the grade and quality of polyethylene over the past few years?

Correlations between clinical observations and laboratory data need to be expanded.

General Opinions

Ex vivo assessments (quantification) must be developed to prospectively follow clinical material.

Investigations of biomaterials, designs, and applications to significantly decrease wear and increase attachment to tissues need to be emphasized.

Discussion of the current understanding of the influence of bacteria on the growth/resorption process is needed.

CERAMICS (CALCIUM PHOSPHATES)

The subcategories for ceramics include:

1. Particulates;
2. Device designs;
3. Tissue interface;
4. Characterization, fabrication, and technology;
5. Definitions and general opinions.

A detailed discussion was conducted regarding hydroxylapatite. This included the biochemistry, clinical experience, basic research, histology of retrieval material, and influence of loose particles on the articulation. Following this, additional discussion resulted in the following conclusions.

Consensus

Device Design

Calcium phosphate ceramic coatings are not in and of themselves solutions for unacceptable device designs or surgeries.

Characterization, Fabrication, and Technology

All of the available calcium phosphate ceramics have not been adequately characterized.

It is not clear whether $CaPO_4$-coated implants last for a long time. With coatings, the difference in batch appears critical.

Definitions and Opinions

Investigations of hydroxylapatite coatings represents a situation in which it is advisable to proceed slowly.

Hydroxylapatite-coated implants (designed for permanent maintenance of coating) should only be investigated in clinical centers participating in prospective, controlled studies with informed consent.

Contention

Particulates

Since there is no osteolysis in recent French devices constructed of alumina bearings, there is a need for detailed evaluations.

What is known about $CaPO_4$-coated devices? Do they result in "early incorporation" and are they of value if "early incorporation" is needed?

Characterization, Fabrication, and Technology

Plasma-sprayed hydroxylapatite coatings as multiphase surfaces may not be adequately reliable. Is there adequate bonding to metallic substrates and will it degrade as a plasma-sprayed coating?

Is it possible to fully control and assess the quality of $CaPO_4$-sprayed coatings?

Definitions and Opinions

Based on present knowledge, the general use of $CaPO_4$-coated implants should be limited to specifically designed conditions.

Future Needs

Tissue Interfaces

What is the nature of the metallic surface beneath the $CaPO_4$ coatings? Does bone actually fill in where $CaPO_4$ coatings have been lost?

Does the bone formed on $CaPO_4$ coatings have the right factors to allow later bone remodeling cycles, e.g., osteocalcin.

Characterization, Fabrication, and Technology

There is a need for quality control and standards for plasma spraying, including starting powders, spraying parameters, and surface of the target (e.g., etched, grit, blasted).

If $CaPO_4$ coatings fail in the long run, will the risk be significantly worse than for uncoated devices?

Definitions and Opinions

What is the clinical utility we are seeking for coated devices?

Study of alternative processing routes to achieve calcium phosphate-type coatings or other surface modifications is needed.

There is a need for long-term trials (i.e., 5 years) which is particularly important for $CaPO_4$-coated total joint replacement devices.

*Biological, Material, and Mechanical
Considerations of Joint Replacement,*
edited by B. F. Morrey.
Raven Press, Ltd., New York © 1993.

13

Clinical Experience with the Anatomic Medullary Locking (AML) Prosthesis for Primary Total Hip Replacement

Charles A. Engh, Thomas F. McGovern, C. Anderson Engh, Jr., and Grace E. Macalino

Anderson Orthopaedic Research Institute, Arlington, Virginia 22206

Clinical trials using a fully porous-coated anatomic medullary locking (AML) femoral prosthesis and a cemented acetabular prosthesis began in 1977. One hundred and fifty-nine primary arthroplasties were done using this method. In 1983, the inventory of femoral prostheses was increased from one to six sizes, and the porous coating was removed from the distal 5 cm of the six new implants. The chrome-cobalt femoral head remained 32 mm in size and nonmodular. In 1982 the senior author began using the porous-coated AML acetabular component. The metal shell had three porous-coated fixation spikes and the polyethylene bearing surface was not modular. Between December 1982 and December 1984, the senior author used these porous-coated femoral and acetabular components for all primary total hip arthroplasties. Two hundred and twenty-seven arthroplasties were performed. Twenty-three of these patients have since died, and 11 femora containing these prostheses were retrieved from these patients at autopsy. Several studies have been performed on these retrieval specimens including a quantitative analysis of implant stability (7) densitometric analysis of periprosthetic bone remodeling (6), and quantitation of changes in strain patterns caused by bone remodeling (7). Transverse sections of methylmethacrylate-embedded specimens were examined by light and scanning electron microscopy to determine the amount of bone ingrowth into the porous surfaces. The results of these studies have been used to assess the accuracy of serial clinical radiographs for predicting bone ingrowth, implant stability, and femoral bone remodeling.

This chapter attempts to summarize some of the most important clinical and laboratory observations following primary total hip arthroplasty with the AML prosthesis (DePuy, Warsaw, Indiana); it is divided into three sections. The first summarizes the authors' experience using plane radiographs to predict osseointegration of the components. The second section summarizes recent information regarding resorptive bone remodeling. The final section describes the current clinical status of the early cases that were treated with both a porous-coated femoral and acetabular component.

RADIOGRAPHIC ASSESSMENT OF THE BIOLOGIC FIXATION OF THE AML PROSTHESIS

The Femoral Component

Osseointegration of the AML femoral component is described using direct and indirect radiographic signs (4). Direct signs refer to bone remodeling changes that occur adjacent to the porous-coated portion of the implant. The indirect signs refer to bone remodeling changes that occur at areas other than the porous-coated interface.

There are two direct signs. First, when endosteal bone appears to become dense adjacent to the porous coating, osseointegration is presumed to have occurred. These areas of densification are termed endosteal spot welds. These spot welds frequently occur near the termination of the porous coating on the implant. Above this area of densification cortical osteoporosis occurs. Below the densification, a sclerotic demarcation line develops adjacent to the portion of the implant that does not contain porous coating. Figure 1 is a clinical radiograph showing this response. Figure 2 is a slab radiograph of a femur containing a porous-coated implant. This slab radiograph was obtained from the level near the termination of the porous coating on the implant. Also shown in Fig. 2 is a scanning electron photomicrograph at this same level.

The other direct sign denotes failure of osseointegration. Demarcation lines separated from the porous-coated implant by a radiolucent space indicates failed osseointegration. Figure 3 is a radiographic view of a femur containing an AML prosthesis in which this sign is present. Figure 4 is a slab radiograph from this same case. To confirm that these signs were good predictors of implant stability, the intact autopsy-retrieved femora were tested for implant stability. Electrical displacement trans-

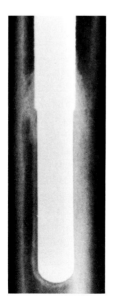

FIG. 1. An osseointegrated implant with local densification or endosteal spot weld near the termination of porous coating. A sclerotic demarcation line adjacent to the smooth surfaced portion of the implant is also present.

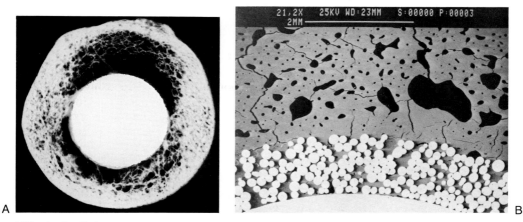

A   B

FIG. 2. A: Slab radiograph of a transverse section obtained near the termination of porous coating on the implant. **B:** Backscatter scanning electron micrograph of the porous surface-metal interface from the section shown in A. A substantial amount of bone has grown into the porous surfaces shown at the bottom of the photomicrograph.

ducers were connected to each implant and each femur at multiple levels. Testing was performed in a device developed by Burke et al. (2). Transverse and axial micromotion were measured in simulated stance and stair climbing. Motion between the porous-coated implant and bone from the cases showing endosteal spot welds averaged less than 20 μm. Micromotion between the implant and bone in the cases showing demarcation lines around the porous coating exceeded 150 μm (7).

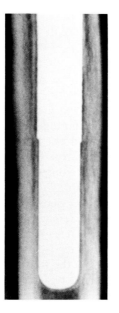

FIG. 3. A direct sign that indicates failure of osseointegration is the presence of demarcation lines separated from the porous-coated implant by a radiolucent space.

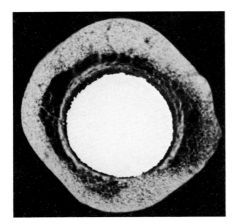

FIG. 4. Slab radiograph of a transverse section obtained from the femur shown in Figure 3. The demarcation line and radiolucent space surround the entire porous surface of the implant at this level.

Three groups of indirect signs have been helpful for predicting osseointegration. These signs occur in the medial femoral neck and intramedullary canal adjacent to the uncoated part of the stem. Atrophy of the medial femoral neck suggests that the implant has become osseointegrated at a level below the femoral neck. Hypertrophy of the femoral neck beneath the collar is a sign that the porous-coated portion of the implant below the collar has not become osseointegrated. Widening of the intramedullary canal around the uncoated distal part of the prosthesis or the presence of demarcation lines in this area indicates that this part of the implant is mechanically unstable. When these signs are present, osseointegration of the proximal porous coated part is less likely to be present. Conversely, if the uncoated distal portion of the implant appears stable, proximal osseointegration is more likely to be present. The presence of an intramedullary pedestal that appears to support the uncoated end of the prosthesis is an indirect sign that the prosthesis has not become fixed proximally. Conversely, the absence of an intramedullary pedestal indicating the absence of end loading is a good indirect sign that the implant has become proximally fixed. Figure 5 shows the immediate postoperative, 2-year postoperative, and 5-year postoperative radiographs of a femur containing a proximally porous-coated implant that has become osseointegrated. Many of the direct and indirect signs that the authors have just mentioned are present in this case.

In some cases, the signs of osseointegration illustrated in Fig. 5 are less clear. In other cases, the signs on the radiographs clearly indicate failed osseointegration. Although these implants may not be as stable *in vivo* as osseointegrated ones, they can be clinically stable. The authors have also developed and tested a method to grade clinical stability of the components (4). This method requires the comparison of serial annual radiographs over at least a 2-year interval. Clinically stable implants maintain a radiographically stable interface, one that does not change its appearance on radiographs from year to year. When an interface is unstable, new demarcation lines frequently develop. Existing demarcation lines also become further separated from the implant and metal particles may be shed from the implant. Clinically stable implants also do not migrate. If there has been no measurable change in the implant position on annual radiographs over a 2-year interval, the implant could be considered clinically stable even if it had migrated at an earlier time interval. Figure 6

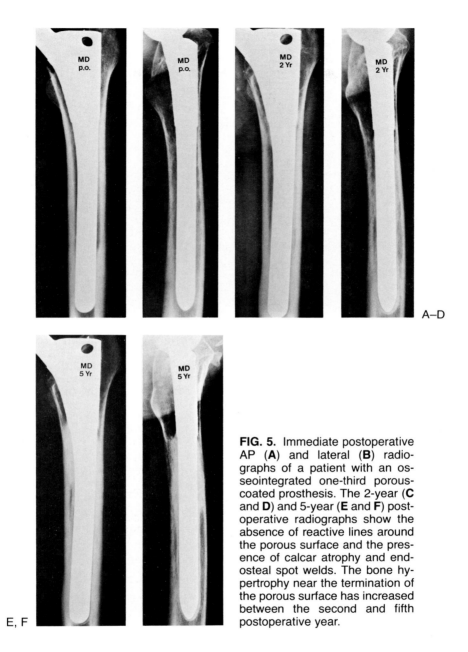

A–D

E, F

FIG. 5. Immediate postoperative AP (**A**) and lateral (**B**) radiographs of a patient with an osseointegrated one-third porous-coated prosthesis. The 2-year (**C** and **D**) and 5-year (**E** and **F**) postoperative radiographs show the absence of reactive lines around the porous surface and the presence of calcar atrophy and endosteal spot welds. The bone hypertrophy near the termination of the porous surface has increased between the second and fifth postoperative year.

shows a series of radiographs from a case showing failed osseointegration. The absence of implant migration over a 10-year interval and an absence of change in interface appearance over a 5-year interval indicates that, although this implant is not osseointegrated, it has maintained clinical stability. Figure 7 shows a series of radiographs illustrating a clinically unstable implant.

The autopsy-retrieved femora from three cases, with radiographic signs of osseointegration and long-term implant stability, were transversely sectioned and ex-

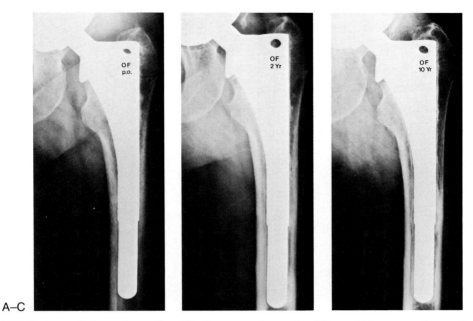

A–C

FIG. 6. Immediate postoperative (**A**), 2-year postoperative (**B**), and 10-year postoperative (**C**) AP radiographs of a patient with a stable, nonosseointegrated four-fifths porous-coated implant. Failed osseointegration is indicated by the presence of a demarcation line separated from the porous surface by a radiolucent space. The implant is considered stable because there has been no change in the appearance of the interface and the position of the implant between the second and tenth postoperative year.

amined by light and scanning electron microscopy. Bone ingrowth was observed throughout the entire porous-coated surface. There was a higher percentage of ingrown fields in the distal half of the porous coating (58%) compared to the proximal half (19%). In the proximal regions, compact bone was most frequently observed on the medial side and medial corners of the components and was joined to the outer cortex by hypertrophied cancellous trabeculae. In the distal regions, compact bone ingrowth frequently occurred circumferentially and was an integral part of the outer cortex.

The Acetabular Component

The authors also studied serial clinical radiographs of porous-coated acetabular components retrieved at autopsy. The microscopic analysis of polished sections in each case confirmed the histologic type of fixation. Based on these studies, a circumferential radiolucency at the bone-porous surface interface was determined to be a sign of failed osseointegration (Fig. 8). Particle shedding or recent measurable change in acetabular component position was found to be indicative of failed osseointegration and component instability. Detection of a delaminated porous surface on an acetabular component requires careful inspection of radiographs (Fig. 9).

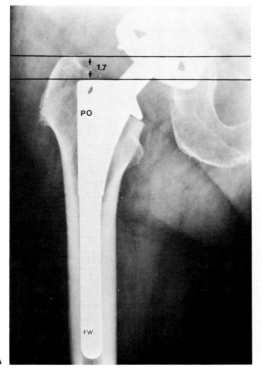

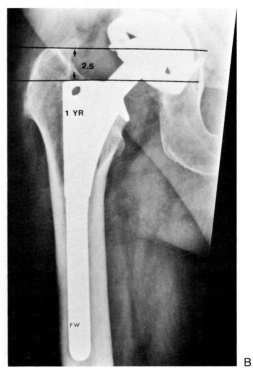

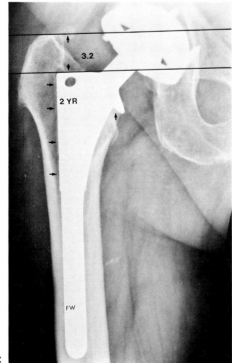

FIG. 7. Immediate postoperative (**A**), 1-year postoperative (**B**), and 3-year postoperative (**C**) AP radiographs of a patient with an unstable one-third porous-coated implant. The increase in vertical distance between the tip of the trochanter and flat horizontal superior edge of the prosthesis indicates subsidence of the implant. The new reactive lines (*arrows*) indicate absence of bone ingrowth into the porous surface in this area.

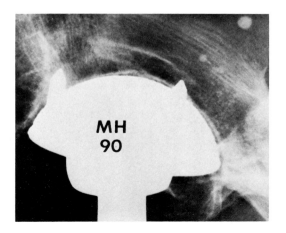

FIG. 8. Radiograph of a porous coated acetabular component with a circumferential radiolucency of the bone-porous surface interface. This is a sign of failed osseointegration. This implant was found at autopsy to be well-fixed by fibrous tissue ingrowth.

The comparison of the histologic and radiographic findings in these cases also convinced the authors that isolated changes in the appearance of the bone-implant interface on serial radiographs can sometimes be an unreliable sign. Analysis showed that bone ingrowth occurred in a random fashion (8). Random areas of bone ingrowth were sometimes directly adjacent to areas where the bone was separated from the porous coating by gaps of fibrous tissue. Therefore, the apparent differences in acetabular interface appearance on serial radiographs may be due to differences in radiographic techniques resulting in different interface areas being visualized, rather than by actual changes in the interface. Only a small portion of the bone-acetabulum interface (that portion of the periphery of the cup that is tangential to the radiographic beam) is visible on any one radiographic view. In addition, anteroposterior (AP) and oblique radiographs of the acetabulum fail to show any of the bone-implant interface on the posterior half of the acetabular component. For these reasons, the

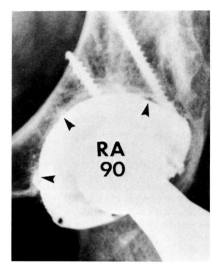

FIG. 9. Radiograph of a porous-coated acetabular component with a delaminated porous surface (*arrows*). This is a sign of failed osseointegration and component instability.

appearance of new radiolucent gaps and deterioration or absence of bone ingrowth in other porous-coated areas are not visualized on the radiograph.

The autopsy studies of the authors' clinical cases also demonstrate that radiographs tend to overestimate the amount of contact that actually occurs between the acetabular component and the host bone (8). Radiographs are two-dimensional representations of a three-dimensional structure. Bone present in planes other than the plane at which the peripheral interface of the cup is visible also appears on the radiograph. Because bone at levels above and below the plane of the visible interface is superimposed, this bone clouds the interface appearance and complicates reading the radiographs. Taking into account all of these limitations associated with radiographic assessment of acetabular fixation, the authors are less confident at grading the stability of the acetabular component in comparison to the femoral component.

BONE REMODELING

Orthopaedic surgeons are concerned about the bone resorption resulting from insertion of porous-coated implants. Engh and Bobyn (3) developed a method to grade the extent of resorptive bone remodeling. The method involved careful comparison of the immediate postoperative and 2-year postoperative radiographs. They emphasized the importance of standardized radiographic techniques. Patient positioning and image contrast and brightness were nearly identical for the radiographs of each of their cases. The femur surrounding the implant was divided into four levels and four quadrants (16 sites). The number of these sites showing visible resorptive bone remodeling at 2 years was recorded and used to quantitate stress shielding. The severity of the stress shielding (mild, moderate, or severe) was based on the total number of sites with resorptive bone remodeling. The study concluded that the factors affecting bone resorption were predominantly mechanical and that the extent of resorptive bone remodeling could be predicted by a stress-shielding formula. The formula was based on implant diameter and the proximal femoral dimensions. Although this method proved valuable for measuring the effects of different mechanical parameters on bone remodeling, it was not quantitative. The extent of changes in radiographic bone density at different postoperative time intervals was not described.

A more quantitative evaluation of radiographic bone remodeling was achieved with computer-assisted video densitometry (5). The method involved converting radiographs into digital computer images. Computer-assisted image processing techniques were used to compensate for the slight differences in contrast and brightness between the radiographic images. Analysis of the digital images allowed quantitative description of the change in postoperative radiographic bone density at individual Gruen zones (9). Figure 10 is a series of radiographs from a case in which extensive stress shielding occurred. The values shown in the 5- and 10-year postoperative radiographs represent changes in the mean radiographic bone density from that recorded on the immediate postoperative radiograph. This method was used to study a series of radiographs from 26 cases similar to one shown in Fig. 10. These cases were randomly selected with the only criterion being a similarity of radiographic technique. Among the cases in which a stem 13.5 mm diameter or larger was used, loss of radiographic density was observed in the proximal and mid-stem Gruen zones. A mean loss of 13% was observed in the proximal zones and 10% in the mid-stem zones. Most of this loss occurred in the first 2 postoperative years. When ex-

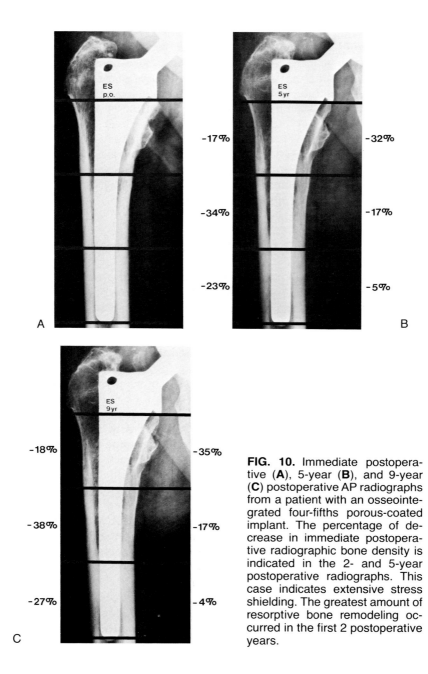

A

-17%
-34%
-23%

B

-32%
-17%
-5%

C

-18%   -35%
-38%   -17%
-27%   -4%

FIG. 10. Immediate postoperative (**A**), 5-year (**B**), and 9-year (**C**) postoperative AP radiographs from a patient with an osseointegrated four-fifths porous-coated implant. The percentage of decrease in immediate postoperative radiographic bone density is indicated in the 2- and 5-year postoperative radiographs. This case indicates extensive stress shielding. The greatest amount of resorptive bone remodeling occurred in the first 2 postoperative years.

tensively porous-coated implants smaller than 13.5 mm in diameter were used, loss of radiographic bone density in the same Gruen zones was minimal.

It is important to recognize that changes in radiographic bone density are different than changes in bone mineral content. Although a relationship between radiographic bone density and bone mineral content does exist, this relationship is complex and is certainly influenced by several factors including soft-tissue overlay. Fortunately, clinicians now have a method to determine changes in bone mineral content by radiography. This method is termed dual energy x-ray absorptiometry (DEXA). The technique, first introduced to study metabolic bone disease, removes the influence of soft-tissue coverage to provide a direct *in vivo* measure of bone mineral content (12). DEXA has been modified recently to determine *in vivo* changes in bone mineral content adjacent to hip prostheses (13). Although this method appears promising, it still is in a rapid stage of development. Investigators are currently collecting prospective data on periprosthetic bone remodeling using this technique, but it will be many years before long-term prospective data will be available (10).

The authors have taken advantage of this technique to study changes in periprosthetic bone mineral content in their long-term autopsy cases. The autopsy cases analyzed by this method involve patients with unilateral hip disease in which radiographs of both femora appeared identical prior to total hip replacement. Both femora were removed at autopsy and a prosthesis of identical size was positioned in the nonoperated femur, which was used as a control. It was then possible to measure changes in periprosthetic bone mineral content between the remodeled and control femur. This method eliminated many variables currently associated with clinical DEXA studies. The loss of periprosthetic bone mineral content in these specimens was similar to the changes in radiographic bone density found by examination of the authors clinical radiographs. Total loss of periprosthetic bone mineral averaged 25% in the five autopsy cases. The total amount of bone loss varied from as little as 7% to as much as 52%. In addition there was a gradient of bone loss from proximal to distal. The mean bone loss in Gruen zones 1 and 7 (the bone adjacent to the upper one-third of the prosthesis) was 45%. In Gruen zones 2 and 4, the mean loss was 28%. Changes in bone density adjacent to the lower third of the stem varied from either slight bone losses to slight increases in periprosthetic bone mineral in this area. These cadaver studies also demonstrated one other potentially important finding. There was a very strong correlation between the amount of bone mineral present in the control femur and the amount of periprosthetic bone loss that occurred as a result of bone remodeling. Patients with very low bone mineral content in their proximal femur at the time of surgery appear to be prone to lose more bone as a result of bone remodeling.

Although computer-assisted videodensitometry and DEXA provide physicians with clinical methods for estimating the amount of bone resorption, these methods do not precisely define the location of the bone loss. Computed tomography would be needed to provide three-dimensional remodeling information. Unfortunately this is currently impossible because of radiographic beam scatter from the implant. To circumvent this problem, the authors have performed calibrated videodensitometric analysis of slab radiograph cases to obtain this same information.

Contact slab radiographs of contiguous 5-mm thick transverse sections were obtained from two of the autopsy-retrieved cases. In both cases the patients were treated for unilateral hip disease and the contralateral normal femur was used as a control. The bone mass surrounding the implant was measured in both the *in vivo* implanted femur and the post mortem implanted control. The results showed that the location and extent of bone mass loss were different in the proximal, mid-stem, and distal sections. Mass loss in the proximal sections occurred medially. In the mid-stem sections the mass loss was more evenly distributed around the implant. Mass loss in the distal sections was predominantly on the lateral side and some increased mass was noted on the medial sides. The overall percentage of mass loss and the proximal-to-distal gradient of loss were similar to the DEXA and videodensitometric results described above.

RESULTS OF LONG-TERM CLINICAL TRIALS

Clinical Material

Between October 1982 and December 1984, 227 primary arthroplasties were performed using porous-coated femoral and acetabular components. Fourteen patients died before their 5th postoperative year. An additional 21 cases did not return for 5-year follow-up. These cases are included in the survivorship analysis, but are otherwise excluded from the description of the results. One hundred ninety-two cases in 180 patients with unilateral arthroplasties and six with bilateral arthroplasties have been evaluated by the authors within the past 2 years. The group includes 98 female and 94 male patients. The mean age for the women was 54.9 years and for the men 54.4 years. Thirty-four of the patients were under 40 years of age at the time of the arthroplasty. Forty were over the age of 65. One hundred and sixty-one cases were performed for osteoarthritis, 15 were performed for avascular necrosis, and 16 were performed for inflammatory arthritis. The mean time interval from the arthroplasty until the last clinical evaluation by the authors was 87.4 months. Data on all of the patients were collected prospectively. The authors' protocol included preoperative functional assessment using the Charnley modification of the D'Aubigne and Postel pain and walking score. Patients were reevaluated postoperatively at annual intervals for the first 5 years and then at 2-year intervals between 5 and 10 years. At each follow-up interval, functional outcome was reassessed using the same scoring system. Four standard radiographs were also obtained at each time interval. These included an AP view of the pelvis to measure acetabular component migration (11) and an iliac oblique view of the acetabulum to evaluate the porous-coated interface of the acetabular component and polyethylene wear. AP and lateral views of the femur were used to evaluate the femoral component. The two femora radiograph views were used to grade bone remodeling and the stability of the components. Osteolytic reactions were recorded. Femoral bone remodeling data have already been presented. This section summarizes the results of the other aspects of the radiographic study as well as the description of functional outcome. Results are presented at 2 years and at last follow-up.

2-YEAR RESULTS

Complications and Reoperations in the First 2 Postoperative Years

At the end of the second postoperative year, one of the 186 patients had required a component exchange. The porous-coated acetabular component in this case had been malpositioned, resulting in recurrent dislocation. This component was revised at the end of the first postoperative year. At the end of the second postoperative year, the patient was asymptomatic and no further dislocations had occurred. No other patients required reoperation in the first 2 postoperative years.

Radiographic Evaluation at 2 Years

The 2-year postoperative radiographs of the remaining 191 acetabular components were analyzed. In 183 cases the radiographs showed no radiolucent gaps in any of the three Charnley and DeLee zones. The interface in these cases was characterized as optimal. In seven cases, isolated radiolucent gaps were noted in some areas. These components were considered to have suboptimal but stable interfaces. None of the 191 components appeared unstable.

In the assessment of the femoral component, the AP and lateral radiographs of the 192 porous-coated stems demonstrated in 175 cases clear signs of osseointegration. Eleven stems were considered to probably not be osseointegrated. A comparison of the immediate and 2-year postoperative radiographs indicated that none of these implants had subsided. Although demarcation lines were present around the porous coating, these had not changed in appearance between the first and second postoperative year. These implants, therefore, were considered not osseointegrated but stable. Six components had migrated in the first postoperative year. Although three of these implants did not migrate in the second year, all six components were considered clinically unstable because our evaluation method requires a component not to migrate for at least a 2-year period to be considered clinically stable. None of the 17 patients in which the radiographs at 2 years showed failed osseointegration of the femoral component was sufficiently dissatisfied at that time to consider reoperation. In none of the cases was there evidence of change in the femoral head position within the acetabular components suggesting polyethylene wear. There were also no osteolytic reactions in any of the 192 cases at 2 years.

CURRENT RESULTS

Reoperations and Complications after 2 Years

At a mean time interval of 87.4 months after arthroplasty, five patients required exchange of one component. In addition to the acetabular component that was exchanged for malposition in the first postoperative year, two other acetabular components required exchange for the same reason. One was exchanged in the fourth postoperative year and the other in the sixth. A fourth patient required exchange of their acetabular component for loosening. This patient, who had severe rheumatoid arthritis, sustained a pathologic fracture of the acetabulum causing a change in the cup orientation. After fracture healing had occurred, the patient became a recurrent dislocator. At the time of revision (in the seventh postoperative year), the component was also found to be loose. All four of the cup exchanges have been successful. On the most recent radiographs, all four components appeared stable. There are at present no patients who are recurrent dislocators.

The fifth component exchange involved a femoral component. This patient was one of the three patients noted to have femoral component subsidence in both the first and second postoperative years. At 5 years, this patient became symptomatic, and femoral component exchange was performed in the sixth postoperative year. It has been 3 years since this femoral revision. The new femoral component is osseointegrated, and the patient now has a good functional result.

Five other operative procedures were performed after the second postoperative year. One patient, who was a chronic subluxator, was treated by changing the polyethylene liner of the acetabular component to one with an elevated rim in the sixth postoperative year. There was no osteolysis observed in this case. Two patients with worn polyethylene surfaces from their acetabular components developed osteolytic reactions in their proximal femur and required bone grafting as well as exchange of the polyethylene liner of the acetabular component. These procedures were done in the sixth and eight postoperative years, respectively. One patient underwent successful excision of heterotopic bone in the fourth postoperative year. All of the above described operative procedures were performed by the senior author. One patient, whose athroplasty had been performed for a congenital dislocated hip, developed postoperative restricted hip abduction caused by an abnormally prominent greater trochanter. A portion of the greater trochanter was removed by another surgeon in the fourth postoperative year. This procedure has been complicated by trochanteric nonunion. Two other patients who had a trochanteric osteotomy done by the senior author also have trochanter nonunions. There were other complications that did not require revision. In total, five patients developed heterotopic ossification sufficient to restrict range of motion, but only one patient required excision. One patient developed an ischial fracture through a region of osteolysis in the ninth postoperative year. The fracture healed uneventfully and the patient is currently asymptomatic. Because the osteolytic process did not affect a weight-bearing area, it has not been surgically treated.

Using component exchange as the end point, the probability that both the femoral and acetabular components that were inserted at the index arthroplasty would still be *in situ* at completion of the patients' eighth postoperative year was 96.8%, with a standard error of 0.08. The probability that the stem would remain in place through the eighth postoperative year was 99.3%. The probability that the cup would remain in place at 9 years was 97.5%. Using any operative procedure as an end point for a survivorship analysis, the probability that the patient would not require another operation to his or her hip in the first 9 years after the index arthroplasty was 93.0%, with a standard error of 0.13. This gave us an assessment of all operative procedures required to bring this study group to their current status.

Current Status Regarding Implant Stability

At final radiographic evaluation of the 192 arthroplasties, 176 of the femoral components appear to have signs of osseointegration, which includes the one case of the femoral component exchanged for loosening in the sixth postoperative year. Of the remaining 16 cases, the radiographs of 14 show signs that the femoral component is not osseointegrated, but stable. Only two femoral components are unstable. These two patients are pain free with good functional results. The changes in femoral component stability between the second postoperative year and final evaluation can be summarized as follows: all of the femoral implants graded as bone ingrown at 2 years remained bone ingrown and all of the femoral components graded as not bone ingrown but stable at 2 years remained stable. Of the six implants noted as unstable at 2 years, three migrated in the first postoperative year, but showed no interface change and no migration in the second postoperative year and have remained stable. They have shown no further interface change and have not migrated. These three were not as unstable as the other three that continued to migrate in the second year. Among the three that were progressively unstable in the first 2 years, one was revised in the sixth year. The other two implants remain classified as unstable because they have continued to subside. The one that subsided 4 mm in the first 2 years subsided an additional 6 mm by the end of the eighth year. In the other case the stem had subsided 3 mm in the first 2 years and subsided an additional 3 mm at the time of last follow-up (9 years).

The most recent radiographs of the 192 acetabular components demonstrate 146 components (including the four that were revised) to have optimum-appearing interfaces. None of these components has shown signs of migration. Radiographs of 43 cases show isolated radiolucent gaps, indicating a less than perfect interface appearance. In many of these cases, isolated gaps were not seen on the immediate postoperative or 2-year postoperative radiographs. Although the interface is not optimal, the radiolucencies are small and indicate overall that the components have shown no signs of interface deterioration. None of these components has migrated. Two components are currently considered unstable. Both components have shown circumferential radiolucencies and a loss of metal particles from the porous surface; neither of the patients is symptomatic.

Femoral osteolytic reactions have been observed in 38 cases. In 29 of these, the area of osteolysis has not increased in size within the last 2 years. In nine cases, the lesions appear to be increasing in size. The typical appearance of a femoral osteolytic reaction is shown in Fig. 11. Femoral osteolytic reactions were confined to osteoporotic areas within the greater and lesser trochanter adjacent to the joint space. No osteolytic reactions have been noted below the level of the lesser trochanter.

The typical appearance of an acetabular osteolytic reaction is shown in Fig. 12. Acetabular osteolytic lesions were observed in 16 cases. In seven cases, the osteolytic reaction appeared to involve part of the acetabular implant-bone interface in

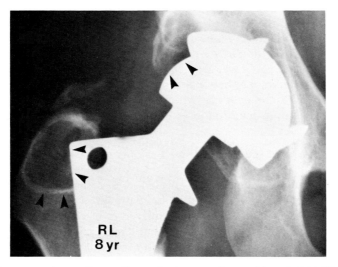

FIG. 11. Eight-year postoperative radiograph shows a femoral head eccentrically positioned within the acetabular component (*arrows*). There is an osteolytic defect in the greater trochanter (*arrows*). The absence of a portion of the medial femoral neck was not caused by osteolysis.

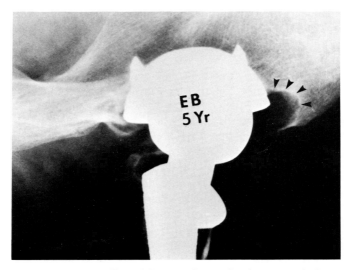

FIG. 12. Five-year postoperative iliac oblique radiograph of an acetabular component. The 32-mm head is not centered in the metal acetabular shell. An osteolytic defect has developed in the ilium (*arrows*).

either Charnley and DeLee zone 1 or 3. In nine cases, the osteolysis did not appear to affect the bone-implant interface. These osteolytic reactions extended from the rim of the acetabular component to the ilium, ischium, or pubis. Ten of the cases with acetabular osteolysis had concurrent femoral lesions. Of the 192 cases, 44 had osteolytic reactions in the femur, pelvis, or both.

A change in the femoral head position within the acetabular component, presumed to be caused by a measurable amount of polyethylene wear, has been observed in 25 cases. An association seems to exist between the presence of polyethylene wear and the presence of osteolytic reactions. Among the 25 cases in which signs of polyethylene wear occurred, either femoral or acetabular osteolytic reactions were present in 19 cases (76%). Although we note a causative relationship between polyethylene wear and osteolysis, we are led to believe that a gradient exists. The assumption is not being made, however, that polyethylene wear is the sole cause of osteolysis. Among the 167 cases in which there was no evidence of polyethylene wear, osteolytic reactions occurred in 25 cases.

Comparison of the Preoperative/Postoperative Clinical Function

Preoperatively, patient function was graded as excellent, good, or fair based on the patient's combined D'Aubigne and Postel pain and walking score. Patients with a combined score greater than 10 were considered to have excellent function. These patients do not require an assistive device and deny experiencing pain sufficient to interfere with normal activities. Patients with scores of 9 or 10 were considered to have good function. They occasionally require canes when walking long distances and usually have a detectable limp when walking without a cane. These patients are also occasionally restricted in normal activities by pain. Patients with a score below 9 are considered to have fair function. These patients frequently use canes or crutches and are always restricted in normal activities because of pain and/or limp. Four of the 186 patients were assessed to have postoperative function similar to that in their preoperative status. The reasons for lack of improvement in their functional status include a cerebrovascular aneurysm leading to hemiparalysis in one case. Two patients have severe rheumatoid arthritis, and one has a loose acetabular component. In three of the four cases clinical failure was, therefore, due to causes other than the hip arthroplasty. None of the patients functions at a lower level. Twenty patients function at least one level better than preoperatively. One hundred and sixty-two patients function two levels better than prior to their total hip arthroplasty.

CONCLUSIONS

Since 1984, there have been significant improvements in the methods used by the senior author to perform cementless total hip arthroplasty. A great deal has been learned from these early cases. This chapter describes the senior author's current clinical and laboratory experience with the AML prosthesis. This experience is placed in the context of a consecutive nonselected group of patients that all received extensively porous-coated femoral and acetabular components.

Radiographic

Radiographic direct and indirect signs of femoral osseointegration have been confirmed with *in vivo* laboratory studies of autopsy specimens. It is apparent that determination of early implant stability is useful for predicting long-term implant outcome. The acetabular component is difficult to evaluate radiographically because of component geometry. *In vivo* studies demonstrate that radiographs overestimate the amount of component contact with host bone. No correlation has been noted by the authors between the results of their *in vivo* studies and useful radiographic predictors of stability unless gross migration or recent metal particle shedding was visible.

Bone Modeling

Studies of bone remodeling, such as the initial mechanical formula for predicting stress shielding, which is elaborated by computer-assisted videodensitometry, DEXA, and densitometry of transverse sections of autopsy-retrieved femora, have shown that changes in radiographic bone density visible on serial radiographs can be quantitated. Large-diameter, extensively porous-coated implants cause bone remodeling changes, resulting in as much as 52% of periprosthetic bone mineral loss. There is a gradient of this bone loss in the frontal plane with the greatest loss occurring proximally. This loss appears to occur primarily in the first 2 postoperative years. The DEXA results suggest that preoperative bone mass is one of the important factors governing the extent of postoperative bone loss. Despite definite bone remodeling, the cortical strain analysis studies that compared *in vivo* remodeled femora with post mortem implanted controls suggest that bone remodeling did not result in an appreciable change in strain patterns. These results demonstrate that factors other than strain reduction affect bone remodeling (1). In addition, a three-dimensional finite element model based on the authors' autopsy cases is currently being developed. Comparison of this information with actual changes in bone mass as determined by analysis of slab radiographs should provide important new information. Understanding bone remodeling is critical and allows orthopedic surgeons to make informed decisions. However, no patients have been revised for severe bone loss nor have problems been created by bone loss at the time of revision for other reasons.

Clinical

The authors have presented new clinical data on a consecutive, nonselected, prospectively studied group of patients with a mean follow-up of 87.4 months. None of the patients' functional status deteriorated over a 9-year follow-up period. Using Kaplin-Meyer survivorship analysis, the probability that a patient would require reoperation for any reason in the first 8 postoperative years is 93.0%, with a standard error of 0.13. The probability that the cup would remain in place through 8 years is 97.5% and that the femoral component would be in place through 8 years is 99.3%.

Wear of the bearing surface leading to osteolytic reactions has been the most serious complication. Two patients were reoperated on for osteolysis secondary to worn polyethylene. In each case, only the polyethylene was exchanged. The components in these cases were found to be stable and were left *in situ* with bone graft placed in the osteolytic defects. It is hoped that decreasing the femoral head size, improving the surface finish of the femoral head, and improving polyethylene quality combined with a more critical selection of patients will lessen this complication.

REFERENCES

1. Beaupre GS, Orr TE, Carter DR. An approach for time dependent bone modeling and remodeling theoretical development. *J Orthop Res* 1990;8:662–670.
2. Burke DW, O'Connor DO, Zalenski EB, Jasty M, Harris WH. Micromotion of cemented and uncemented femoral components. *J Bone Joint Surg [Br]* 1991;73:33–37.
3. Engh CA, Bobyn JD. The influence of stem size and extent of porous coating on femoral resorption after primary cementless hip arthroplasty. *Clin Orthop* 1988;231:7–28.
4. Engh CA, Massin P, Suthers KE. Roentgenographic assessment of the biologic fixation of porous surfaced femoral components. *Clin Orthop* 1990;257:107–128.
5. Engh CA, McGovern TF, Schmidt LM. Roentgenographic densitometry of bone adjacent to a femoral prosthesis. *Clin Orthop (in press)*.
6. Engh CA, McGovern TF, Bobyn JD, Harris WH. A quantitative evaluation of periprosthetic bone remodeling following cementless total hip arthroplasty. *J Bone Joint Surg [Am]* 1992;74:1009–1020.
7. Engh CA, O'Connor D, Jasty M, McGovern TF, Bobyn JD, Harris WH. Quantification of implant micromotion, strain shielding, and bone resorption with porous coated AML femoral prostheses. *Clin Orthop* 1992;285:13–29.
8. Engh CA, Zettl-Schaffer KF, Kukita Y, Sweet D, Jasty M, Bragdon C. Histologic and radiographic assessment of well functioning porous coated acetabular components: a human postmortem retrieval study. *J Bone Joint Surg (in press)*.
9. Gruen TA, McNeice GM, Amstutz HC. Modes of failure of cemented stem type femoral components. *Clin Orthop* 1979;141:17–21.
10. Kilgus DJ, Shimaoka EE, Eberle RW. Quantification of peri-prosthetic femoral stress remodeling. *Transactions of the 38th Annual Meeting* 1992;17:311.
11. Massin P, Schmidt L, Engh CA. Evaluation of cementless acetabular component migration. An experimental study. *J Arthroplasty* 1989;4:245–251.
12. Mazess R, Collick B, Trempe J, Barden H, Hanson J. Performance evaluation of a dual energy x-ray bone densitometer. *Calcif Tissue Int* 1989;44:228–232.
13. McCarthy CK, Steinberg CG, Agnew M, Leahey D, Wyman E, Baran DT. Quantifying bone loss from the proximal femur after total hip arthroplasty. *J Bone Joint Surg [Br]* 1991;73:774–778.

Biological, Material, and Mechanical Considerations of Joint Replacement, edited by B. F. Morrey. Raven Press, Ltd., New York © 1993.

14

Retrieval: Successful Uncemented Implants

Joshua J. Jacobs, Dale R. Sumner, Robert M. Urban, and Jorge O. Galante

Department of Orthopedic Surgery, Rush-Presbyterian-St. Luke's Medical Center, Chicago, Illinois 60612

The importance of implant retrieval programs has been increasingly recognized by the orthopedic community (4) and the biomaterials community in general (11). Additional impetus to such programs has recently been stimulated by federal regulations established in the midst of the silicone breast implant controversy (15). Systematic, comprehensive, and correlative retrieval studies provide unique and critical information with regard to the long-term performance of implantable devices.

In this chapter, the authors discuss the available information on cementless total joint replacement components retrieved from patients with successful implants. As will become apparent, there is little such information.

IMPLANTS RETRIEVED AT REVISION SURGERY

The first histologic studies of porous-coated total joint components were based mainly on implants retrieved at revision surgery. These studies were undertaken primarily to determine how much bone ingrowth occurs in prostheses implanted in human patients under functional loading. These investigations have ranged from case reports to larger series (Tables 1 and 2). Some of these studies have found bone ingrowth in fewer than one-half of the components and in most studies the maximum amount of bone ingrowth has been reported to be two to three times less than the average amount typically observed in animal experiments.

Three relatively large studies of acetabular components retrieved at revision surgery have been reported. Bone ingrowth was observed in nine of 58 cases (16%) by Collier and co-workers (5), 28 of 42 cases (67%) by Cook (6), and 18 of 25 (72%) cases by Sumner et al. (21). Cook et al. (7,10) reported no cases with more than 10% of the void space within the porous coating occupied by bone, whereas in the series of Sumner et al., there were two cases with more than 20% of the void space occupied by bone ingrowth. In fact, the values for these cases were comparable to those observed in some canine models (25–35%), although the average for all of the longer term cases was only 6.9%. When only components with adjuvant screw fixation from the study of Cook et al. (9) were considered, the proportion of implants with bone ingrowth increased to 77% (17 of 22), which is more consistent with our retrieval studies in which adjuvant screw fixation had also been used (20,21).

TABLE 1. *Incidence and amount of bone ingrowth in components retrieved from patients with cementless total hip arthroplasty*

Component	Incidence	Amount[a]	Center (ref.)
Acetabular	9/58 (16%)	n/a	Dartmouth (5)
Acetabular	28/42 (67%)	0.0–<10.0% <5%: 22/28 >5%: 6/28	Tulane (6)
Acetabular	18/25 (72%)	0.0–35.2% <5%: 13/18 >5%: 5/18 (2 >10%)	Rush-Presbyterian-St. Luke's, Massachusetts General Hospital (21)
Acetabular[b]	10/11 (91%)	0.0–27.6% <5%: 3/10 >5%: 7/10 (all 7 >10%)	Rush-Presbyterian-St. Luke's (20)
Acetabular[b]	9/9 (100%)	0.5–35.9%	Anderson Clinic (25)
Femoral	28/104 (27%)	n/a	Dartmouth (5)
Femoral	32/45 (71%)	0.0– <10.0% <5%: 25/32 >5%: 7/32	Tulane (6)
Femoral	12/12 (100%)	3.0–64.8% <5%: 2/12 >5%: 10/12 (5 >10%)	Rush-Presbyterian-St. Luke's (16)
Femoral[c]	9/11 (82%)	n/a	Anderson Clinic (12)
Femoral[b]	11/14 (79%)	0.0–37.4% <5%: 1/11 >5%: 10/11 (9 >10%)	Rush-Presbyterian-St. Luke's (24)

[a]Amount of bone ingrowth refers to the volume of void space within the porous coating occupied by bone. This is often called the "volume fraction", "area fraction" or "area density" of bone ingrowth.
[b]Autopsy cases only.
[c]Ten of the 11 were autopsy cases.
n/a, not available.

TABLE 2. *Incidence and amount of bone ingrowth in components retrieved from patients with cementless total knee arthroplasty*

Component	Incidence	Amount[a]	Center (ref.)
Femoral	19/33 (58%)	0.0–<10.0% <5%: 15/19 >5%: 4/19	Tulane (6)
Patellar	21/33 (64%)	0.0–<10.0% <5%: 16/21 >5%: 5/21	Tulane (6)
Tibial	(<10%)	n/a	Dartmouth (18)
Tibial	18/41 (44%)	0.0–<10.0% <5%: 15/18 >5%: 3/18	Tulane (6)
Tibial	13/13 (100%)	0.5–30.1% <5%: 4/13 >5%: 9/13 (6 >10%)	Rush-Presbyterian-St. Luke's (22)
Tibial	10/10 (100%)	8–22%[b] >5%: 10/10 (6 >10%)	V.A. Salt Lake City (3)

[a]Amount of bone ingrowth refers to the volume of void space within the porous coating occupied by bone. This is often called the volume fraction, area fraction, or area density of bone ingrowth.
[b]These figures may include autogenous bone graft chips within the porous coating.
n/a, not available.

The incidence of bone ingrowth into total hip replacement (THR) femoral components retrieved at surgery has been reported to vary from 27% to 100% (Table 1). In addition, the amount of bone ingrowth has been found to vary significantly within and between studies. For instance, Cook (6) found that 32 of 45 femoral components had bone ingrowth, but in only seven of these 32 cases did the bone occupy more than 5% of the void space within the porous coating. In contrast, Jacobs et al. (16) found bone ingrowth in all 12 femoral components analyzed, and in five of these cases the bone occupied more than 10% of the void space of the porous coating, with one case having 64.8% of the void space occupied by bone (Fig. 1). Both of these centers have noted lower incidences and amounts of bone ingrowth in revision stems compared with primary stems (8,16,24).

At the knee joint, large numbers of femoral and patellar components have been studied only by Cook (6), who found 58% of the femoral components and 64% of the patellar components with bone ingrowth (Table 2). The data for the tibial component are considerably more variable, with Mayor and Collier (18) reporting an incidence of bone ingrowth of less than 10%, Cook (6) reporting 44%, Bloebaum et al. (3) reporting 100%, and Sumner et al. (22) reporting 100%. As with the femoral component of THR, there is considerable variability in the amount of bone ingrowth: Cook (6) found that less than 5% of the void space was occupied by bone in 15 of the 18 components with bone ingrowth, whereas Sumner et al. (22) found that nine of 13 components had more than 5% of the void space occupied by bone, and six of these nine had more than 10%

In addition to observations on the incidence and amount of bone ingrowth, these early retrieval studies shed some light on the qualitative character of the interface. Most of the studies have noted that areas not occupied by bone are typically filled with loose to dense fibrous tissue or fatty marrow. Other tissue types, notably fibrocartilage, have been found at limited foci. The presence of lymphocytic infiltrates and particulate debris has also been noted in components that were not loose or infected.

Most of the retrieval studies have included a variety of component types removed for various reasons. Even when cases removed for loosening are excluded, the reported incidence and amount of bone ingrowth have varied widely. In many cases, particularly involving retrieved acetabular components, no or small amounts of bone ingrowth were found, but the surgeon reported that the component was grossly stable. Thus, the question of how much bone ingrowth is needed is still open.

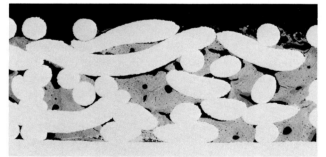

FIG. 1. Backscattered scanning electron micrograph of a femoral component (Harris-Galante I [HG]) retrieved at revision surgery at 54 months postoperative. The implant was removed for progressive femoral osteolysis. Note the extensive bone ingrowth with nearly the entire pore area occupied by mature lamellar bone. ×16.

Many factors can affect bone ingrowth and some of these factors presumably contributed to the variability observed both within and between the studies reviewed here. In some instances it has been argued that reliable radiographic signs of bone ingrowth can be ascertained, whereas other authors have found this not to be the case. The limited number of studies performed to date have been insufficient to elucidate fully how factors such as the length of implantation, the type of surgery (primary as opposed to revision), surgical technique and implant design affect bone ingrowth.

The inherent limitation of retrieval studies performed on components obtained at revision surgery must be kept in mind. The devices analyzed in these studies have failed clinically and as such may not have been subjected to normal physiologic loads. Clearly, this may affect the local bone response. In addition, these implants may have been exposed to adverse conditions (i.e., inflammatory cells and tissue fluids, particulate wear debris, eccentric loading) that could influence the character of the implant-tissue interface or the implant itself. Therefore, the findings of the above-mentioned studies may not reflect the status of implants in patients with well-functioning devices. These concerns are partially, but not completely, addressed by those studies that have been performed on components removed for reasons other than loosening or infection (3,6,7,10,16,21,22).

An additional consideration is that, whereas insights into the failure mechanisms can be gleaned from devices retrieved at revision surgery, the information obtained is at the end stage of what may have been a complex cascade of events leading up to the failure.

It is in light of these considerations that autopsy-retrieval studies are crucial to facilitate the understanding of the character of the clinically successful implant and also provide insights into failure mechanisms early on in the cascade of events. Not only are autopsy retrievals potentially more representative of patients with well-functioning devices, but the implant can be retrieved with the surrounding interfacial and skeletal tissues undisturbed, providing a unique source of histomorphological information.

IMPLANTS RETRIEVED AT AUTOPSY

Total Hip Replacement

The largest published study to date on post-mortem specimens with well-functioning total joint replacements is a multicenter effort under the aegis of the Hip Society (4). The material consisted of more than 85 specimens with THR, more than 70 of which were uncemented implants. Of these, the vast majority were porous-coated devices with only two hydroxyapatite (HA)-coated implants. Although one center (S. D. Cook, Tulane Medical Center) reported that the results for bone ingrowth in post-mortem specimens were comparable to those implants previously analyzed obtained from nonloosened, cause-related revisions, our center (D. R. Sumner and J. O. Galante) found that the variability of bone ingrowth was less in autopsy retrievals.

Several of the centers agreed that the harvesting of the periprosthetic tissues, including the adjacent skeleton, provided valuable information. For example, J. D. Bobyn (Montreal General Hospital) and S. D. Cook (Tulane Medical Center) observed clear evidence of increased porosity in femurs with implants in comparison to the contralateral nonimplanted femurs suggestive of stress shielding. J. P. Collier and M. B. Mayor (Dartmouth Biomedical Engineering Center) observed direct bonding of bone without an intervening fibrous layer to a "smooth-surfaced" titanium implant. L. A. Whiteside (DePaul Biomechanical Research Laboratory) performed biomechanical tests on a retrieved porous ingrowth component and used as a control the contralateral femur that was implanted post mortem with an identical component. His study suggested that tissue ingrowth provided rigid fixation of the femoral stem compared to the press-fit fixation in the contralateral femur.

Much of the information in this report was anecdotal in the form of case reports. In addition, there was no standardized evaluation protocol among the different centers, making comparisons somewhat difficult.

Hydroxyapatite

Bauer et al. (1) reported on five HA-coated femoral components retrieved at autopsy from three patients. These implants were in place 4.5, 6, 9, 14, and 25 months prior to death. The 6-month implant was in place in a patient on chronic immunosuppression for psoriasis, whereas the two longest term cases were in a patient on high-dose corticosteroids for chronic autoimmune liver disease. These authors determined the thickness of the HA coating, chemical composition of the coating, and linear extent of bone apposition. They found that the retained HA was of relatively uniform thickness but was not present in all locations. Neither the thickness of the HA nor the linear extent of retained HA correlated with the duration *in vivo*. The authors did observe "remodeling canals," suggesting the occurrence of focal cell-mediated resorption through osteoclasts. They did not believe that direct dissolution of the coating was a major cause of HA loss, nor did they observe delamination of the coating. HA granules were observed within histiocytes/macrophages, and this was considered to be part of a normal remodeling phenomenon. The pattern of bone apposition, condensation, and remodeling—with bone deposition most prominent at the anterior and medial aspects and at the lateral-oblique corners—was thought to be governed by Wolff's law.

Although this represents one of the first studies of its kind, there still are a number of unanswered questions concerning HA-coated implants. First, the longest term implant was only 25 months postoperative, so that little can be said about longer term performance. Second, two of the three patients had medical problems necessitating the administration of immunosuppressants in one case and high-dose corticosteroids in the other. These agents may well affect the metabolic activity of the bone-implant interface. Third, this report concerns a very small number of cases. The finding of phagocytosed HA within histiocytes raises the specter of particulate-induced osteolysis, although this was not observed in this series.

Porous-Coated Acetabular Components

Zettl-Schaffer et al. (25) reported on post-mortem analysis of nine uncemented acetabular components (three titanium Arthropor components, two titanium Trilock components, and four anatomic medullary locking [AML] cobalt alloy components) and their surrounding hemipelves *in situ* for 12 to 99 months. All components were clinically and radiographically stable and demonstrated bone ingrowth. On average, 32% (range 3–84%) of the surface area and 13.9% (range 0.5–36%) of the void space demonstrated bone ingrowth. Furthermore, intimate bone contact was observed adjacent to pegs and screws. The incidence and extent of bone ingrowth in this autopsy study were significantly higher than those reported from cause-related retrievals (5,6,7,10,21).

Our laboratory recently reported on 11 primary uncemented titanium fiber-metal acetabular components (Harris-Galante I, Zimmer) from eight autopsy retrievals (20). The focus of the analysis was on the distribution of tissue ingrowth into the porous coating, nature of the tissue at the bone-prosthesis interface, distribution of particulate wear debris, and correlation between clinical radiographs and histology. The patients had well-functioning prostheses up to the time of their death. The prostheses were *in situ* for 41 months (range 5 weeks to 75 months) with seven implanted for more than 45 months (all of which had the procedure done at our institution) and four in place for 8 months or less. The average age was 56 years (range 33.5–82.5). The cause of death was metastatic carcinoma in five and septicemia, renal failure, and pneumonia in the remaining patients. Prior to death, the Harris Hip Score in the seven longer term cases was greater than 80 (good to excellent) in all but one patient who had diffuse bone pain due to renal osteodystrophy.

Tissue ingrowth was quantitated using two measures: (i) extent, defined as the percentage of 1-mm fields occupied by the tissue of interest (determined by light microscopy), and (ii) volume fraction, the ratio of the mineralized bone within the pores to the pore area (determined with backscattered scanning electron microscopy and image analysis). Particulate wear debris and cellular response was quantitated using the Mirra scale (19).

Bone ingrowth was present in 10 of 11 acetabular components. The mean extent was 20.9% (range 0–55%), whereas the mean volume fraction was 12.1% (range 0–27.6%). These values are similar to those reported by Zettl-Schaffer et al. (25), discussed above. There was significantly more bone around holes with adjuvant fixation screws than around unfilled screw holes (35% vs 20% extent, $p < 0.05$) (see Fig. 2), and there tended to be more bone ingrowth at the rim than at regions away from the rim. Within the porous coating, there was a gradient of bone ingrowth with more at the bone-coating interface and progressively less toward the coating-substrate interface.

Correlation with clinical radiographs revealed that there was a statistically significant inverse correlation between the number of radiolucencies at the interface and the extent of bone ingrowth ($r = -0.76$, $p < 0.05$).

Small amounts of fibrocartilage were observed in 10 of the 11 cups and, interestingly, fibrocartilage was observed neither in the specimen with the greatest extent of bone ingrowth nor in areas adjacent to fixation screws. Retained articular cartilage was seen at the interface in two cases, and in each instance no bone was present in the subjacent porous coating. Lymphocyte and plasma cells were uncommon and polymorphonuclear leukocytes were rarely observed.

Metal debris at screw holes was present in 10 hips. However, the amount of debris was similar in empty holes and holes filled with screws, suggesting that fretting between the fixation screws and metal shell may not be the dominant source of such debris. If it were, one would expect more debris adjacent to holes with screws. Polyethylene debris was seen in three cases in holes without screws. Both the metal and polymer debris were associated with histiocytes, but overall the amount of debris

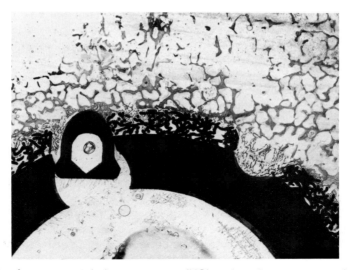

FIG. 2. Section from an acetabular component (HG) retrieved post-mortem after 1 month *in situ*. There is evidence of early bone ingrowth into the porous coating with porous areas adjacent to the filled screw hole demonstrating greater ingrowth than those adjacent to the unfilled screw hole. ×2.4.

and the associated histiocytic response were small and tended to be localized. No granuloma formation was evident.

As with Zettl-Schaffer's study, our work has demonstrated larger amounts of bone ingrowth than in studies performed on retrievals obtained at revision surgery. Nevertheless, the ingrowth was quite variable. As yet, the optimal amount of bone ingrowth has not been determined. In our study, the presence of screws influenced the pattern of bone ingrowth—50% more bone was seen adjacent to screws. However, empty screw holes could serve as conduits for migration of particulate wear debris to the bone-prosthesis interface.

Porous-Coated Femoral Stems

We have also performed a post-mortem evaluation on 14 cementless titanium fiber-metal femoral stems (11 Harris-Galante [HG], two BIAS, one Gustillo-Kyle [GK], Zimmer) and their surrounding tissues in 10 patients (24). These implants were noncircumferentially porous coated and had a modular cobalt-alloy femoral head (except for the GK prosthesis, which had a nonmodular titanium-alloy head). Twelve implants were used in primary total hip arthroplasty and two in revision total hip arthroplasty. All patients had well-functioning implants retrieved after an average of 35 months *in situ* (range 1–75 months). For the 11 primary cases of the HG design (nine of which had bone ingrowth), the mean extent of bone ingrowth was 42.8% (range 0–91.6%) with a mean volume fraction of 13.8% (range 0–37.4%). The primary BIAS stem had 58.7% extent and 24.1% volume fraction of bone ingrowth. For the two revisions, the extent measurements were 0.0% and 6.1%, with volume fraction measurements of 0.0% and 3.2%. In addition to this quantitative information, the study also illustrated that bone ingrowth occurred through the early formation of woven bone as had been suggested from numerous animal studies (Fig. 3). Although extensive bone ingrowth was typically observed in the primary cases, contiguous nonporous coated region of the stem demonstrated a fibrous membrane (Fig. 4). This membrane was often separated from the surface by a gap of 50 to 250 μm, which was filled with amorphous eosinophilic debris and histiocytes. Several of the retrieved modular devices exhibited corrosion at the head-neck junction.

This study demonstrated potential migratory pathways for articular wear debris adjacent to uncoated regions of the femoral stem and may help to explain the relatively high incidence of diaphyseal femoral osteolysis with noncircumferentially coated femoral stems (17,23). The importance of corrosion at the head-neck junction is a subject of continuing investigation.

Engh et al. (13) studied 14 femurs containing AML prostheses retrieved at autopsy and found that the stems, which were classified roentgenographically as bone ingrown (11 of 14), were mechanically very stable with a maximum of 40 μm of relative motion under the most adverse loading condition. Increasing the amount of stem coverage by the porous coating reduced micromotion at the distal tip of the prosthesis. In addition, the medial subperiosteal strains did not return to control values despite extensive bone remodeling. In a separate study of five paired cadaver femurs

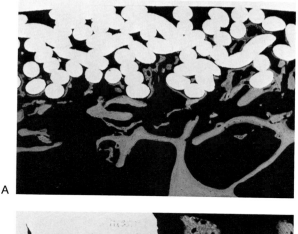

A

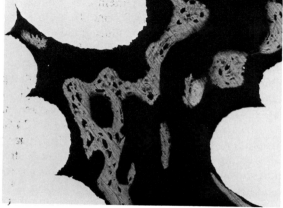

B

FIG. 3. Section from a femoral component (HG) retrieved post-mortem after 1 month *in situ*. Note at this early stage ingrowth of fine trabeculae of woven bone into the fiber-metal coating. **A,** ×12.5; **B:** ×75.

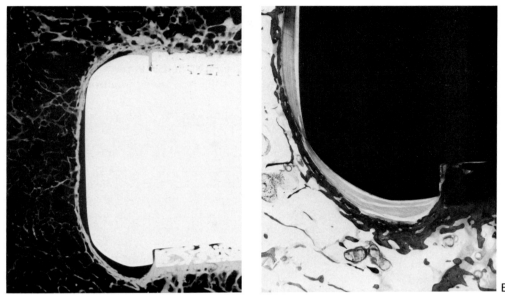

A   B

FIG. 4. Section from a femoral component (HG) retrieved post-mortem after 63 months *in situ.* **A:** Cross-section microradiograph demonstrating a trabecular shell circumscribing, but separated from, the lateral uncoated surface of the stem. Note bony condensation adjacent to anterior and posterior fiber-metal pads and contiguous with the bone within the porous coating. ×2.75. **B:** Corresponding histologic section reveals a fibrous membrane in the gap between the trabecular shell and the surface of the implant. These gaps are potential conduits for migration of articular wear debris. ×5.5.

in which an AML prosthesis had been implanted unilaterally from 17 to 84 months prior to the patient's death, Engh et al. (14) found that there was 7% to 52% less periprosthetic bone mineral content (BMC) in the operated femur compared to comparable regions of the intact femur. Furthermore, the decrease in BMC was inversely correlated with the post-mortem control BMC (contralateral femur).

Total Knee Replacement

Information available on autopsy-retrieval analysis of cementless total knee arthroplasty is limited to case reports. For example, Bloebaum et al. (2) reported on two post-mortem retrievals from a patient with bilateral cementless total knee replacement. On one side, the patient had a sintered bead-coated, cobalt-alloy implant; on the other side, the patient had a cancellous-structured, titanium-coated implant. Although both implants were clinically successful, only the titanium implant had appreciable bone ingrowth.

This group has a more recent study analyzing 10 retrieved cementless tibial components, four of which were obtained post-mortem (3). In all cases, autograft bone chips were implanted between the cancellous tibial bed and tibial tray. The four post-mortem cases were retrieved 1 week, 3 weeks, 13 months and 19 months after implantation. The volume fraction of bone ingrowth in both the longer term post-mortem cases (13 and 19 months) was 18%. Comparable values were obtained in the cause-related retrievals in components *in situ* for longer periods (24–48 months), although the authors did not specifically compare autopsy with revision retrievals. The authors concluded that autograft bone chips enhanced the degree of bone ingrowth based on a comparison with previous reports in the literature, primarily from cause-related retrievals.

FUTURE DIRECTIONS

Many centers now have active autopsy recruitment programs, and the next decade should witness a plethora of autopsy-retrieval studies on a variety of implant designs. Clearly, as the number of cases accumulate and the data base expands, the role of various clinical features (e.g., bone quality, underlying diagnosis, nonsteroidal anti-inflammatory usage), specific design features (e.g., the use and placement of pegs or screws, location and extent of ingrowth surfaces), manufacturing processes (e.g., surface hardening treatments, surface finish, coating application), and surgical technique (e.g., fill of the femoral canal, orientation of the acetabular component, level of resection of the tibial component) on the nature of the implant-bone interface as well as long-term device performance can be elucidated. Although some of these variables are amenable to study in animal models, continued analysis of retrieved implants is critical to determine if the principles gleaned from experimental studies are useful for improving clinical outcome.

More sophisticated characterization of the tissue and cellular response to the implant will be forthcoming. Utilization of modern immunohistochemical techniques as well as molecular biological methods on tissues retrieved at autopsy should enhance our fundamental understanding of the nature of the host-prosthesis interaction.

In addition to histologic assessment, further studies will also focus on degradative phenomena (e.g., corrosion, wear, oxidation) of the implant itself. By performing biomechanical tests on retrieved successful implants, the degree of implant fixation can be quantitated and histologic-mechanical correlations can be established. Analysis of long-term autopsy retrievals may also shed significant light on long-term periprosthetic bone remodeling phenomena when a contralateral unoperated bone is available for comparison. Also, analysis of remote tissues including lymph nodes and reticuloendothelial organs will provide insight into possible remote and systemic effects of implanted prostheses.

Finally, it is important to point out that, although autopsy retrievals do provide a unique source of information, the subjects may have been chronically ill for some time before their ultimate demise. The presence of metabolic bone disease or other systemic disorders could potentially influence the character of the bone-implant interface. Future post-mortem retrieval studies should take this into account by selecting those subjects that are least likely to be prone to this sort of artifact and therefore are the most representative of healthy patients with well-functioning devices.

ACKNOWLEDGMENTS

This work was supported by NIH grant AR39310 and Zimmer, Inc.

REFERENCES

1. Bauer TW, Geesink RCT, Zimmerman R, McMahon JT. Hydroxyapatite-coated femoral stems: histological analysis of components retrieved at autopsy. *J Bone Joint Surg [Am]* 1991;73:1439–1452.
2. Bloebaum RD, Rhodes DM, Rubman MH, Hofmann AA. Bilateral tibial components of different cementless designs and materials. Microradiographic, backscattered imaging, and histologic analysis. *Clin Orthop* 1991;268:179–187.
3. Bloebaum RD, Rubman MH, Hofmann AA. Bone ingrowth into porous-coated tibial components implanted with autograft bone chips. Analysis of ten consecutively retrieved implants. *J Arthroplasty* 1992;7:483–493.
4. Collier JP, Bauer T, Bloebaum RD, et al. Results of implant retrieval from post-mortem specimens in patients with well-functioning long term THR. *Clin Orthop* 1992;274:97–112.
5. Collier JP, Mayor MB, Chae JC, Surprenant VA, Surprenant HP, Dauphinais LA. Macroscopic and microscopic evidence of prosthetic fixation with porous-coated materials. *Clin Orthop* 1988;235:173–180.
6. Cook SD. Clinical radiographic and histologic evaluation of retrieved human noncement porous coated implants. *J Long Term Effects Med Implants* 1991;1:11–51.
7. Cook SD, Barrack RL, Thomas KA, Haddad RJ. Quantitative analysis of tissue growth into human porous total hip components. *J Arthroplasty* 1988;3:249–262.
8. Cook SD, Barrack RL, Thomas KA, Haddad RJ. Tissue growth into porous primary and revision femoral stems. *J Arthroplasty* 1991;6:S37–S46.
9. Cook SD, Thomas KA, Barrack RL, Whitecloud TS. Tissue growth into porous-coated acetabular components in 42 patients: effects of adjunct fixation. *Clin Orthop* 1992;283:163–170.
10. Cook SD, Thomas KA, Haddad RJ. Histologic analysis of retrieved human porous-coated total joint components. *Clin Orthop* 1988;234:90–101.
11. Duncan E. Implication of implant retrieval: goals and objectives. *Trans Soc Biomater* 1992;15:9.
12. Engh CA, Bobyn JD, Glassman AH. Porous-coated hip replacement: the factors governing bone ingrowth, stress shielding, and clinical results. *J Bone Joint Surg [Br]* 1987;69:45–55.
13. Engh CA, O'Connor D, Jasty M, Harris WH. Quantitation of implant micromotion, strain shielding and bone resorption with porous coated AML cementless femoral prosthesis retrieved at autopsy. Transaction of the 20th Open Scientific Meeting of the Hip Society, February 1992, Washington, DC.
14. Engh CA, McGovern TF, Bobyn JD, Harris WH. A quantitative evaluation of periprosthetic bone-remodeling after cementless total hip arthroplasty. *J Bone Joint Surg [Am]* 1992;74:1009–1020.
15. Frisch EE. Implication of implant retrieval: logistics and economics of medical device tracking. *Trans Soc Biomater* 1992;15:13.1–13.5.
16. Jacobs JJ, Sumner DR, Turner TM, Urban RM, Galante JO. A quantitative assessment of bone ingrowth into titanium total hip femoral components removed for reasons other than loosening. Presented at the American Academy of Orthopaedic Surgeons, 1989.
17. Jacobs JJ, Urban RM, Schajowicz F, Garvrilovic J, Galante JO. Particulate-associated endosteal osteolysis in titanium-base alloy cementless total hip replacement. In: St. John DR, ed. *Particulate debris from medical implants: mechanisms of formation and biological consequences. ASTM STP 1144.* Philadelphia: American Society for Testing and Materials, 1992:52–60.
18. Mayor MB, Collier JP. The histology of porous coated knee prostheses. *Orthop Trans* 1986;10:441–442.
19. Mirra JM, Amstutz HC, Matos M, Gold R. The pathology of the joint tissues and its clinical relevance in prosthesis failure. *Clin Orthop* 1976;117:221.
20. Pidhorz LE, Urban RM, Jacobs JJ, Sumner DR, Galante JO. A quantitative study of bone and soft tissue in cementless porous coated acetabular components retrieved at autopsy. *J Arthroplasty (in press)*.
21. Sumner DR, Jasty M, Jacobs JJ, et al. Histologic analysis of cementless porous-coated acetabular components retrieved from one week to 35 months post-operatively in patients. *Acta Orthop Scand (in press)*.
22. Sumner DR, Kienapfel H, Jacobs J, Urban RM, Turner TM, Galante JO. Bone in-growth into cementless porous-coated tibial components removed from patients: a quantitative histomorphometric analysis and correlation with technical factors *(submitted)*.
23. Tanzer M, Maloney WJ, Jasty M, Harris WH. The progression of femoral cortical osteolysis in association with total hip arthroplasty without cement. *J Bone Joint Surg [Am]* 1992;74:404–410.
24. Urban RM, Sumner DR, Gilbert JL, Pidhorz LE. Autopsy retrieval: analysis of noncircumferentially porous coated cementless femoral stems. Presented at the American Association of Orthopaedic Surgeons Annual Meeting, February 1993, San Francisco.
25. Zettl-Schaffer KF, Engh CA, Sweet D, Bragdon C. Histologic and roentgenographic assessment of well functioning porous coated acetabular components. A human post-mortem retrieval analysis. *Trans Soc Biomater* 1992;15:43.

Biological, Material, and Mechanical Considerations of Joint Replacement, edited by B. F. Morrey. Raven Press, Ltd., New York © 1993.

15

The Interface Between Host and Unsuccessful Cementless Prostheses: The Knee

John P. Collier, Ian R. Williams, Michael B. Mayor, Helene P. Surprenant, and Kathleen Kidd

Dartmouth Biomedical Engineering Center, Dartmouth College, Hanover, New Hampshire 03755

Cementless orthopaedic prostheses were introduced in the mid-1970s as a response to the need for a more durable interface between host and prosthesis than could be provided at that time by bone cement. Examination of early retrieved, porous-coated prostheses (1–3,8) indicated that a combination of bone and fibrous tissue provided sufficient mechanical stability and relief from pain that a more extensive use of the technology was warranted. Shortly thereafter, porous-coated acetabular components and porous-coated knees became commercially available. The major expectation then, as now, was that over time Wolff's law would prevail, and more bone would grow into the porous coating in response to the increased stress, resulting from increased patient activity, thereby permitting the application of joint replacement in younger and more active patients. However, concurrently the development of more modular designs, the requirement for the use of a metal backing to provide a substrate upon which to put the porous coating, and the lack of recognition of the importance of a careful design rationale led to components whose structural and biomechanical differences from their cemented counterparts led to an unexpected number of failures. Therefore, any focus on the interface between the host and uncemented, porous-coated prostheses must segregate those components whose failure can be attributed primarily to mechanical failure from those devices whose failure was primarily interface related.

There is a general consensus today that a cementless acetabular component, properly designed, is the state of the art in orthopaedics for the younger and more active patient. Although not all cementless acetabular component designs are without concerns, the overall risk/benefit ratio supports their use where the loads are expected to be high. There is less of a consensus for the femoral side of the hip. Whereas cementless stems have demonstrated the ability to reliably permit bone and fibrous tissue ingrowth for fixation, a percentage of the patients still experience pain, which, combined with improved cemented implant design and cementing technique, has led to a resurgence in enthusiasm for cemented femoral hip components. Additionally, the cementless femoral prosthesis inherently provides a dilemma. Because the stems need to be long enough to find support in the diaphysis, the question of how much of the component should be porous coated arises. Concerns about proximal stress shielding and difficulty in removal suggest proximal porous coating would be beneficial to alleviate these concerns. However, the work of Engh et al. (7), which demonstrated an improvement in the reduction of pain with fully porous-coated prostheses compared to an identical design with less porous coating, would suggest that more porous coating would tend to decrease the incidence of pain. Less has been done to analyze the risk/benefit ratio for the use of porous coating to provide a biological ingrowth fixation in the knee.

KNEE DESIGN ISSUES

The development of cementless, porous-coated knee components was first successfully realized in the Howmedica PCA knee. In retrospect, the importance of many of the design decisions that were made in the development of the cementless knee can be seen to have dramatically influenced the clinical success rate. Cemented knees were typically provided with thick, all-polyethylene tibial plateaus and all-polyethylene patellar buttons. Cementless designs required a metal substrate for the porous coating to be adhered to. Therefore, both patellar and tibial components required metal backings, which reduced the available thickness of the polyethylene considerably. Additionally, the difficulty in securing the polyethylene to the metal backing was not well addressed in the patella and was subject to conflicting concerns of secure fixation and the desire for modularity in the tibial component. Many metal-backed designs sacrificed the integrity of the polyethylene-metal bond in the interests of modularity in the tibial component and struggled for sufficient fixation of the polyethylene to the limited metal backing in the patellar component. The outcome was that many designs of both components failed with unnerving regularity. By the early 1980s, metal-backed patellar designs had all but been eliminated due to the need for thicker polyethylene and elimination of the polyethylene-metal separation that plagued many of the designs. Metal-backed tibial components are still seen as beneficial in that they permit a more rigid structure that will provide a more uniform stress distribution to the underlying tibial bone or bone cement, as well as providing a tray upon which modular polyethylene tibial inserts may be affixed. High contact stress design, thin polyethylene tibial bearings, and the variable quality polyethylene led to many fatigue failures of the tibial components (4). These mechanical failures and those of the metal-backed patellar components could contaminate the joint with large amounts of polyethylene (and occasionally metal) wear debris (5,6). Not surprisingly this led in many cases to a breakdown of the host-implant interface. Tibial components suffered from an additional concern associated with the degree of difficulty of consistently achieving bone and fibrous tissue ingrowth. The flexibility of the proximal tibial bone, combined with the variability from compartment to compartment, resulted in a component that was subject to rocking and tilting. Further, the biomechanical design of the knee, which requires the contact area to move from an anterior to a posterior position during normal gait, exacerbates the tendency toward tipping of a poorly fixed device. The early components did not meet the need for rigid initial fixation. More recent components, provided with multiple screws as well as pegs, have done a better job of providing rigid fixation to the tibial bone stock but had been plagued with the problems of both polyethylene-metal debris caused by fretting of screws and bearing inserts against the metal backing. Screw holes provide an easy path for this material, which can then attack the host-implant interface, causing eventual loosening and significant bone resorption.

The frequency and variety of problems associated with cementless knee components have led to a resurgence of cementing. On the femoral side this probably makes little difference. It is not clear that cemented femoral knees were at significant risk nor that cementless femoral knees would permit more reliable or durable fixation. Flawed cementless patellar designs were prone to failure, although some cleverly designed, low-contact-stress prostheses have performed well. Properly designed components should provide little to choose from between cemented and cementless components other than the increased polyethylene thickness permissible with all polyethylene designs.

The tibial component provides both the greatest challenge and the greatest potential benefit for the use of cementless fixation. Concerns for the breakdown of the cement-bone interface in young active patients provide a significant risk against which the potential benefit of biological fixation can be weighed. However, as previously discussed, the design of many of the available tibial components makes them subject to early fatigue failure, resulting in large amounts of polyethylene and metal debris, which contaminate the joint and break down the biological interface. It is apparent, however, from the analysis of retrieved components that properly designed prostheses will not suffer from fatigue failure or provide undue wear and can be successfully affixed to the proximal tibia, permitting bone and fibrous tissue interdigitation in the absence of the screws that are so problematic. The question of the durability and performance of cementless knee components in the absence of mechanical breakdown remains. It is the goal of this chapter to provide some light on this topic.

METHODS

Four hundred and sixty-four uncemented, total knee prostheses, 96% of which were retrieved at the time of revision (the remainder being recovered from post mortems or amputations) (13 post mortems, five amputations) and had been made available for histological examination, were included in the study. The reason(s) for retrieval, taken from the implant retrieval form sent with each prosthesis, were integrated with an initial visual examination in an attempt to determine the cause of failure.

Each component was examined and scored for wear using a Nikon binocular dissection microscope at $10 \times$ magnification. Wear damage and other characteristics were assessed using a 0 to 3 scoring system. The ratings were developed as follows: 0 = no wear, 1 = less than 10% of the surface involved, 2 = 10% to 50% of the surface involved, and 3 = greater than 50% of the surface is involved or severe, localized wear is present. The articular and nonarticular surfaces for each component were analyzed and scored for wear characteristics, and then an overall wear score for each was calculated. Metal components were scored for burnishing, scratching, abrasion, and fretting. The surfaces of the polyethylene inserts were likewise scored for burnishing, scratching, abrasion, pitting, delamination, creep, cracking, and fusion defects. Transilluminating the inserts with ordinary light enhanced the detection of the cracking and fusion defects.

Subsequently each component was photographed and studied (we are not at present mapping) for areas of tissue adherence. Those components that presented regions of significant tissue adherence were dried in solutions of alcohol and acetone, embedded in ethylmethacrylate, and sectioned into 200- to 500-μm thick wafers. Each thick section was then hand ground to 20-μm, stained with hematoxylin-eosin, and subjected to histological evaluation using the Zeiss Photomicroscope III.

RESULTS

An initial examination of the 464 retrieved, uncemented knee components revealed that 227 components were retrieved due to mechanical failure including wear through of the bearings, disassociation of the polyethylene from the metal backing, fracture of the components, dislocation, subluxation, or malposition. Because the goal of the study was to investigate the interface of well-functioning yet failed cementless knees (Figs. 1 and 2), those devices that failed mechanically were eliminated from the study. Those components retrieved for pain, looseness, subsidence, instability, bone fracture, amputation, or retrieved post mortem were maintained in the study. In cases in which two or more components of a total knee were retrieved due to mechanical failure of one or more of the components, all of the components were eliminated. Data on the initial 464 components and the 237 that remained after eliminating the 227 that failed for mechanical reasons can be seen in Tables 1 and 2.

The 237 knee components retrieved for reasons other than mechanical failure included those that showed evidence of significant wear (ratings from 2 to 3 on the 0 to 3 scale) that was interpreted as evidence that these components had contributed large amounts of polyethylene debris to the interface. As the tissue response to the debris could confound this study in its effort to determine the characteristics of pain-free and painful biological interfaces in well-functioning knee components, those

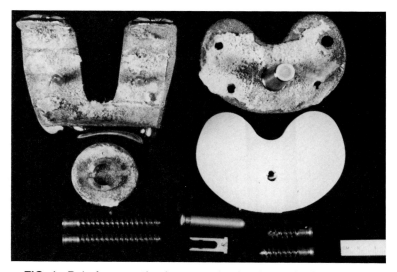

FIG. 1. Pain-free prosthesis was revised at 9 months for infection.

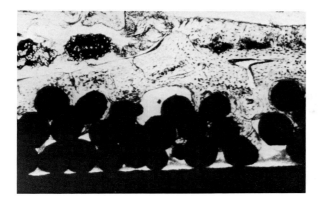

FIG. 2. Bone ingrowth of the tibial plateau (Fig. 1) provided pain-free service.

TABLE 1. *Total available retrieved components*

Component	Total number	Bone ingrown and painful	Bone ingrown and not painful	Bone not ingrown and painful	Bone not ingrown and not painful
Femoral	146	45	26	28	47
Tibial	183	38	26	60	58
Patellar	135	26	37	34	38
Total	464	109	89	122	143

TABLE 2. *Components retrieved for reasons other than mechanical failure (all wear ratings included)*

Component	Total number	Bone ingrown and painful	Bone ingrown and not painful	Bone not ingrown and painful	Bone not ingrown and not painful
Femoral	77	35	8	18	16
Tibial	98	29	5	44	20
Patellar	62	22	4	24	12
Total	237	86	17	86	48

TABLE 3. *Components retrieved for reasons other than mechanical failure (no wear ratings of 2 or 3)*

Component	Total number	Bone ingrown and painful	Bone ingrown and not painful	Bone not ingrown and painful	Bone not ingrown and not painful
Femoral	30	11	4	8	7
Tibial	30	7	1	15	7
Patellar	12	6	0	4	2
Total	72	24	5	27	16

TABLE 4. *Nonworn, noncemented knee components retrieved for reasons other than mechanical failure*

Component	Total number	Bone ingrown and painful	Bone ingrown and not painful	Bone not ingrown and painful	Bone not ingrown and not painful
Femoral	8	2	2	3	1
Tibial	7	2	1	4	0
Patellar	4	2	0	1	1
Total	19	6	3	8	2

components with wear ratings of 2 or 3 were eliminated from the study. Once again, if any of a total knee's components were ranked 2 or 3, all of the components of that knee were excluded from the data set. The data for the remaining 72 total knee components can be seen in Table 3. Of the 72 remaining components, it was determined that some of them had been sent without the polyethylene bearing inserts and others had been mated to known cemented components. When these were eliminated from the study, only 19 components remained. Data on these 19 components are shown in Table 4.

DISCUSSION

The goal of this chapter is to assess the interface between host and unsuccessful cementless knee prostheses. In order to do so a large number of total knee implants were initially examined. Almost half of these components were retrieved for mechanical failure, which appeared to be more a function of design and polyethylene material properties than whether the knee was implanted without cement. Therefore, these devices were eliminated from the study because it was considered that no useful insight could be made from examination of their interfaces. Specifically, knee components retrieved for dislocation, subluxation, malposition, polyethylene or metal wear, or implant fracture were eliminated from the study, and those components retrieved for pain, looseness, subsidence, instability, bone fracture, or amputation or retrieved post mortem were maintained in the study.

Examination of wear of the articular surfaces of the knee components indicated that many of the devices had been subjected to significant wear and had generated visible wear debris. Due to the known relationship between wear debris and osteolysis, those components with wear greater than 2 on a scale of 0 to 3 were eliminated from the study as well. An examination of the remaining 72 components revealed that many of the devices had been sent to us without the polyethylene bearings or had been mated to cemented components, and therefore it was unclear whether the reason for retrieval was related to wear debris or related to pain of the cemented interface. These cases were also eliminated from the study. Of the final 19 components that remained, nine were bone ingrown and 10 were not. Six of the nine bone-ingrown implants were painful, whereas eight of the 10 nonbone-ingrown implants were painful.

Implant retrieval studies such as this one are valuable for determining the viability of new concepts such as whether porous coating will permit bone ingrowth and whether there are any differences in the body's response to material type or pore

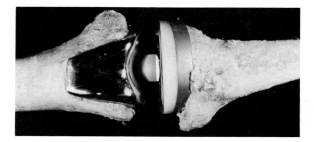

FIG. 3. Pain-free total knee was made available upon the patient's death 18 months postoperatively.

size. Additionally, these studies highlight various mechanisms that can lead to implant failure such as poor implant design resulting in high contact stress or implant fracture and questionable material properties that can lead to high rates of bearing wear. Unfortunately, these studies have much greater difficulty in determining the overall characteristics of either well- or poorly functioning prostheses. This is primarily due to the fact that more than 95% of the retrievals in this study were revision cases in which the patient was unsatisfied with the prosthesis. Only 5% of the implants arrived as the result of amputation or patient death (Figs. 3 and 4).

An effort was made in this study to determine which of the three knee components, femoral, patellar, or tibial, was typically the source of pain requiring implant revision (Fig. 5). Unfortunately, the data did not support any strong conclusion. Very few knee components are retrieved alone. Typically multiple components are retrieved at the time of revision surgery. It also appears that the surgeon has great difficulty in determining which knee component is responsible for the generation of the sensation of pain requiring the revision. Additionally, we sought to determine whether bone-ingrown interfaces could reliably be determined to be more pain free than fibrous-ingrown interfaces. Unfortunately, we were unable to do so. In no component type, femoral, patellar, or tibial, were more than 60% of the retrieved implants bone ingrown. It was impossible to statistically determine that bone-ingrown interfaces would be more pain free than fibrous tissue-ingrown interfaces (Fig. 6). It appears that either bone or fibrous tissue ingrowth is sufficient to provide pain-free

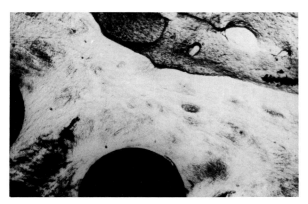

FIG. 4. Fibrous tissue ingrowth of the tibial plateau (Fig. 3) provided pain-free service.

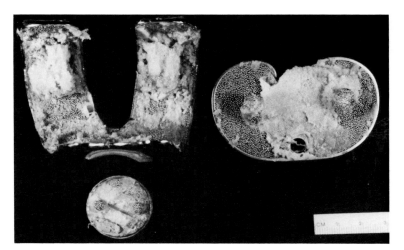

FIG. 5. Painful prosthesis was revised at 42 months.

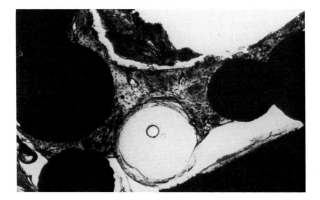

FIG. 6. Bone ingrowth of all three components, including this tibial plateau, was not sufficient to eliminate pain.

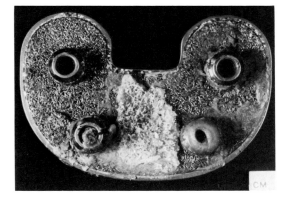

FIG. 7. Painful prosthesis was revised at 30 months.

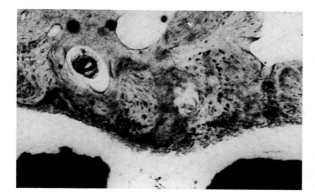

FIG. 8. Fibrous tissue ingrowth of the tibial component and bone ingrowth of the femoral and patellar components provided pain.

performance in some patients, although neither will eliminate the possibility of pain in all patients (Figs. 7 and 8). The difficulty in distinguishing a painful interface is due to the lack of any significant histological characteristic that can reliably be associated with the pain.

It should be noted that it was apparent that implants that had been *in situ* for longer periods of time often had greater amounts of bone ingrowth than those that were in for short periods of time. However, it would also appear, as seen in Table 5, that those devices with longer durations and removed for reasons other than mechanical failure are more often removed for reasons associated with pain than for nonpain reasons. Perhaps a painful device can be endured longer than, for example, a loose device. Significance tests, specifically the unpaired t test, were calculated for each set of means. This test requires the assumption that the data fit a normal distribution, and for duration this is perhaps unsatisfactory. However, the data set of $n = 237$ provided a highly significant result at the $p < 0.01$ level. The other means did not offer significant differences.

Independent of the reason for failure it becomes apparent that bone ingrowth is more reliable in the femoral and patellar components than in the tibial component. This is likely an indication that fixation of the tibial component is more difficult than either patellar or femoral components and perhaps tibial component looseness is the source of much of the pain in these knees. However, an extensive study of functioning implants in which a technique would need to be developed to specifically locate the source of pain is required in order to document this determination.

TABLE 5. *Mean duration in months for components in each data set that did and did not exhibit pain*

Data set (n)	Mean duration in months	
	Painful	Not painful
464	26.1	27.1
237	24.1	15.2
72	21.6	16.9
19	14.3	12.7

In this study we have not made an effort to segregate patients by age, weight, or activity, but rather have taken the entire series of retrieved components in order to assess whether a characteristic of the interface could be attributed to painful or pain-free operation. In this effort we were foiled.

CONCLUSIONS

Nearly half of all of the revised total knee components that we examined were retrieved for reasons of mechanical failure, which indicates that implant design and material properties of the bearings need careful attention. If mechanical failures and severely worn components are removed from the study, the interfaces between host and prostheses of painful and pain-free components cannot be assessed from the histology. Bone ingrowth was seen to provide pain-free performance in some prostheses, but other bone-ingrown components were revised for pain. Fibrous tissue ingrowth was seen to be sufficient to provide pain-free performance in some patients, while other patients complained of pain with fibrous tissue-ingrown interfaces. In every data set, bone ingrowth of femoral and patellar components was seen in more than 40% of the cases, whereas bone ingrowth of tibial components was seen in less than 45% of the cases. Components were retrieved in sets; single components were the exception. Post-mortem specimens are probably more valuable than revision specimens for determining the characteristics of pain-free versus painful interfaces in cementless prostheses.

ACKNOWLEDGMENTS

We would like to acknowledge the support of the Veterans Affairs Rehabilitation Research and Development Grant #A-473DA in this research. We would also like to thank the more than 500 surgeons who have provided us with retrieved devices for this study.

REFERENCES

1. Collier JP, Mayor MB, Bobyn JD, Engh CA, Orr T. The histology of tissue ingrowth into porous-metal coated femoral hip prostheses in five humans. *Trans Soc Biomater* 1983;6:79.
2. Collier JP, Mayor MB, Chae JC, Surprenant VA, Surprenant HP, Dauphinais LA. Macroscopic and microscopic evidence of prosthetic fixation with porous-coated materials. *Clin Orthop* 1988;235:173–180.
3. Collier JP, Mayor MB, Engh CA, Brooker A. Bone ingrowth of porous-coated Moore prostheses. *Trans Soc Biomater* 1984;7:113.
4. Collier JP, Mayor MB, McNamara JL, Surprenant VA, Jensen RE. Analysis of the failure of 122 polyethylene inserts from uncemented tibial knee components. *Clin Orthop* 1991;273:232–242.
5. Collier JP, Mayor MB, Surprenant VA, Surprenant HP, Jensen RE. Examination of porous-coated patellar components and analysis of the reasons for their retrieval. *J Appl Biomater* 1991;2:95–99.
6. Collier JP, McNamara JL, Surprenant VA, Jensen RE, Surprenant HP. All-polyethylene patellar components are not the answer. *Clin Orthop* 1991;273:198–203.
7. Engh CA, O'Connor D, Jasty M, Harris WH. Quantitation of implant micromotion, strain shielding and bone resorption with porous-coated AML cementless femoral prostheses retrieved at autopsy. Charnley Award Paper presented at the 20th Open Scientific Meeting of the Hip Society, February 23, 1992, Washington, DC.
8. Tronzo RG. A microporous coated hip implant infected 11 years after insertion. *Orthop Rev* 1983;12:85.

Biological, Material, and Mechanical Considerations of Joint Replacement,
edited by B. F. Morrey.
Raven Press, Ltd., New York © 1993.

16

Histological and Biochemical Aspects of Failed Femoral Implants

*Kang Jung Kim, *Jungi Chiba, and †Harry E. Rubash

*Institute of Rheumatology, Tokyo Women's Medical College, Tokyo 162, Japan;
†Department of Orthopaedic Surgery, University of Pittsburgh,
Pittsburgh, Pennsylvania 15213*

Research on the cellular composition and biochemical effects of tissue surrounding loosened hip prostheses has led to a better understanding of the cellular process underlying deterioration of the prosthesis-bone interface and aseptic loosening. Previous investigators have characterized the interface membranes obtained from failed cemented femoral prostheses (cemented membranes) as an infiltration of histiocytes associated with polymethylmethacrylate (PMMA) and polyethylene debris in a fibrous tissue stroma (15,20,28). Several biochemical factors found in the activated membrane have been associated with bone resorption and are believed to play an important role in osteolysis around cemented prostheses (10,17).

Cementless prostheses were developed in part to diminish the adverse effects of PMMA and to reduce the incidence of aseptic loosening. Nonetheless, these prostheses are reported to have a high incidence of early aseptic loosening (3,8). In addition, a histiocytic reaction associated with numerous metal and polyethylene particles has been observed in interface membranes obtained from failed cementless implants (cementless membranes) (16,19,21). Furthermore, femoral osteolysis, which previously had been reported to occur around only cemented implants, more recently was observed around both loosened and stable cementless femoral components (Fig. 1) (16,21,22). Several investigations, including our previous study, have found that chemical factors with the ability to induce bone resorption are often present in the interface membranes around failed cementless prostheses (7,11,16). These various findings suggest that the histological and biochemical behavior of these membranes holds clues to understanding, and thus avoiding, the process of aseptic loosening and osteolysis associated with failed cemented and cementless implants.

HISTOLOGY

Histological findings in cemented membranes have been well documented. The predominant features are marked infiltrates of histiocytes and multinucleated foreign-body giant cells, large accumulations of cement and polyethylene, and an underlying fibrous tissue stroma (Fig. 2) (15,19,20,28). We have found that the ce-

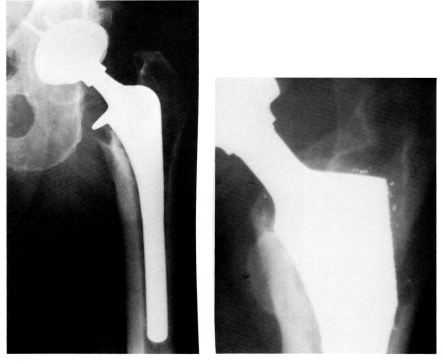

FIG. 1. A: Anteroposterior radiograph of a failed titanium prosthesis with marked proximal femoral osteolysis. **B:** Anteroposterior radiograph of a chrome-cobalt total hip arthroplasty with implant loosening and marked proximal femoral osteolysis.

mentless membranes from loosened femoral components with a polyethylene articulation frequently contain polyethylene and metal debris with a notable histiocytic reaction (Fig. 3) (16). Even membranes obtained from nonpolyethylene endoprostheses often contained metal particles and histiocytes; however, the histiocytic infiltrates were not as severe as those seen in cementless prostheses with a polyethylene articulation. In contrast, Kozinn et al. (18) described the membrane surrounding failed smooth-surface implants (nonpolyethylene endoprostheses) as dense connective tissue with rare inflammatory cells.

Whether porous coated or nonporous coated, the membranes we retrieved contained substantial amounts of minute (<10 μm in diameter) metal particles (16). Based on the grading system of Mirra et al. (23), the cementless membranes had significantly more of these metal particles than the cemented membranes. In addition, membranes from implants made of titanium alloy tended to contain more metal debris than did those from implants made of cobalt-chromium alloy.

Compared to histological analyses with hematoxylin and eosin staining, immunohistochemical analysis is a more sensitive method to investigate the cellular content of the interface membranes. Santavirta et al. reported that membranes around cemented femoral components (25) and cementless acetabular components (26) contained many macrophages stained by macrophage-specific monoclonal antibodies. They found few lymphocytes in the interface tissues using immunohistochemical

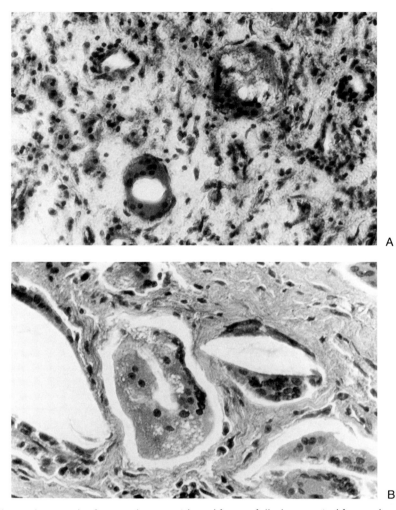

FIG. 2. Photomicrograph of a membrane retrieved from a failed cemented femoral component with infiltrates of histiocytes, multinucleated foreign-body giant cells, and accumulations of cement (**A**) and polyethylene (**B**).

methods. We performed an immunohistochemical analysis of cementless femoral membranes using anti-CD68 monoclonal antibody for macrophages as well as anti-CD3 and anti-CD22 for T and B lymphocytes, respectively (5). The results showed the presence of numerous macrophages that had phagocytized birefringent polyethylene, metal particles, or both (Fig. 4). As in the studies by Santavirta et al. (25,26), lymphocytic infiltrates in the membrane were very rare.

BIOCHEMICAL ANALYSIS

Goldring et al. (10) were one of the first to identify significant levels of prostaglandin E_2 (PGE_2) and collagenolytic activities in the culture media of membranes from

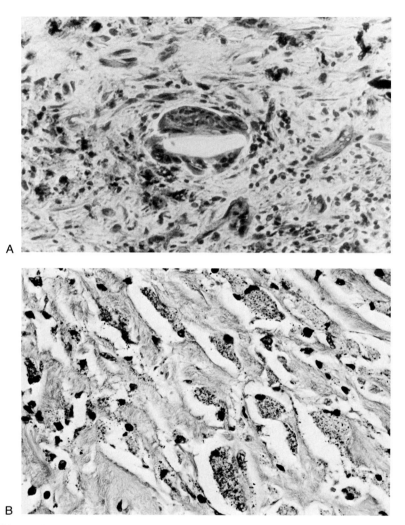

FIG. 3. Photomicrograph of a membrane obtained from a failed cementless femoral component with a histiocytic reaction, multinucleated foreign-body giant cells, and large accumulations of polyethylene (**A**) and metal debris (**B**).

the bone-PMMA interface of failed cemented prostheses. Kim et al. (17) later described the presence of significant PGE_2 levels in interface membranes as well as an osteoclast-activating factor. On the other hand, Goodman et al. (11) demonstrated the absence of interleukin-1 (IL-1) and collagenase in the membranes from both cemented and cementless prostheses, although they examined only a few cementless membranes. Recently, we reported finding significant levels of collagenase, PGE_2,

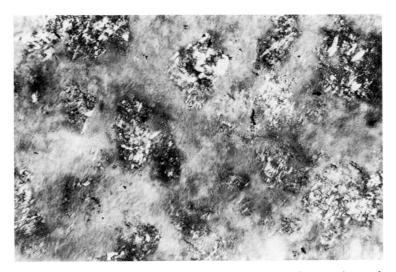

FIG. 4. Photomicrograph of the immunohistochemical staining of a membrane from a failed cementless component using anti-CD68 for macrophages. Predominantly macrophages and histiocytes with rare lymphocytes are shown.

and IL-1 in the interface membranes around failed cementless femoral components; these levels were similar to those found in failed cemented femoral components (16). We also compared the biochemical properties of cementless femoral membranes from patients with titanium-alloy, cobalt chromium-alloy, and nonpolyethylene endoprostheses to investigate the effects of the implant composition on the production of bone resorbing factors. The levels of collagenase, IL-1, and other factors in the membranes from titanium and cobalt-chromium implants were significantly higher than those in the membranes from nonpolyethylene endoprostheses (16).

Osteolysis or endosteal erosion around loosened and stable cementless femoral components has been described in several reports (7,16,22). Dorr et al. (7) noted significant levels of collagenase, PGE_2, and IL-1 in cementless membranes. Nevertheless, they suggested that biomechanical factors such as implant motion might play a more important role in inducing osteolysis around cementless femoral components. Maloney et al. (22) also suggested that implant motion might cause focal osteolysis. Among our own series of patients, we compared the biochemical findings for membranes from those who had endosteal erosion or focal osteolysis with those for patients without osteolysis. The membranes from patients with osteolysis released significantly higher levels of cytokines such as IL-1, IL-6, and tumor necrosis factor-α (TNF-α) into culture media. However, there were no significant differences between the two groups in the levels of collagenase and PGE_2. Histological and immunohistochemical analyses of the membranes from the patients with osteolysis showed a more intense histiocytic infiltrate associated with polyethylene and metal debris as compared to membranes from patients without osteolysis (5).

DISCUSSION

Cementless prostheses apparently are not immune to the adverse effects of implant materials. A histiocytic reaction to polyethylene and metal particles in a fibrous-tissue stroma is a common finding in histiological studies of interface membranes. The significantly greater amounts of metal debris in cementless membranes compared to cemented membranes (16) may be the result of metal wear, fretting, and corrosion of loosened cementless implants as they are abraded by the surrounding tissues (2,21). The poor wear performance of titanium and titanium alloy (6) may be responsible for the larger amounts of metal debris found in the titanium implants in comparison to the cobalt-chromium implants. The results of immunohistochemical analysis (25,26) suggest that a lymphocyte-mediated immune response to the metal debris is an unlikely cause of the inflammatory membranes around failed cementless implants (4). Instead, these membranes might be caused by excessive wear debris and other factors and the infiltration of macrophages that are activated by these factors.

Our biochemical comparison of the composition of these implants suggests that polyethylene particles might play a role in promoting the production of collagenase and IL-1 by the cells in cementless membranes. Interestingly, the levels of PGE_2 in the membranes from nonpolyethylene endoprostheses were similar to those from the implants with a polyethylene articulation, despite relatively little particulate material in the latter. Moreover, immunohistochemical analysis showed that the membranes from patients with and without osteolysis contained similar amounts of PGE_2, whereas the membranes from patients with osteolysis contained more macrophages and fewer fibroblasts. These findings indicate that PGE_2 could be produced by cells such as fibroblasts, as well as by histiocytes in the membranes. Although PGE_2 has been implicated in bone resorption (24,29), our studies have demonstrated that cytokines such as IL-1, IL-6, and TNF-α might be more important factors in the osteolysis around failed cementless prostheses. Willert and Semlitsch (28) suggested that polyethylene alone can be responsible for osteolysis around prostheses. Current theory suggests that osteolysis around cementless implants may be enhanced by the production of cytokines (IL-1, IL-6, TNF-α) after the phagocytosis of polyethylene particles by macrophages.

Given the clinical evidence of osteolysis around cementless femoral components, several *in vitro* studies were conducted to confirm the effects of different implant particles on the cellular production of chemical factors associated with bone resorption (4,5,9,13). These studies demonstrated that monocytes and macrophages apparently can produce chemical factors associated with bone resorption, such as PGE_2 and IL-1, via the phagocytosis of implant particles. In addition, fibroblasts are reported to be able to produce PGE_2 in response to metal particles *in vitro* (1,4). The results of these and other studies suggest that fibroblasts may also contribute to the process of osteolysis. The accurate characterization of wear particles in retrieved membranes is needed to further define the response of cells to implant particles.

SUMMARY

Several studies confirm the ability of cementless and cemented membranes to release into culture media similar amounts of the chemical factors associated with bone resorption (collagenase, PGE$_2$, and IL-1) (12). In view of the clinical evidence of osteolysis around cementless femoral components, these factors may play a role in the bone resorption associated with aseptic loosening of cementless femoral components. After the implantation of a cementless prosthesis, surrounding cells are influenced by various kinds of mechanical and biochemical factors. A fibrous membrane may be formed if implant motion takes place or if the osteogenic response to the implant material is weak. Continuous implant motion and the resultant fretting and corrosion produce metal particles that may stimulate and enhance the growth of a fibrous membrane. The cells comprising the fibrous membrane are predominantly macrophages and fibroblasts. In addition, polyethylene particles generated from the joint articulation can migrate into the bone-implant interface and be phagocytized by macrophages in the membrane (14). A continuous supply of metal and polyethylene particles can accelerate and perpetuate the inflammatory process with the release of biochemical agents associated with bone resorption. Once bone resorption occurs at the endosteal surface of cortical bone, further implant motion and migration can occur, and more wear debris can be generated. The high concentrations of polyethylene and metal particles in the region of the membrane may induce the cellular production of cytokines such as IL-1, IL-6, and TNF-α, as well as other chemical factors (PGE$_2$ and collagenase). There is increasing evidence that these factors play an important role in the osteolysis that occurs around cementless implants.

Much is currently known about the histological and biochemical characteristics of membranes around loosened implants. Further characterization of the cellular response and the size, shape, and content of the particles will continue to unravel the process of osteolysis and aseptic loosening. Understanding the process of aseptic loosening will have a great impact on implant design and longevity.

ACKNOWLEDGMENTS

The authors would like to thank Helga I. Georgescu, B.S., and Lori McIntyre, B.S., for their assistance in the histological and biochemical aspects of this project. We also thank Christopher H. Evans, Ph.D., for his valuable discussions, Robin L. Evans, R.N., M.S.N., for assistance in preparation of this manuscript, and Helene Marion for her helpful editorial comments.

REFERENCES

1. Bennett NE, Wang JT, Manning CA, Goldring SR. Activation of human monocyte/macrophages and fibroblasts by metal particles. Release of products with bone resorbing activities. *Trans Orthop Res Soc* 1991;37:188.
2. Buchert PK, Vaughn BK, Mallory TH, Engh CA, Bobyn JD. Excessive metal release due to loosening and fretting of sintered particles on porous-coated hip prostheses. *J Bone Joint Surg [Am]* 1986;68:606–609.
3. Callaghan JJ, Dystart SH, Savory CG. The uncemented porous-coated anatomic total hip prostheses. Two-year results of a prospective consecutive series. *J Bone Joint Surg [Am]* 1988;70:337–346.
4. Chiba J, Doyle JS, Noguchi K. Biochemical and morphological analyses of activated human macrophages and fibroblasts by particulate materials. *Trans Orthop Res Soc* 1992;17:343.
5. Chiba J, Iwaki Y, Kim KJ, Rubash HE. The role of cytokines in femoral osteolysis after cementless total hip arthroplasty. *Trans Orthop Res Soc* 1992;17:350.
6. Clark IC, McKellop HA, McGuire P, Okuda R, Sarmiento A. Wear of Ti-6A1-4V implant alloy and ultrahigh molecular weight polyethylene combinations. In: Luckey HA, Kubli F, eds. *Tita-*

nium alloy in surgical implants, ASTM STP 796. Philadelphia: American Society for Testing and Materials, 1983:136–147.

7. Dorr LD, Bloebaum R, Emmanuel J, Meldrum R. Histologic, biochemical, and ion analysis of tissue and fluids retrieved during total hip arthroplasty. *Clin Orthop* 1990;261:82–95.

8. Engh CA. Hip arthroplasty with a Moore prosthesis with a porous coating. A five-year study. *Clin Orthop* 1983;121:52–66.

9. Glant TT, Jacobs JJ, Tabith K, Galante JO. Particulate-induced bone resorption in organ culture. *Trans Orthop Res Soc* 1992;17:44.

10. Goldring SR, Schiller AL, Roelke M, Rourke CM, O'Neill DA, Harris WH. The synovial-like membrane at the bone-cement interface in loose total hip replacements and its proposed role in bone lysis. *J Bone Joint Surg [Am]* 1983;65:575–584.

11. Goodman SB, Chin RC, Chiou SS, Schurman DJ, Woolson ST, Masada MP. A clinical-pathologic-biochemical study of the membrane surrounding loosened and nonloosened total hip arthroplasties. *Clin Orthop* 1989;244:182–187.

12. Gowens M, Wood DD, Ihrie EJ, McGuire MKB, Russel RGG. An interleukin-1-like factor stimulates bone resorption in vitro. *Nature* 1983;306:378–380.

13. Howie DW, Haynes DR, Hay S, Rogers SD, Pearcy MJ. The effect of titanium alloy and cobalt chrome alloy wear particles on production of inflammatory mediators IL-1, TNF, IL-6, and prostaglandin E2 by rodent macrophages in vitro. *Trans Orthop Res Soc* 1992;17:344.

14. Howie DW, Vernon-Roberts B, Oakeshott R, Manthey B. A rat model of resorption of bone at the cement-bone interface in the presence of polyethylene wear particles. *J Bone Joint Surg [Am]* 1988;70:257–263.

15. Johanson NA, Bullough PG, Wilson PD Jr, Salvati EA, Renawat CS. The microscopic anatomy of the bone-cement interface in failed total hip arthroplasties. *Clin Orthop* 1987;218:123–135.

16. Kim KJ, Greis PE, Wilson SC, D'Antonio JA, McClain EJ, Rubash HE. Histological and biochemical comparison of membranes from titanium, cobalt-chromium, and nonpolyethylene hip prostheses. *Trans Orthop Res Soc* 1991;16:191.

17. Kim WC, Nottinghan P, Luben R, Amstutz HC, Mirra JM, Finerman GAM. Mechanism of osteolysis in aseptic loose total hip replacements. *Trans Orthop Res Soc* 1988;13:500.

18. Kozinn SC, Johanson NA, Bullough PG. The biologic interface between bone and cementless femoral endoprostheses. *J Arthroplasty* 1986;1:249–259.

19. Lennox DW, Schofield BH, McDonald DF, Riley LH Jr. A histologic comparison of aseptic loosening of cemented, press-fit and biologic ingrowth prostheses. *Clin Orthop* 1987;225:172–191.

20. Linder L, Carlsson A. Aseptic loosening of hip prostheses. A histological and enzyme histochemical study. *Clin Orthop* 1983;175:93–104.

21. Lombardi AV Jr, Mallory TH, Vaughn BK, Drouillard P. Aseptic loosening in total hip arthroplasty secondary to osteolysis induced by wear debris from titanium-alloy modular femoral heads. *J Bone Joint Surg [Am]* 1989;71:1337–1342.

22. Maloney WJ, Jasty M, Harris WH, Galante JO, Callaghan JJ. Endosteal erosion in association with stable uncemented femoral components. *J Bone Joint Surg [Am]* 1990;2:1025–1034.

23. Mirra JM, Amstutz HC, Matos M, Gold R. The pathology of the joint tissues and its clinical relevance in prosthesis failure. *Clin Orthop* 1976;117:221–240.

24. Robinson DR, Tashjian AH Jr, Levine L. Prostaglandin-stimulated bone resorption by rheumatoid synovia. A possible mechanism for bone destruction in rheumatoid arthritis. *J Clin Invest* 1975;56:1181–1188.

25. Santavirta S, Konttinen YT, Eskola A, Bergroth V, Tallroth K, Lindholm S. Aggressive granulomatous lesions associated with hip arthroplasty. *J Bone Joint Surg [Am]* 1990;72:252–258.

26. Santavirta S, Konttinen YT, Hoikka V, Eskola A. Immunopathological response to loose cementless acetabular components. *J Bone Joint Surg [Br]* 1991;73:38–42.

27. Willert HG, Bertram H, Buchhorn GH. Osteolysis in alloarthroplasty of the hip. The role of ultrahigh molecular weight polyethylene wear particles. *Clin Orthop* 1990;258:95–107.

28. Willert HG, Semlitsch M. Reactions of the articular capsule to wear products of artificial joint prostheses. *J Biomed Mater Res* 1977;11:157–164.

29. Yoneda T, Mundy GR. Monocytes regulate osteoclast-activating factor production by releasing prostaglandins. *J Exp Med* 1979;150:338–350.

*Biological, Material, and Mechanical
Considerations of Joint Replacement,*
edited by B. F. Morrey.
Raven Press, Ltd., New York © 1993.

17

Basic and Clinical Investigations of Osseointegrated Hip and Knee Replacements

*T. Albrektsson, *†L. V. Carlsson, *M. Jacobsson, and *‡W. Macdonald

*Departments of *Handicap Research and †Orthopaedic Surgery, University of
Gothenburg, S-413 12 Gothenburg, Sweden; ‡King's College Hospital,
London SE5 9RS, United Kingdom*

BACKGROUND

The most frequently used mode of anchorage for hip and knee replacements is poly-methylmethacrylate (PMMA) bone cement that, for instance, in Scandinavia is used in more than 90% of all hip arthroplasties. The general outcome of cemented replacements is quite acceptable, exemplified by reported 10-year success rates of 90% or higher (1,24) for hip replacements. These high success rates indicate that bone cement is the material of choice for the majority of arthroplasties to date. This statement is based on our awareness that the most important part of the introduction of new biomaterials designs and principles is the clinical long-term testing: to our knowledge no clinical follow-ups of cement-free implants have been reported that can match those of the cemented devices. Problems associated with disuse osteoporosis, and an observed sparse bone ingrowth in porous-coated cement-free prostheses have led many authors to remain sceptical to currently available designs of cement-free prostheses (2,9,10,15).

However, having said this, it is our conviction that we must constantly strive to replace bone cement with a biological type of anchorage that can be reliably achieved and maintained in the long term. Bone cement contains many toxic substances, of which PMMA is only one example (19). Emboli have been frequently observed during experimental (4) as well as clinical administration of bone cement (23). In a series of experiments performed at our laboratory, we documented cement side effects such as long-term disturbances in the remodeling pattern of the host bone, long-term impairment of new bone formation as well as a remaining soft-tissue coating around cemented test pieces, despite control for monomer leakage and heat trauma (19). In addition, even if the reported clinical results with cemented arthroplasties so far have been reasonable, there are limitations in most clinical studies. This is because statistics are generally limited to patients over 60 years of age, dropout figures are high for various reasons, and reported clinical survival figures have often been mistaken as success data.

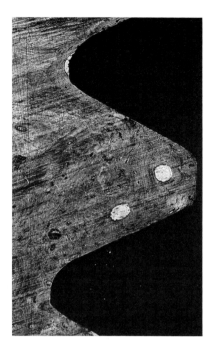

FIG. 1. Craniofacial implant retrieved from a female patient more than 1 year after insertion. The implant had been clinically loaded and was removed despite an undisturbed anchorage function. Such implants have demonstrated more than 80% (average) cortical bone to implant contact.

Members of our research group have actively investigated direct bone anchorage of osseointegrated implants since the 1960s, with both animal experiments and clinical trials. This work has resulted in clinical product innovations in the fields of oral and extraoral craniofacial implants to treat edentulousness and facial malformations as well as certain types of hearing disorders (5,6,8,16) (Fig. 1). For more than 10 years we have been involved in experimental work to translate to the orthopaedic field our experimental and clinical observations in the craniofacial skeleton, work that has resulted in the successful animal tests of new principles for the anchorage of arthroplasties. Ten Ph.D. projects on these topics have been completed at our laboratories since 1984. Our clinical trials with the newly developed hip and knee arthroplasties have begun but are at a very early stage. The purpose of this chapter is to report on our current standpoint with respect to osseointegrated arthroplasties. We will discuss the basis for our choice of materials for the anchorage and gliding surfaces of hip and knee joints, the importance of controlling not only the hardware but the software with respect to osseointegration, and our intended mode of follow-up of the clinical devices.

IMPLANT FACTORS: BASIC INVESTIGATIONS

Currently, the preferred metallic materials for joint arthroplasties are stainless steel, cobalt-chrome alloys, and $TiAl_6V_4$ alloy. In the porous-coated type implants, cobalt-chrome and titanium alloys have been seen as advantageous, as the stainless steels are suspected to have an unacceptably high tendency to corrode in the human body (2) (Fig. 2). Johansson (17) compared bone-tissue reactions to various metals

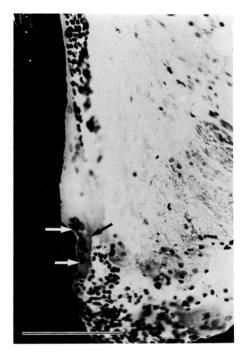

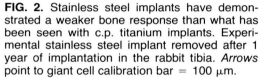

FIG. 2. Stainless steel implants have demonstrated a weaker bone response than what has been seen with c.p. titanium implants. Experimental stainless steel implant removed after 1 year of implantation in the rabbit tibia. *Arrows* point to giant cell calibration bar = 100 μm.

and reported a direct bone to metal interface (at the light microscope level of resolution) for several different metals (including the above-cited alloys). However, in quantified investigations with commercially pure (c.p.) titanium as a control material, significantly more bone was observed in the c.p. titanium interface compared to any of the common alloys used in arthroplasties. In part, these findings could be related to inevitable differences in surface topography of hard metal such as cobalt-chrome and a softer metal such as c.p. titanium. However, even in cases when the surface topography was controlled, as in the investigation of bone-tissue reactions to c.p. titanium and Ti6Al4V alloy, there was significantly more bone formed in the interface of the c.p. titanium. Johansson (17) postulated that a demonstrated ionic leakage was the reason for the inhibited bone response to the alloy. Recent investigations on hard-tissue reactions to c.p. titanium confirm the notion that this metal is the optimal choice for a clinical implant material from a biocompatibility point of view (22).

However, c.p. titanium has been regarded as too weak a material to be suitable for major arthroplasties, and it has clear disadvantages when used as a gliding surface. With respect to the mechanical characteristics, c.p. titanium is as notch sensitive as its alloys, and less stiff and less strong than most other implant materials. Balanced against these disadvantages is the possibility of true bone-implant mechanical integration as discussed below, which leads to the possibility of a novel design solution to the implant requirements.

Such a novel design solution has undergone all the usual engineering design processes and verifications of those designs. The proposed design was submitted to stress analysis to confirm initial estimations of strength. Further analyses with finite

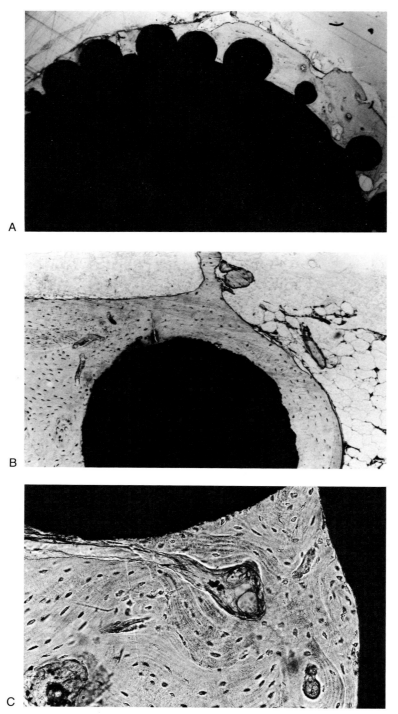

FIG. 3. Porous-coated implants, such as this Lord prosthesis removed after more than 7 years of clinical function, may demonstrate a high proportion of bone to implant contact at certain locations (**A**). In this retrieved case, however, irrespective of the substantial bone to implant contact in this section, the great majority of the implant length was completely encapsulated in soft tissue (**B**). The cortical bone demonstrated signs of ongoing creeping substitution (**C**).

element modeling was undertaken to estimate the magnitude of bone loading and check structural integrity under monotonic and fatigue loading conditions. The reliance of the design on the bone mechanical support meant that such modeling needed to take more accurate account of the bone morphology and distribution of mechanical properties (18). These calculations were confirmed by mechanical testing: both gross strength tests and under physiologic conditions, including repetitive stresses to investigate fatigue and fretting behavior.

Calcium phosphates such as hydroxyapatite (HA) have recently gained some popularity as a new material for the anchoring surface of a joint. Theoretical advantages of HA include reports of a quantitatively, as well as qualitatively, superior bone attachment in comparison to the uncoated metal. A disadvantage of ingrowth-type prostheses with porous coating or mesh-type surfaces is that the increased surface area causes increased ionic leakage, which may be harmful to the tissues (7). HA coating has been regarded as a barrier to such leakage and as minimizing its effect, even if this mode of action has been questioned with respect to titanium-type metals (11). With our joint design and surfaces we have indications that the ionic leakage is of a minor proportion and unlikely to result in tissue problems. Furthermore, based on the findings of Gottlander (14), we have not been convinced that the HA material is the optimal one for implantation purposes. Gottlander did not find any obvious long-term advantages with HA, at least not when combined with threaded implants. Because our new hip and knee joints are dependent primarily on threaded fixation, the proposed advantage of HA being able to more rapidly bridge a gap than c.p. titanium has not been a strong argument for our introduction of HA. Furthermore, in the field of oral implants where HA was introduced more than 5 years ago, there is now an increasing body of evidence that shows a gradually developing bone resorption in many clinical cases. Whether this bone resorption is a general finding or is related to accidental loss of the coating is, at present, difficult to state with certainty. Therefore, we have found the present state of knowledge insufficiently clear to support the inclusion of HA in our present joint designs.

Carlsson's (9) thesis compared design and surface parameters of anchoring screws. The screw had some clear advantages with respect to implant take compared to other designs, and a certain implant roughness was found important for implant acceptance, whereas an artificially enhanced surface energy (in comparison to the surface energy of ordinary metal implants) did not improve the bone response. We are continuing to study the "ideal" geometry, topography, and surface energy of the threaded type of implants that we have preferred in our new hip and knee designs. We believe that one major reason for the relative lack of clinical success with many cement-free implants is that the choice of implant hardware in many cases has been dominated by engineering and manufacturing know-how rather than by knowledge of the cellular response to implant materials and designs (Fig. 3).

HOST BED, SURGICAL TECHNIQUE, AND LOADING CONDITIONS

Another major reason for current clinical long-term problems with many cement-free arthroplasties is failure to treat the tissues in a biologically acceptable manner. In many cases, instruments and surgical techniques used when inserting a cemented implant are preferred when inserting a cement-free one. We believe this is misconceived as success, with a cement-free implant, in contrast to the cemented device, depending on regenerating tissues. The surgical fit (9) is of great importance and needs to be controlled for reliable integration of the implant. However, the press-fit advocated in some modern cement-free implants may not improve the situation if the subsequent bone remodeling around a stem-design implant results in a deteriorating fit with time. Furthermore, the press fit does not necessarily mean a total contact fit of the implant to the bone but, in the practical situation, rather a point contact. We have not been convinced by the extant literature that it is possible to achieve proper osseointegration with such prostheses and maintain it during clinical loading conditions. The surgical trauma unavoidable with most current cement-free designs is another reason for unwanted bone resorption. Bone tissue can tolerate no more than 47°C for 1 min, without subsequent necrosis (12).

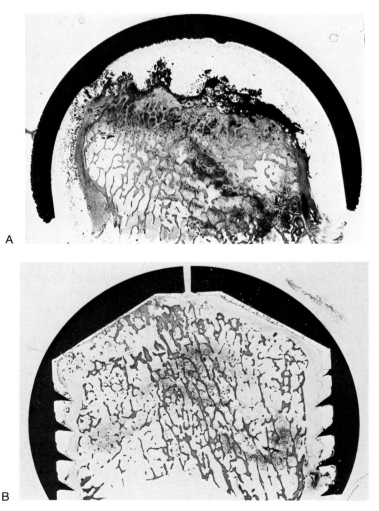

FIG. 4. Surface hip replacements, irrespective of cemented (**A**) or uncemented (**B**), have generally demonstrated a soft-tissue interface between bone and metal. Many such implants have had to be removed due to instability.

Uncemented stem-design hip prostheses have often been demonstrated to result in unwanted bone resorption, in many cases due to disturbed bone remodeling or endosteal erosion (13). The reasons for unwanted bone resorption vary, but include early implant movements (3) and disuse osteoporosis (15). The most reliable way to avoid bone resorption would be to allow a healing period for the implant before actual loading takes place (3). However, in clinical cases two-stage surgery may be impractical. Osseointegration has been demonstrated with immediate loading (20), but this depends presumably on joint design as well as on the likelihood of rotational forces, which seem to be particularly harmful to early implant stability.

All previous designs have followed the Charnley principles including initial stability due to mechanical fit and long-term tolerance by the tissues. Many have attributed failure of cemented designs to the acrylic cement and assumed that a similar design with alternative fixation would give comparable results. But all, including different surface hip replacements, have been inhibited by the uncertainty of long-term fixation and the need to provide reserve stability (Fig. 4).

In contrast, the assurance of long-term reliable bone interaction with the implant has enabled a truly novel conceptual approach to implant design. For the first time, implants could be designed as skeletal replacements for the failed anatomical parts. Since the bone serves its normal function in supporting the implant, disuse osteoporosis and fibrous membrane reactions are avoided. The conditions of true mechanical integrity in the skeleton and the assurance of a stable long-term bone reaction have led to a design with an expected improving stability as clinical life progresses.

GLIDING SURFACES

Röstlund (20) investigated the wear behavior of nitrogen-implanted titanium alloy against ultrahigh molecular weight polyethylene (UHMWPE). The polymer wear rate was not affected by the ion implantation, but the metal wear was significantly reduced by this treatment. Ion implantation, furthermore, resulted in good protection of the metal surface against third-body wear by PMMA. The wear properties of c.p. titanium were likewise improved by ion implantation. It was speculated that a better polishing technique, in combination with a method that enables a more profound penetration depth of the nitrogen ions, would further improve the wear properties of c.p. titanium. It is our opinion that the potentially most problematic part of the articulation of a new joint is the UHMWPE side and that specifically treated metals and ceramics such as zirconia will minimize the unavoidable wear debris production. Röstlund (20) presented mathematical and graphic data of the geometry of the lower end of the femur, knowing that a detailed knowledge of the femoral joint surfaces would be instrumental in the construction of a new knee arthroplasty aimed at osseointegration.

CLINICAL SURVEILLANCE

The clinical follow-up of any inserted implant should ideally continue at regular intervals over the remaining life span of the patient. Stringent clinical and radiographic protocols must be outlined to ensure early detection of failures. Ideally, the patients should be randomized into test groups and controls. The studies should be prospective and initially cover 3-year follow-up, with continuing annual follow-up indefinitely. We use a modified version of Hip and Knee Scores, as we believe that statistical evaluation alone is not sufficient for analysis. Visual analogue and verbal rating scales for pain, general physical examination, and registration by independent observers of any adverse effects attributable to the new method or device are most important.

Conventional radiographic evaluations include anteroposterior and lateral exposures as well as a pelvic overview preoperatively, postoperatively, and at every scheduled follow-up. Prosthetic position and bone remodeling are examined as well as any signs of subsidence or bone resorption. Roentgenstereophotogrammetry (RSA) is being utilized as this is the best method to register minute movements between the implanted device and the host bone bed. The RSA analysis can be separated into four parts (21): (a) implantation of tantalum markers, (b) radiographic examination, (c) measurements on radiographs, and (d) mathematic calculations. Special tantalum balls with a diameter of 0.8 or 1 mm are inserted in the bone and prosthesis. Tantalum has a high atomic number, which facilitates identification on radiographs, and is highly resistant to corrosion. This is an established approach because more than 20,000 tantalum markers have been implanted in more than 2,000 patients in different follow-up studies since 1972. Simultaneous exposures are taken by two roentgen tubes with the patient in a plexiglass calibration cage fitted with tantalum markers at an exactly known position. Two exposures are taken simultaneously. Radiation doses at RSA examinations have proved to be low compared to similar conventional radiographic examinations. Relative positions of all the markers are calculated by three-dimensional trigonometry, using a computer. Movements can thus be detected down to an accuracy of 10 to 150 μA or 0.03 to 0.6°. In the case of hip joint prostheses evaluations, the accuracy is usually 0.3 to 0.4 mm and 0.4 to 0.6°.

CONCLUDING REMARKS

The Gothenburg osseointegrated hip and knee replacements have been developed from more than 20 years of applied experimental and clinical research. The material, design, and surface topography of our implants do not resemble any other hip and knee replacements with which we are familiar. The insertion of our hip and knee designs is dependent on the use of specially constructed directional guides and newly developed surgical instruments that, according to our research, enable a more exact and less traumatizing insertion. Despite our efforts and the fact that we have seen most promising results in animal experiments, the future role of any novel arthroplasty should be determined primarily on clinical documentation performed according to established protocols. In the absence of adequate follow-up data, as in our case, any new devices should be regarded as being of an experimental nature only.

ACKNOWLEDGMENTS

The Gothenburg hip and knee replacements have been constructed in a combined research effort with Björn Albrektsson, M.D., Ph.D., and Tord Röstlund, M.D., Ph.D., of the Orthopaedic Clinic of Mölndal, Sweden, and with Stig Wennberg, engineer. Our work has been supported by grants, gratefully acknowledged here, from the Swedish Medical Research Council, the Eyvind and Elsa K:son Sylvan Foundation, the Ågren Foundation, the Wilhelm and Martina Lundgren Foundation, and the Astra Tech Company, Mölndal, Sweden.

REFERENCES

1. Ahnfeldt L, Herberts P, Malchau H, Andersson GBJ. Prognosis of total hip replacement. A Swedish multicenter study of 4664 revisions. *Acta Orthop Scand* 1990;61(suppl 238):1–26.
2. Albrektsson T. The reactions of bone to non-cemented implants. In: Hall BK, ed. *Bone: a treatise. Fracture repair and regeneration.* Boca Raton: CRC Press, 1992:153–208.
3. Albrektsson T, Brånemark PI, Hansson HA, Lindström J. Osseointegrated titanium implants. Requirements for ensuring a long-lasting direct bone anchorage in man. *Acta Orthop Scand* 1981;52:155–170.
4. Albrektsson T, Linder L. Bone injury caused by curing bone cement. Vital microscopic study in the rabbit tibia. *Clin Orthop* 1984;183:280–287.
5. Albrektsson T, Brånemark PI, Jacobsson M, Tjellström A. Present clinical applications of osseointegrated percutaneous implants. *Plastic Reconstr Surg* 1987;79:721–730.
6. Albrektsson T, Dahl E, Embom L, et al. Osseointegrated oral implants. A Swedish multicenter study of 8139 consecutively inserted Nobelpharma implants. *J Periodontol* 1988;59:287–296.
7. Albrektsson T, Carlsson LV, Morberg P, Wennerberg A. Directly bone-anchored implants with special emphasis on the concept of osseointegration in orthopaedic surgery. In: Cameron HU, ed. *Implant-bone interface.* St. Louis: CV Mosby, 1992.
8. Brånemark PI, Hansson BO, Adell R, Breine U, Lindström J. Hallén O, Öhman A. Osseointegrated implants in the treatment of the edentulous jaw. Experience from a 10 year period. *Scand J Plast Reconstr Surg* 1977;suppl 16:1–132.
9. Carlsson LV. *On the development of a new concept for orthopaedic implant fixation.* Ph.D. thesis. Biomaterials Group, University of Gothenburg, Sweden, 1989:1–112.
10. Coventry MB. Lessons learned in 30 years of total hip arthroplasty. *Clin Orthop* 1992;274:22–29.
11. Ducheyne P, Bianco PD, Kim C. Bone tissue growth enhancement by calcium phosphate coatings on porous titanium alloys: the effect of shielding metal dissolution products. *Biomaterials* 1992;13:617–624.
12. Eriksson RA. *Heat-induced bone tissue injury. An* in vivo *investigation of heat tolerance of bone tissue and temperature rise in the drilling of cortical bone.* Ph.D. thesis, Biomaterials Group, University of Gothenburg, Sweden, 1984:1–91.
13. Galante JO, Lemons J, Spector M, Wilson P Jr, Wright TM. The biologic effects of implant materials. *J Orthop Res* 1991;9:760–775.
14. Gottlander M. *On hard-tissue reactions to hydroxyapatite-coated titanium implants.* Ph.D. thesis. University of Gothenburg, Sweden, 1992.
15. Harris WH. The first 32 years of total hip arthroplasty. *Clin Orthop* 1992;274:6–11.
16. Jacobsson M, Tjellström A. Clinical applications of percutaneous implants. In: Szycher M, ed. *High performance biomaterials.* Lancaster, Basel: Technomic, 1991:207–229.
17. Johansson C. *On tissue reactions to metallic implants.* Ph.D. thesis, University of Gothenburg, Sweden, 1991:1–109.
18. Macdonald W. Bone mechanical properties for the design of prosthetic systems. In: *Proceedings of the international symposium on computer methods in biomechanics and biomedical engineering, 1992.*
19. Morberg P. *On tissue reactions to acrylic cement.* Ph.D. thesis, University of Gothenburg, Sweden, 1991:1–101.
20. Röstlund T. *On the development of a new arthroplasty with special emphasis on the gliding elements in the knee.* Ph.D. thesis, University of Gothenburg, Sweden, 1990:1–133.
21. Selvik G. A roentgen stereophotogrammetric method for the study of the kinematics of the skeletal system. *Acta Orthop Scand* 1989;60(suppl 232).
22. Sennerby L. *On the bone tissue response to titanium implants.* Ph.D. thesis, University of Gothenburg, Sweden, 1991:1–111.
23. Ulrich C, Heinrich H. Intrafemoral pressure in total hip replacement. In: Older J, ed. *Implant-bone interface.* New York: Springer, 1990:95–98.
24. Wroblevski BM. 15–21 year results of the Charnley low-friction arthroplasty. *Clin Orthop* 1986;211:30–39.

*Biological, Material, and Mechanical
Considerations of Joint Replacement,*
edited by B. F. Morrey.
Raven Press, Ltd., New York © 1993.

18

Interface Zone

Factors Influencing Its Structure for Cementless Implants

R. M. Pilliar, J. M. Lee, and J. E. Davies

Centre for Biomaterials, University of Toronto, Toronto, Ontario, Canada M5S 1A1

Clinical experiences to date suggest that long-term success of cementless bone-interfacing implants in any major load-bearing application (orthopaedic or dental) requires the formation of an intimate bone-biomaterial interface capable of sustaining significant load transfer with a minimal amount (if any) of interposed fibrous connective tissue. Of particular importance in the establishment of such an interface are the conditions prevailing during the healing period following implant placement. Although the use of biocompatible materials is necessary for the fabrication of successful implantable devices, it is by no means sufficient. A number of studies have demonstrated the overriding importance of relative movement between implant and host tissues during the healing phase in determining success. Sufficient stability of implant relative to bone is necessary during this period to allow bone to form in close apposition to the implant surface. Despite the significance of this factor, few quantitative data have been reported on the limits of acceptable relative motion to allow bone formation at an implant surface. In this chapter we review our current understanding of this important issue and, further, explore the significance of implant surface topography on the sensitivity to relative motion during healing.

To understand the effect of relative movement on the formation of the "interface zone" it is necessary to define the formation of that zone in the absence of movement. Recent studies using both *in vitro* and *in vivo* methods have provided new information in this regard (4,5,7). A brief review of these studies is included.

PREVIOUS STUDIES ON RELATIVE MOVEMENT AND THE INTERFACE ZONE

Except for one recent report (12), only retrospective analysis of results of *in vivo* studies have been used to provide information on the limits of allowable relative motion for achieving bone ingrowth and close apposition to an implant surface. Pilliar et al. (22) suggested that for porous-coated implants made by sintering CoCrMo-alloy particles in the size range of 50 to 150 μm (yielding interconnected pores of 50 to 100 μm in cross section after sintering), relative movements greater than 150 μm inhibited bone formation and ingrowth, whereas bone ingrowth occurred despite some movement below 28 μm (no firm maximum being suggested). The studies by Hollis et al. (12) were consistent with these results.

The 150-μm quantity was determined from analysis of load-displacement curves of porous-coated segmental replacement implants placed in dog femurs (14,15). The implants had become attached by fibrous tissue forming and interdigitating with the surface pores during a 6- to 12-month period of function. The fibrous-tissue layer was characterized by collagen fibers oriented more or less obliquely to the implant surface (Fig. 1). The layer was approximately 0.3 to 1.0 mm thick and formed around the porous-coated parts of the implant in contrast to an encapsulating membrane with collagen fibers running parallel to the surface next to uncoated regions. The obliquely oriented fibers formed a union with a peripheral bone shell comprising part of a trabecular bone network attached at points to the endosteal cortical bone surface. The junction of the collagen fibers and bone was morphologically similar to Sharpey's fiber attachments seen at normal ligament-bone junctions (Fig. 1) and, indeed, the implant-fibrous tissue-bone construct resembled a normal tooth-periodontium structure with periodontal ligament attachment of tooth to alveolar bone. Although the shape of the load-displacement curve varied somewhat from specimen to specimen (a reflection of the degree of organization of the fibrous tissue), for some cases (the looser fibrous tissue structures) it could be represented by a bilinear curve with a low stiffness region ($k_1 = 0.003$–0.004 N/μm) for loads below approximately 1 N and a higher stiffness region ($k_2 = 0.3$–0.7 N/μm) for applied loads above 1 N (compression and tension) (15). The more organized, denser fibrous-tissue layers had a less pronounced low stiffness region, particularly when loaded in tension with $k_1 = 0.006$ to 0.2 and $k_2 = 0.12$ to 0.17 N/μm. These stiffness values are an order of

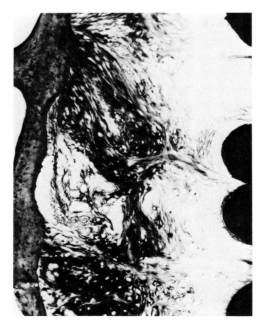

FIG. 1. Transmitted light micrograph showing obliquely oriented fibrous tissue between the porous coating (*right*) and part of the shell of bone that forms around the porous-coated region (*left*). Field width = 500 μm.

magnitude lower than reported intrusive stiffness values for human teeth measured *in vivo* as reviewed by Brunski (2). Those values ranged from $k_1 = 0.1$ to 0.2 N/μm and $k_2 = 1.0$ to 3.0 N/μm. The maximal displacements during test loading between 20-N tension and compression equaled approximately 180 μm for the denser fibrous-tissue samples and 500 μm for the looser structures. Because of the steep slopes of the load-displacement curves at higher loads (tensile and compressive), the maximal displacements measured during cyclic loading between -20 and $+20$ N probably were representative of maximal displacements experienced during normal function.

Due to uncertainties related to the contribution of trabecular bone element deformation to the measured displacements, it was not possible to precisely define the stiffness of the fibrous-tissue interface zone. For the bone-ingrown samples, the overall stiffness was determined to range between 0.8 and 1.7 N/μm with displacements between 20 and 40 μm for applied loads of -20 to $+20$ N. This suggests that the shear distortion of the fibrous-tissue layer for the more organized, denser structures is equal to approximately 150 μm. It seems reasonable to assume that the displacements occurring during healing would be greater than those measured in samples retrieved and tested just after sacrifice following a period of *in vivo* function. (All mechanical tests were conducted on fresh tissue specimens in saline at 37°C immediately after sacrifice.) Hence, it was concluded that relative motion greater than approximately 150 μm gave rise to fibrous-tissue formation and attachment with porous-coated implants (22).

The observation of bone ingrowth into a porous-coated endosseous endodontic implant (17), despite limited relative motion at the implant-bone interface, provided some insight on acceptable levels of movement that could be tolerated and still allow bone formation and ingrowth. The analysis required knowledge of (i) periodontal ligament stiffness and (ii) levels of axial loads applied to the tooth. The intrusion characteristics of teeth, as reported by Parfitt (19) and others (2), suggested stiffness values for periodontal ligaments of $k_1 = 0.1$ to 0.2 N/μm and $k_2 = 1.0$ to 3.0 N/μm. Hipp and Brunski (11) reported axial forces acting on canine teeth during chewing between 4 and 32 N with an average load of 8 N. Using this range of properties and assuming an applied load of 8 N, the axial displacement of the porous-coated implant relative to its host alveolar bone would be equal to approximately 7 to 21 μm. These values would be higher for higher loads, but it seems reasonable to assume that such high loads would not be imposed during the early healing phase. Therefore, this retrospective analysis provided some speculative values for acceptable relative movement for bone ingrowth to occur. The observation made by Hollis et al. (12) that 25-μm relative displacements resulted in full ingrowth to porous-coated titanium cylindrical plugs placed transcortically is in line with this conclusion. Further studies planned specifically to test the hypothesis that relative motion greater than 25 μm, for example, will inhibit bone formation at an implant surface are required.

It is of interest to consider the effective shear strains resulting from the suggested degree of relative movement resulting in fibrous-tissue formation and attachment (segmental replacement experiment [20]) and bone formation (endosseous endodontic implant model [17]). As noted above, the thickness of the fibrous-tissue layer observed in the segmental replacement study was fairly constant and equal to 0.3 to 1.0 mm. Assuming no torsion and shear displacement due to axial loading only within the interface zone (porous coating-fibrous tissue-peri-implant bone shell), and relative displacements of 150 μm, the shear strain acting within the interface zone would be equal to 0.15 to 0.5. During the healing phase, strains of this order would

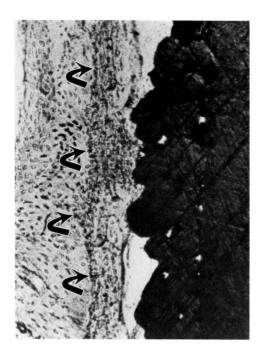

FIG. 2. Transmitted light micrograph of transapical region of a porous-coated endosseous endodontic implant-bone interface region. A reversal line is indicated by the *arrows*. Width of healing zone is approximately 300 μm. Field width = 1.2 mm.

act on differentiating cells in the interface zone. As proposed by Carter and Giori (3), imposition of shear and tensile strains above some critical level would cause differentiating cells to alter their phenotypic expression from osteoblast-like to fibroblast-like. An indication of the magnitude of these critical strains is suggested by *in vitro* cell culture studies in which imposition of known strains on osteoprogenitor cell lines has been studied (13). At 0.01 shear strain a change in phenotypic expression was observed. This value suggests that strains greater than 0.01 could result in fibrous-tissue formation as was the case in our *in vivo* study. From the endosseous endodontic implant study, based on an initial interface zone width of approximately 300 μm (distance from the porous coating to the observed reversal line [see Fig. 2]) and the estimated relative displacement using assumed maximal loads and reported tooth intrusion stiffness properties (i.e., 7–21 μm), shear strains below 0.1 (= 0.02 to 0.07) would have occurred within the interface zone. Considering the assumptions used in these *in vivo* and *in vitro* studies (or perhaps because of the assumptions), the agreement is reasonable and provides a first approximation of the critical shear strain (≈0.01).

EFFECTS OF TOPOGRAPHY

The primary objective of the endosseous endodontic implant experiment referred to above (17) was to compare the bone fixation and resulting implant stability with porous-coated and threaded implants used for this application. Since the implants were loaded soon after placement (the dogs returned to a normal diet within 2 to 3 days), significant relative motion as determined by the stiffness of the periodontal ligament could have occurred during the healing period. The porous-coated and threaded implants were loaded equally. However, a surprising observation was that while the early imposed loading caused bone resorption followed by fibrous-tissue formation with the threaded design (fibrous-tissue encapsulation), the porous-coated implants became fixed by bone ingrowth. The single variable that appeared responsible for this different behavior was the surface geometry of the two implant types. It was suggested that the porous surface resulted in an environment conducive to early bone formation despite the early loading, perhaps because of its three-dimensional interconnected porosity. The initial fibrin-fibrous tissue matrix that forms within the interface zone would become interdigitated with the three-dimensional interconnected pore structure of the porous-coated implants, thereby resulting in resistance to shear, tensile, and compressive forces acting at the interface. This type of attachment would not result with the threaded geometry so that resistance to tensile forces would not occur. As a result, greater resistance to movement during early loading would be expected with the porous-coated implants, thereby reducing displacements (and shear strains) to the point at which bone formation could occur. Replacement of fibrous connective tissues by bone following reduced loading (and shear strains) has been reported in other situations (25) and is consistent with the hypothesis presented by Carter and Giori (3). Thus, it appears that surface geometry can have a profound effect on tissue formation within the interface zone when significant loads are applied to an implant shortly after placement. Other more subtle implications related to implant topography and bone bonding have been suggested more recently (8,21).

ULTRASTRUCTURAL CHARACTERIZATION OF THE INTERFACE ZONE

Our recent studies have provided new information on the extracellular matrix synthesis by bone-derived cells at a biomaterial surface (4,5,7). Using rat bone-marrow cells obtained from femurs of young adult animals and cell culture methods developed by Maniatopoulos et al. (18) we showed that an early stage of cell-substrate interaction involved the attachment of differentiating bone cells to the substrate, presumably already covered by a protein conditioning film (16), and cell-mediated elaboration of a collagen-free sulfur-containing fine filamentous organic substance. This organic material forms a scaffold for subsequent deposition of a calcium phosphate phase (within 11 days in the cell culture system reported by Davies et al. [4,5,7]). Seeding of calcium phosphate continues (assuming appropriate local conditions) to form a continuous cement-like layer over the substrate surface covered by bone cells (Fig. 3). The next phase of cell activity involves the secretion of collagen and its mineralization, thereby forming a structure similar to that found at reversal lines in bone with new bone apposed to the "cement" line. The use of cell culture methods allowed the preparation of thin sections of the interface zone for ultrastructural examination using transmission electron microscopy (TEM). The studies were conducted using a variety of substrate surfaces including normal polymer culture dishes and dishes sputter-coated with thin layers of commercially pure titanium and Ti6Al4V. Other studies involved use of bulk substrates and freeze fracture methods to provide samples for scanning electron microscopy (SEM) and TEM examination of the interface region (5).

A major limitation of these *in vitro* studies is the uncertainty that the observations made are representative of bone healing around implants *in vivo*. A significant find-

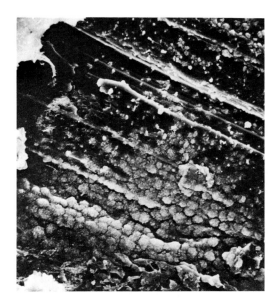

FIG. 3. SEM appearance of calcium phosphate globular deposits formed *in vitro* on a titanium substrate. The globules are agglomerates of finer particles. Field width = 15 μm.

ing in this regard was the results obtained from another retrospective study (6) involving small disk-shaped implants placed in rabbit mandibles (a part of a dental implant study within our laboratory). Implants were placed for periods ranging from 2 weeks to 6 months, ostensibly to examine changes to biomaterial surfaces during these periods of implantation and study trace ion release and uptake by tissues (24). Retrospective examination of retrieved porous-coated Ti6Al4V and porous Al_2O_3 disks, and dense hydroxyapatite disks showed evidence of an approximately 0.5 μm thick collagen-free amorphous layer between the implant surface and bone. For the porous-coated Ti6Al4V disks, calcified globular deposits similar to those seen in the *in vitro* experiments were observed, with a suggestion that thermal etching lines (formed during the high-temperature sintering process used to form the samples) served as foci for the deposition of the calcium phosphate globules (Fig. 4). An example of the interface zone is shown in Fig. 5. The cement layer appears next to the titanium alloy surface (region A). The close apposition of the layer is implied despite the apparent gap at the interface (an artefact due to sample preparation). Comparison to SEM examination of interface bone cells on cell culture dishes showed a striking morphological similarity of globular deposits formed *in vitro* (Fig. 3) and those observed on the retrieved implants (Fig. 4).

From these studies it was concluded that the interface zone formed during bone healing of a *stationary* implant placed into a properly prepared bone site consisted of a cement-like layer of approximately 0.5 μm in thickness in contact with the implant (and any adsorbed conditioning film) and new bone juxtaposing and intimately associated with this layer. Formation of this structure by differentiating bone cells requires a degree of relative stability at the bone-implant interface. Excessive relative movement could inhibit the formation of the afibrillar cement-like substance, perhaps because of excessive mechanical straining of cells attached to the biomaterial surface. These cells would then differentiate to form fibroblast-like cells resulting in fibrous-tissue rather than bone formation at the implant surface. Alternatively,

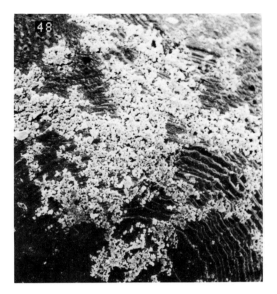

FIG. 4. SEM appearance of mineral deposits formed *in vivo* on a Ti6Al4V particle that is part of a porous-coated disk implant. Thermal etch lines are evident on the powder particle surface. Field width = 15 μm.

excess loading and relative motion following cement deposition and the initiation of bone formation as described above could result in adhesive failure at the implant-cement or cement-bone interface or the prevention of mineralization of collagen because of excessive strains imposed on bone-forming cells in this region resulting in a change in phenotypic expression.

It should be noted that the description of the interface zone at a well-stabilized implant in bone, as presented by Davies et al., is significantly different from an ear-

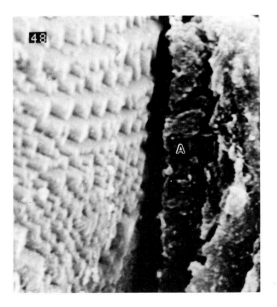

FIG. 5. SEM of interface zone of disk implant placed *in vivo*. Region A is the cement layer. The gap at the implant-cement layer interface is believed to be an artefact due to critical point drying in preparation for SEM examination. Field width = 3.5 μm.

lier proposal presented by Albrektsson et al. (1). Those researchers described a non-mineralized proteoglycan-rich layer separating bone from the implant surface. It was proposed that commercially pure titanium provided a preferred substrate for osseointegration as a result of a thinner proteoglycan layer forming next to it. The studies by Davies et al. suggest that this layer is in fact a calcium phosphate layer formed by mineral deposition within an unidentified loose, afibrillar, organic matrix. No unequivocal evidence favoring any one biomaterial composition over another for forming a rigid interface has yet been presented (considering only the accepted biocompatible materials for bone-interfacing implant fabrication). However, the effect of surface geometry and topography on a much finer scale than previously considered is thought to significantly influence the nature of this interface (8). It appears that submicron-size irregularities can act significantly to promote mechanical keying of the initial calcium phosphate globular deposits and the resulting cement-like layer (see Fig. 4). The possible beneficial effect of elemental interdiffusion with surface oxide layers (specifically TiO_2) is suggested by the studies of Hanawa (10), but further research is required.

SURFACE GEOMETRY AND SENSITIVITY TO RELATIVE MOTION

The cement-like layer-bone interface zone that forms *in vitro* under appropriate culture conditions has been referred to as a "reference" interface "formed in the absence of extrinsic mechanical forces" (7). As discussed above, imposition of loads and resulting strains and relative motion can either prevent the formation of or disrupt such an interface, leading to fibrous-tissue encapsulation (smooth or threaded implants) or attachment (porous-coated implants characterized by three-dimensional interconnected pore channels). From earlier studies (17), different surface designs appear to be more or less sensitive to relative motion. It is interesting to attempt to relate the proposed stages of healing at a bone-implant site, as outlined above, to surface geometry in order to rationalize the observations made on porous versus threaded implants subjected to early loading.

A schematic illustration of an implant interface zone for the situation in which excessive early loading and relative motion have prevented direct bone apposition to the implant surface is shown in Fig. 6. A layer of fibrous tissue is represented between the implant and "new bone" that has formed by appositional growth at the host bone surface. This fibrous-tissue layer is assumed to be attached to the implant surface and forms the interface zone (a pseudo ligamentous attachment). It is assumed that the load acting on the implant causes shear displacement of the implant relative to the bone. A shear strain will develop within the interface zone, its magnitude dependent on the applied load, the shear modulus of the interface zone, and its thickness T. Assuming a uniform strain across the interface zone, the shear strain $\gamma = \Delta/T$, where Δ = the relative displacement and T = the fibrous-tissue layer thickness. It is proposed that initially a relatively thin region of nonmineralized tissue exists between the implant and host bone. For a fixed load and relative displacement, the cells within the fibrin-fibrous tissue matrix in the "gap" region will experience high shear strains. As a result, osteoblast formation and activity may be discouraged resulting in net bone resorption due to osteoclast activity not in balance with osteoblast activity. The resulting widening of the gap region will result in lower shear strains (for the same loads) until the point is reached at which bone-forming cells

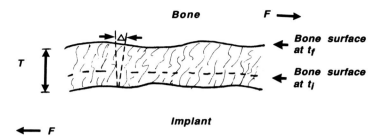

FIG. 6. Schematic illustration of the interface zone for a fibrous tissue-attached implant.

can form and synthesize new bone matrix. This defines an equilibrium thickness of the fibrous-tissue zone. This argument assumes attachment of the fibrous-tissue layer at the implant surface. If fibrous-tissue attachment does not occur at the implant surface, a nonmineralized layer will again form, but mimicking in this case a synovial-like membrane. Such layers have been described in association with cemented and noncemented implants (9,23). The factors determining the thickness of this layer are uncertain. Presumably, compressive deformation would predominate in such layers and the magnitude of compressive dilatational strains would determine membrane thickness, as implied by the differentiation hypothesis of Carter and Giori (3).

For a nonplanar surface (such as a threaded or porous-coated surface), partial mechanical keying of the early fibrin-fibrous tissue interface region with the implant would result in compressive deformation of this layer in addition to shear. As a result, distortion of the fibrous tissue would be reduced, leading to lower strains acting within the interface zone. This would result in thinner equilibrium fibrous tissue layers. Mineralization of the peripheral region might result in mechanical interlock of mineralized tissue with the implant protuberances, thereby resulting in still greater resistance to motion, more bone formation, and greater interlock until the total interface zone is bone filled. Critical to the formation of new bone is the development locally of sufficiently low shear strains (below γ_c). An added benefit of a porous surface structure exhibiting a three-dimensional interconnected pore network is that not only shear and compressive stresses but also tensile stresses can be transferred across the interface zone. Such structures provide more secure anchorage for fibrous tissues, thereby promoting the formation of pseudo ligamentous structures, as described above. With maturation of this ligamentous layer would come an increased resistance to deformation, leading to the possibility of mineralization of the interface zone with time.

CONCLUSION

Whereas other factors such as metal ion release, particulate wear debris, and vascularity are known to affect bone formation around implants, this chapter has focused on the effect of relative movement between implant and host bone during the early postimplantation healing phase. Gross relative movements result in significant fibrous-tissue formation within the interface zone, whereas bone apposition can occur despite some relative motion. *In vivo* studies and *in vitro* experiments suggest that the development of bone within the interface zone requires local strains to be below a critical value, which appears to be equal to approximately 0.01. Implant surface geometry is important in achieving conditions for bone formation. The development of an interface healing zone in which bone formation and rigid fixation can occur requires (i) the formation and suitable attachment of a cement layer (probably by mechanical interlock) at the implant surface, (ii) collagen-fiber attachment to the implant (either through the cement layer or by some other means such as interweaving with a porous-surface coating), (iii) maintenance of this attachment during normal implant loading, and (iv) development of shear strains below a critical level (approximately 0.01) in the interface zone. Maturation of a well-attached fibrous-tissue layer can lead to reduced shear strains that will eventually be below the critical level, thereby allowing bone to form. Repeated high loading of the implant can result in repeated healing tissue disruption, thereby preventing rigid implant fixation. Further studies are needed to provide the quantitative information necessary for the design of more reliable implants and procedures for their use.

ACKNOWLEDGMENTS

Financial support for these studies was provided by the Medical Research Council of Canada and Natural Science and Engineering Research Council of Canada.

REFERENCES

1. Albrektsson T, Branemark P-I, Hansson HA, et al. The interface zone of inorganic implants *in vivo:* titanium implants in bone. *Ann Biomed Eng* 1983;11:1–27.
2. Brunski JB. Biomechanical factors affecting the bone-dental implant interface. *Clin Mater* 1992;10:153–201.
3. Carter DR, Giori NJ. Effect of mechanical stress on tissue differentiation in the bony implant bed. In: Davies JE, ed. *The bone-biomaterial interface.* Toronto: University of Toronto Press, 1991:367–379.
4. Davies JE, Chernecky R, Lowenberg B, Shiga A. Deposition and resorption of calcified matrix *in vitro* by rat marrow cells. *Cells Mater* 1991;1:3–15.
5. Davies JE, Lowenberg B, Shiga A. The bone-titanium interface *in vitro. J Biomed Mater Res* 1990;24:1289–1306.
6. Davies JE, Nagai N, Takeshita N, Smith DC. Deposition of cement-like matrix on implant materials. In: Davies JE, ed. *The bone-biomaterial interface.* Toronto: University of Toronto Press, 1991:285–294.
7. Davies JE, Ottensmyer P, Shen X, Hashimoto M, Peel SAF. Early extracellular matrix synthesis by bone cells. In: Davies JE, ed. *The bone-biomaterial interface.* Toronto: University of Toronto Press, 1991:214–228.
8. Davies JE, Pilliar RM, Smith DC, Chernecky R. Bone interfaces with retrieved alumina and hydroxyapatite ceramics. In: Bonfield W, Hastings GW, Tanner KE, eds. *Bioceramics,* vol 4. London: Butterworth-Heinemann, 1991:199–204.
9. Goldring SR, Schiller AL, Roelke M, Rourke CM, O'Neil DA, Harris WH. The synovial-like membrane at the bone-cement interface in loose total hip replacements and its proposed role in bone lysis. *J Bone Joint Surg [Am]* 1983;65:575–584.
10. Hanawa T. Titanium and its oxide film: a substrate for formation of apatite. In: Davies JE, ed. *The bone-biomaterial interface.* Toronto: University of Toronto Press, 1991:49–61.
11. Hipp JA, Brunski JB. An *in vivo* experiment to investigate biomechanical requirements at the interface of endosseous dental implants. *Trans Soc Biomater* 1982;5:116.
12. Hollis JM, Hofmann OE, Stewart CL, Flahiff CM, Nelson C. Effect of micromotion on ingrowth into porous coated implants using a transcortical model. Transactions of the Fourth World Biomaterials Congress, Berlin, 1992:258.
13. Jones DB, Nolte H, Scholubbers J-G, Turner E, Veltel D. Biochemical signal transduction of mechanical strain in osteoblast-like cells. *Biomaterials* 1991;12:101–110.
14. Lee JM, Pilliar RM, Bobyn JD, Cameron HU, Abdulla D, Binnington AG *(submitted).*

15. Lee JM, Pilliar RM, Abdulla D, Bobyn JD. *In vitro* testing of porous-coated orthopedic implant support after 1 year: differences between fibrous tissue and bone ingrowth. Transactions of the Second World Congress on Biomaterials, Washington, DC, 1984:166.

16. Ling RSM. Observations on the fixation of implants to the bony skeleton. *Clin Orthop* 1986; 210:80–96.

17. Maniatopoulos C, Pilliar RM, Smith DC. Threaded versus porous-surfaced designs for implant stabilization in bone-endodontic implant model. *J Biomed Mater Res* 1986;20:1309–1333.

18. Maniatopoulos C, Sodek J, Melcher AH. Bone formation in vitro by stromal cells obtained from bone marrow of young adult rats. *Cell Tissue Res* 1988;254:317–330.

19. Parfitt GJ. Measurement of the physiological teeth mobility of individual teeth in an axial direction. *J Dent Res* 1960;39:608.

20. Pilliar RM, Cameron HU, Welsh RP, Binnington AG. Radiographic and morphologic studies of load-bearing porous surface structured implants. *Clin Orthop* 1981;156:249.

21. Pilliar RM, Davies JE, Smith DC. The bone-biomaterial interface for load-bearing implants. *MRS Bull* 1991;16:55–61.

22. Pilliar RM, Lee JM, Maniatopoulos C. Observations on the effect of movement on bone ingrowth into porous-surfaced implants. *Clin Orthop* 1986;208:108–113.

23. Revell PA, Lalor PA. Synovial cells at the interface with retrieved implants. In: Davies JE, ed. *The bone-biomaterial interface*. Toronto: University of Toronto Press, 1991:438–443.

24. Smith DC, Pilliar RM, McIntyre NS. Surface characteristics of dental implant materials. In: Kawahara H, ed. *Oral implantology and biomaterials*. Amsterdam: Elsevier, 1989:185–192.

25. Uhthoff HK, Germain JP. The reversal of tissue differentiation around screws. *Clin Orthop* 1977;123:248–252.

Biological, Material, and Mechanical
Considerations of Joint Replacement,
edited by B. F. Morrey.
Raven Press, Ltd., New York © 1993.

Discussion of the Uncemented Interface

Jorge O. Galante and Joshua J. Jacobs

Department of Orthopedic Surgery, Rush-Presbyterian-St. Luke's Medical Center,
Chicago, Illinois 60612

The following represents the views of 15 surgeons and scientists regarding areas of agreement, disagreement, and future needs as related to questions of the uncemented bone-prosthesis interface.

CONSENSUS

1. The use of porous-coated cementless devices for fixation of total joint arthroplasty can give satisfactory clinical results in a large percentage of cases. To date, better clinical results seem to have been obtained from more extensive degrees of coating.

2. The absence of bone ingrowth, as determined by analysis of retrieved implants, does not preclude a good clinical result.

3. The degree of bone ingrowth varies with the specific anatomical site. This is most likely related to local mechanical factors such as the shape of the implant and the ability to obtain initial stabilization, the mechanical properties of the underlying bone, the ability to obtain intimate apposition, and the ability to provide adequate immobilization of the implant.

4. Four modes of failure of the uncemented implant were delineated:

a. Fixation failure secondary to the lack of adequate tissue incorporation (this is an early failure mode);
b. Fixation failure secondary to late trabecular fracture;
c. Osteolysis mediated by a granulomatous reaction to particulate corrosion and wear debris;
d. Severe stress-induced bone loss.

The latter three are delayed failure responses.

5. With contemporary cementless designs, all current porous-coating types should yield low loosening rates in properly selected patients, assuming appropriate bone stock, implant apposition, and immobilization.

6. Osteolysis is the major clinical problem with uncemented implants. Prevention of osteolysis will require attention to a number of factors. Circumferential extensive coatings will help in limiting access of articular wear debris to the bone-implant

interface. For acetabular implants, eliminating screw holes should also eliminate access to the bone-prosthesis interface. The apparent higher incidence of osteolysis in cementless compared to cemented arthroplasty is confounded by the concurrent introduction of modularity in most cementless systems.

7. Stress shielding does occur and is potentially a clinical problem, specifically with large metallic implants used in bone-deficient environments.

8. Bone ingrowth into porous coatings is a desirable outcome in patients undergoing cementless total joint arthroplasty.

9. Bone ingrowth can occur into a variety of types and morphologies of surface porosity. Although experimental studies have suggested that there are differences in the incidence of bone ingrowth between implants of different compositions and surface textures, these distinctions have not been observed in clinical experiences.

10. The stability of cementless implants by roentgenstereophotogrammetry (RSA) has shown to be less than cemented devices. It is recommended that more extensive use be made of this technology to properly evaluate the stability of uncemented components.

11. There currently is no evidence to support the contention that cement is a superior barrier to articular wear debris in comparison to a well bone-ingrown interface.

12. It is unreasonable and probably not necessary to expect complete (100%) bone ingrowth from a mechanical point of view.

CONTENTIONS

1. There is disagreement on the surgical indications for the use of cementless devices. Some surgeons think that the use of cementless devices should be restricted to circumstances in which cement has a poor track record, such as patients under the age of 65 or in the revision arthroplasty situation. There are some surgeons who believe that cementless acetabular fixation is indicated in all patients.

2. There is no agreement on the role or value of soluble calcium phosphate coatings to enhance early bone-ingrowth fixation.

3. The role and efficacy of circumferentially proximally coated, second-generation cementless implants have yet to be defined.

4. There is no consensus on the definition of osseointegration. The initial definition (Swedish) has been changed to a more functional one related to implant stability.

5. There is no consensus on the optimal implant geometry on either a macroscopic or microscopic scale in terms of satisfactory incorporation of the implant device.

NEEDS

1. Because of the high specific surface area of these cementless porous-coated devices, there continues to be a need to carefully document and identify the magnitude and toxicological significance of metal ion release.

2. Identification of the relationship between load transfer and bone remodeling needs to be further elucidated. In particular, the significance of implant stiffness on periprosthetic bone loss needs to be characterized, perhaps leading to the development of low stiffness implants such as composites. To achieve this, significant developments in materials technology are required.

3. Continuing evaluation of the effectiveness of hydroxyapatite coatings, bone growth factors, and other enhancing agents in improving the efficacy of bone ingrowth fixation is needed. The use of these agents may be a function of the anatomical site.

4. There is an urgent need to incorporate designs minimizing the formation of particulates. This can be approached in terms of limiting both the access and sources of particulates. In this vein, considerable attention needs to be paid to improving modular connections.

5. There is a need to characterize the behavior of different types of surface textures, both at the tissue and cellular level. The role of porous "ingrowth" surfaces versus "ongrowth" surfaces in obtaining long-term osseointegration needs to be elucidated.

6. There is a continuing need to evaluate the different porous-coating types in long-term prospective studies.

7. There is a need for basic studies on the relationship of micromotion as well as other variables to bone ingrowth at both the tissue and cellular levels.

8. Prospective clinical studies of current designs to evaluate clinical outcome and objectively evaluate device performance are crucial.

Biological, Material, and Mechanical
Considerations of Joint Replacement,
edited by B. F. Morrey.
Raven Press, Ltd., New York © 1993.

19

Hip Wear

Clinical Aspects

*Michael H. Huo and †Eduardo A. Salvati

*Joint Replacement Center, Waterbury Hospital, Waterbury, Connecticut 06708; †Hip
and Knee Service, The Hospital for Special Surgery, New York, New York 10021 and
Cornell University Medical College, New York, New York 10021*

Understanding of total hip replacement (THR) failures has initially focused on the loss of bonding between bone and cement or between bone and prosthesis in cementless THR. This process has been postulated to be primarily mechanical and generally occurs during the first decade after implantation. However, recent data have supported an associated process that is primarily biologic and observed usually in the second decade following implantation. In this biologic process, macrophages stimulated by wear debris infiltrate the bone-cement or bone-prosthesis interface, leading to significant bone resorption. The progressive erosion of skeletal support subsequently results in loss of prosthetic fixation and loosening (Fig. 1).

Improved methods of implant fixation have increased the longevity of *in situ* service, making wear an increasingly important issue to consider, particularly as joint replacements are being performed in younger patients. Wear debris in THR can be generated at the articulating surface and between the prosthesis, cement, and bone. The authors will address currently available clinical data on prosthetic wear and the biologic effects of wear debris.

CEMENT DEBRIS

Sir John Charnley revolutionized prosthetic arthroplasty of the hip by introducing methylmethacrylate for fixation. The largest clinical experience in THR in the world has been with cement fixation over the past three decades. The mechanically *stable* bone-cement interface has been demonstrated to be surrounded by viable bone, calcium deposition in the collagen fibrils, and hydroxyapatite formation (9). There is no evidence of fibrous tissue or macrophage infiltrate.

Jasty and associates (17) recently reported the long-term autopsy-retrieval study results of cemented THR. On the femoral side, long-term bone remodeling occurred around a well-fixed cement mantle, forming a neocortex that encircled the stem without an interposed fibrous membrane, and provided continued stable fixation and no adverse biologic reaction. They, however, observed cracks within the cement in sev-

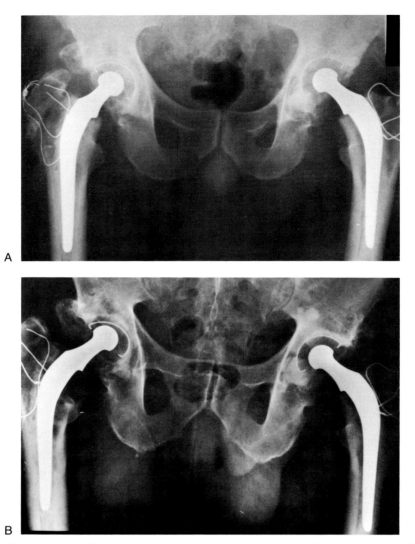

FIG. 1. Radiographs of bilateral Charnley prostheses obtained 2 (**A**) and 14 years (**B**) following implantation at the age of 62 years in a patient with primary osteoarthritis (height 175 cm, weight 99 kg). Both hips had a perfect clinical result until 13 years of follow-up, when the patient noticed progressive right hip pain. The left hip remained asymptomatic. At revision surgery, the femoral stem was well fixed distally, but had undergone proximally a varus, progressive plastic deformation of approximately 5 mm. The severe calcar resorption resulted from the intense histiocytic response, secondary to polyethylene and acrylic debris, as observed histologically. The femoral stem was revised with a long neck prosthesis, the cup was well fixed and left intact, and the result has been excellent.

eral cases and concluded that the initiating event on the femoral side was cement fragmentation, leading to loss of fixation. In two cases with focal bone resorption, electron microscopy of the autopsy specimens demonstrated cement particulate debris.

The histologic features of the bone-cement interface in *loose* THRs are characterized by a layer of fibrous tissue containing macrophages and foreign-body giant cells (10). It has been shown that these cells can produce bioactive cytokines such as collagenase, interleukins, prostaglandins, and tumor necrosis factor, all of which are potential mediators of bone resorption. Cement debris is seen within and around the macrophages. Horowitz and associates (11) demonstrated no evidence of macrophage activation by exposure to methylmethacrylate particles. However, upon phagocytosis of cement particles, macrophage cell death was evident, which led to the release to the tissues of the above-mentioned cytokines and all the intracellular proteolytic enzymes. When cement particles are entrapped in the articulating surface, significant metal and polyethylene debris can occur due to three-body wear. In combination, this particulate wear debris is postulated to activate and accelerate the biologic loosening process.

METAL DEBRIS

Metallic wear in THR can occur in several areas: at the articulating surface between the head and polyethylene; the stem abrading against cement or bone; the metal backing of the cup abrading against cement or bone; the Morse taper between the head and neck; the stem and modular proximal and distal sleeves; and between screws and the metallic shell in cementless acetabular components due to fretting.

We conducted several studies evaluating metallic wear debris in THR using histology and trace element analysis at The Hospital for Special Surgery. Agins and associates (1) first reported nine cases of failed titanium- (Ti) alloy femoral implants. Excessively high tissue levels of titanium, aluminum, and vanadium were found in the periprosthetic tissue in most cases. Histology demonstrated intracellular and extracellular metallic debris. The mean duration from implantation to failure was only 33 months. In another study, we observed gross abrasive wear of the femoral head and stem in 71 all-Ti alloy cemented femoral prostheses retrieved at revision surgery (7). Burnishing of the head was observed in every case with an average 50% of the total surface area. Stem burnishing was seen in 71% of the cases. Femoral endosteal bone erosion was evident in 90% of the hips, and in 51% it was classified as severe. The mean duration *in situ* was 4.5 years. The mean linear polyethylene wear rate in this series was 0.22 mm per year, nearly twice the wear rate reported for stainless steel (SS) and cobalt-chromium- (Co-Cr) alloy prostheses. Furthermore, Lee and associates (19) recently reported that larger polyethylene wear debris was isolated in failed total hips with Ti-alloy articulating surfaces (Table 1).

Brien and associates (5) from our institution demonstrated that there were higher metal and barium levels in the synovial fluid of loose cemented THRs compared to well-fixed hips, based on synovial fluid samples obtained from 44 loose and 37 well-fixed THRs. The femoral components included all three major biomaterials. On average, for the SS group, loose hips had threefold greater Cr and nickel (Ni) levels than well-fixed hips. For the Co-Cr group, loose hips had 10-fold higher Co levels and threefold higher Cr levels. For the Ti-alloy group, loose hips had *21-fold higher*

TABLE 1. *Size of polyethylene debris*

Material	Short dimension	Long dimension
Titanium alloy	4.1 ± 3.2	12.8 ± 11.0
Co-Cr alloy	2.7 ± 1.4	8.1 ± 5.2
Stainless steel	3.1 ± 3.3	8.4 ± 7.5

Values are given as the mean and standard deviation (in micrometers).

titanium levels. Furthermore, for the entire study, loose hips had on average 16-fold higher barium levels representing greater cement debris within the joint. Barium, which is added to bone cement to make it radiopaque, has a hardness similar to stainless steel and can scratch the prosthetic head. The homogeneous distribution of barium sulfate in bone cement is essential to avoid clumps, which, if liberated from the cement and entrapped within the articulating surface, can cause increased three-body wear of the prosthetic head and polyethylene. The higher barium levels can explain in part the greater metal levels and polyethylene wear detected in the loose hips from three-body wear.

Adverse biologic effects of metallic trace elements on cellular function have been documented by several investigators. Rae (25) demonstrated that particulate Co, Cr, and Ni could be toxic to macrophages and fibroblasts in cell cultures. Blumenthal and Cosma (4) demonstrated *in vitro* that titanium levels as low as 0.05 mmol could retard hydroxyapatite formation. The effects of trace elements in cell cultures are generally exaggerated because there is no clearance mechanism, as there is *in vivo*. Nonetheless, these experiments documented the deleterious effects of these elements on cellular biology. It has been shown recently that serum concentrations of titanium were elevated approximately twofold in patients with loose Ti-alloy prostheses, compared to the values for the control patients without hip prostheses (16).

An aggressive and destructive local erosion of the femoral endocortex (femoral endosteolysis [FE]) has been observed to occur with both loose and well-fixed THRs, and with cemented and cementless fixation. We have analyzed the metal and barium levels in 12 consecutive patients with FE associated with loose cemented THRs (13). Histologically, macrophages and cement debris were seen in the FE tissues in every case. Polyethylene debris was present in 92% and metallic debris in 33%. Detectable metal levels were found in all FE tissues. Metal levels were on average 2.5 times higher in FE than in femoral pseudomembrane (PM) from nonlytic areas, and 4.2 times higher than in the pseudocapsular tissue. Barium levels were on average 1.7 times higher in FE than in the femoral PM and 42.2 times higher than in the joint pseudocapsule. Our data demonstrated greater amounts of metal and cement debris in the FE lesions. The greater quantities of wear debris may interact in a synergistic fashion to cause the accelerated bone resorption in these focal sites. This bone resorptive process is also seen on the acetabular side (Fig. 2).

It has been postulated that the size of the wear particles may play an important role in initiating the macrophage biologic response in the bone-prosthesis or bone-cement interface. We recently reported that the particle size was similar for SS, Co-Cr, and Ti-alloy metallic wear debris in periprosthetic tissues retrieved at revision surgery (19) (Tables 2 and 3). It seems that the constituents of the alloy, the amount and speed of debris generation, and the tissue response to them are more likely to be responsible for the bone resorption than the size alone. Shape, surface polarity, and polarity of the particles may also be contributory.

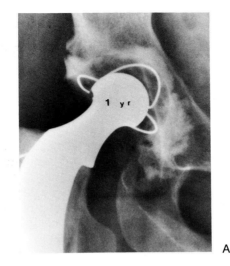

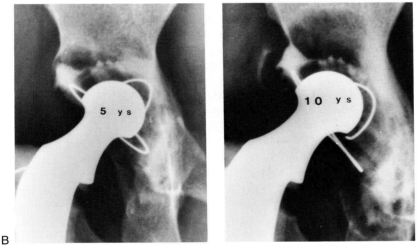

FIG. 2. Radiographs of a Charnley prosthesis, obtained at 1 (**A**), 5 (**B**), and 10 years (**C**) following implantation at the age of 26 years in a patient with juvenile rheumatoid arthritis (height 162 cm, weight 53 kg). Despite the progressive osteolysis of the acetabular dome, the patient refused to consider revision surgery, as the hip was asymptomatic. Eleven years after surgery, she developed acute hip pain and the acetabular cup migrated into the osteolytic lesion. At surgery, the inferomedial acetabular bone cement was intact and well fixed to the bone. The femoral stem was well fixed, despite the 1-cm calcar resorption. The small plastic cup demonstrated 3 mm of superior wear and the histopathology revealed a histiocytic infiltrate, polyethylene, and acrylic debris. The hip was successfully revised with a superolateral acetabular bone graft and the stem was left intact.

Collier and associates (8) recently reported corrosion around the Morse taper in modular femoral components. They analyzed 139 retrieved modular femoral components. In 91 cases the head and stem were made of similar alloy. In another 48 cases, a Co-Cr head was matched to a Ti-alloy stem. A galvanic-accelerated crevice corrosion phenomenon at the Morse taper was observed in 25 of the 48 stems with dissimilar metals. This corrosion was a function of time; in fact, *all* retrieved stems

TABLE 2. *Size of metallic debris with isolation method*

Material	Short dimension	Long dimension
Titanium alloy	0.88 ± 1.01	1.64 ± 1.95
Co-Cr alloy	0.86 ± 1.05	1.57 ± 1.82
Stainless steel	1.06 ± 1.30	1.79 ± 2.07

Values are given as the mean and standard deviation (in micrometers).

with Co-Cr heads impacted onto Ti-alloy stems showed corrosion after 40 months of service. Similar findings have been observed in our laboratory. Available data currently support a corrosive process rather than fretting at this interface. However, corrosion may deteriorate the Morse taper fit with time, leading to micromotion, and excessive metallic debris generation, which could contribute to the loosening process, or mechanical failure of the prosthesis (dissociation or breakage). These observations refute a previous study that concluded that the Co-Cr/Ti-alloy couple was stable (18).

With Dr. Huk we recently completed a prospective study to evaluate the liner-metal cup interface of modular cementless acetabular components as nonarticular sources of ultrahigh molecular weight polyethylene (PE) and metal debris. The PM, which forms at the screw-cup junction and within the empty screw holes of the metal backing, was prospectively harvested at revision surgery in 19 cases after an average implantation time of 22 months (range, 1–72 months). Two of the revised cases had associated acetabular osteolytic lesions that were separately harvested. All the PM underwent histological analysis and atomic absorption spectrophotometry for the trace element titanium. The back surfaces of the retrieved PE liners and fixation screws were evaluated for damage. Scanning electron microscopic examination of the back surface of selected PE liners was also conducted.

The PM from the screw-cup junction revealed amorphous acellular necrotic material containing PE debris in seven specimens (47%) and metal debris in 10 specimens (67%). The PM from empty screw holes revealed acellular necrotic tissue in one-half of the specimens and dense fibroconnective tissue consisting of a proliferative histiocytic infiltrate and foreign body giant cell reaction to particulate debris. PE and metallic debris was present in 14 specimens (88%) and five specimens (31%), respectively. The two specimens from the acetabular osteolytic lesions also showed a foreign body giant cell reaction to particulate debris. The average Ti level in the PM from the screw-cup junction and empty screw hole was 959 μg/g (range, 48–11,900) and 74 μg/g (range, 0.72–331), respectively. The PM from both lytic lesions contained an average Ti level of 143 μg/g (139 and 147). The average damage score of the back surface of the PE liners was 9.6/84 (range, 2/84 to 16/84). Three modes of PE damage were identified: *surface deformation, burnishing,* and *embedded*

TABLE 3. *Size of metallic debris with nonisolation method*

Material	Short dimension	Long dimension
Titanium alloy	0.39 ± 0.13	0.67 ± 0.27
Co-Cr alloy	0.40 ± 0.15	0.69 ± 0.28
Stainless steel	0.36 ± 0.12	0.64 ± 0.26

Values are given as the mean and standard deviation (in micrometers).

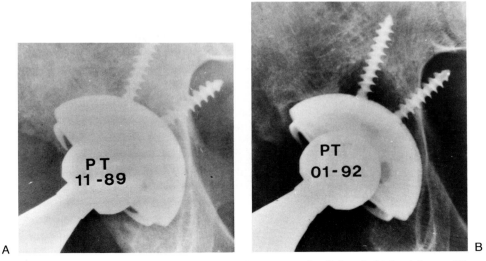

FIG. 3. Radiographs of a Harris-Galante cup with a 28-mm Co-Cr head obtained 1 year (**A**) and 38 months (**B**) following surgery in a patient 37 years of age, with the preoperative diagnosis of osteonecrosis (height 155 cm, weight 93 kg). An asymptomatic, progressive acetabular osteolytic lesion developed during the second year. At revision surgery, which was performed 38 months after implantation, the cup was well fixed, the lesion was curetted and grafted, and the histopathology revealed polyethylene and metal debris. Atomic absorption spectrophotometry demonstrated titanium levels of 138 μg/g of dry tissue in the osteolytic area.

metal debris. All retrieved fixation screws demonstrated fretting at the base of the heads and on the proximal screw shaft.

The identification of PE and metallic debris in the harvested PM and the damage modes identified in the back surfaces of the PE liners and fixation screws retrieved after relatively short implantation times is witness to the fact that each modular junction creates new interfaces for the generation of particulate debris. The particulate debris triggers a foreign body granulomatous reaction with osteolytic potential that will eventually lead to component loosening. The design of modular cementless acetabular components should focus on the minimization of debris generation.

Modularity of acetabular components has provided the surgeon with alternatives for supplemental screw fixation and elevated polyethylene liner. However, micromotion at the liner-cup and screw-cup junctions can lead to wear-debris generation. The empty holes within the cup provide a portal of exit for this debris, which can lead to significant acetabular osteolysis.

POLYETHYLENE DEBRIS

Sir John Charnley's earlier efforts in prosthetic hip arthroplasty using Teflon resulted in severe wear of the cups and rapid bone resorption, which led to the introduction of ultrahigh molecular weight polyethylene (UHMWP). Polyethylene has become the standard biomaterial to fabricate the articulating surface of the cups in cemented and cementless THR. Due to the biomechanical characteristics of this material, wear of polyethylene remains the major source of debris generation in THR.

Bartel and associates (3) outlined three important factors that could influence the stresses arising from contact between the metal and polyethylene in artificial joints: the conformity between the metal and polyethylene, the thickness, and the elastic modulus of the polyethylene. Greater contact stresses are generated in the tibial components of total knee replacements than in THR due to less conformity. Contact stresses in the tibial and acetabular components increase significantly when the thickness is less than 8 mm. Recent data have suggested that there is great variability in the mechanical properties of polyethylene from manufacturer to manufacturer and even from the same manufacturers at different times. This may explain in part the observation of accelerated wear in some hips but not in others with the same implant system performed by the same surgeons (32). Furthermore, the manufacturing and sterilization process may alter the physical properties of the polyethylene, making it more susceptible to wear and biochemical degradation *in vivo*.

Clinical polyethylene wear has been evaluated by serial radiographs and implant-retrieval analysis. It is difficult to differentiate dimensional changes due to creep (cold flow) and wear. Rose and associates (28) reported that wear accounted for no more than 30% of the observed dimensional changes in the polyethylene. Currently, most investigators accept that most of the cup dimensional changes are due to wear rather than creep, a fact that is supported by the wear debris observed in retrieved periprosthetic tissues. The validity of radiographic analysis of cup wear has been questioned. Rimnac and associates (26), from The Hospital for Special Surgery, demonstrated that the radiographic evaluation of maximal change in cup thickness was an accurate indicator of actual wear in 10 retrieved cups. Radiographic analysis of cup wear in metal-backed components is more difficult.

Clinically, polyethylene wear rate by radiographic analysis has been reported to be between 0.07 and 0.15 mm per year. Wroblewski (34) reported radiographic wear rate of 0.096 mm per year in patients with well-fixed Charnley low-friction arthroplasties (LFA) at 15 to 21 years of follow-up. The same author reported in another study a mean rate of 0.19 mm per year in 22 LFA sockets retrieved at revision surgery (33). Our experience at The Hospital for Special Surgery with the first 100 consecutive LFA with a minimum 15 years of follow-up demonstrated a mean radiographic wear rate of 0.121 mm per year (21). The linear direction of maximal wear was vertical in 70% of the hips. Polyethylene wear was positively correlated with calcar resorption. Sixteen percent of the cups showed no measurable wear. Agins and associates (2) reported the 9- to 15-year follow-up in 122 consecutive patients who underwent 244 single-stage bilateral cemented THRs at The Hospital for Special Surgery. Measurable cup wear was seen in 48% of the hips, and 67% of these patients showed cup wear in both hips. The mean wear rate was 1.29 ± 0.14 mm (range 0.5–5.2 mm) for the unilateral cases. The mean wear in the bilateral patients was 1.37 ± 0.16 mm (range 0.5–5.2 mm), which was not statistically different from those that demonstrated unilateral wear.

Some of these clinical studies demonstrated greater wear rate in men, younger patients, and with longer duration of service. However, no statistical correlation has been found between patient weight and cup wear.

Metal backing has the theoretical advantage of distributing surface forces more evenly to the underlying cement and bone and has offered the attractive alternative of changing the polyethylene liner. Metal-backed cups became popular in the 1980s. If the outer diameter of the cup is maintained, plastic thickness must decrease with metal backing and/or larger head size, which may result in greater polyethylene wear and cup loosening.

Clinical data have demonstrated greater cup loosening and revision in THR with metal backing and larger head size. Ritter and associates (27) reported increased radiographic loosening, cup migration, and revision rates in metal-backed cups than in a comparable group of patients with all-polyethylene cups. However, we have not observed any increased cup loosening or revision in metal-backed cups in patients reconstructed using the Charnley system, perhaps because the 22.25-mm prosthetic head maximized plastic thickness (14). Morrey and Ilstrup (22), using survival analysis, reported that the cumulative probability of cup revision rate at 10 years was 0.7% for components with 22-mm heads, 1.5% for 28-mm heads, and 3.5% for 32-mm heads.

Livermore and associates (20) reported that polyethylene wear correlated significantly with head size. The greatest volumetric wear was observed with the 32-mm heads, whereas the greatest liner wear was observed with the 22-mm heads. It is therefore recommended that an intermediate head size (28 or 26 mm) be used. In addition, as the head penetrates further into the cup, the range of motion decreases because of earlier impingement of the prosthetic neck on the edge of the cup. This impingement increases impact stresses on the prosthesis-cement-bone interface, challenging the fixation. This has been supported by Wroblewski (35), who demonstrated a significant correlation between depth of cup wear, cup migration, and loosening. Furthermore, as penetration progresses, the loading direction upon the cup can become eccentric, generating a turning moment on the cup, further challenging the fixation. Wroblewski also showed in an earlier study of 22 retrieved cups that 41% wore laterally to the vertical line, supporting his contention that the loading direction changed as polyethylene wear progressed.

As previously stated, barium from the bone cement can be entrapped in the articulating surface, leading to three-body wear and accelerated generation of polyethylene and metal debris. Isaac and associates (15) recently reported minimal polyethylene wear in eight all-polyethylene cups implanted without cement, concluding by indirect evidence that the cement debris contributing to cup wear probably came from the acetabular side.

Convincing data support polyethylene particulate debris contributing to bone resorption. Howie and associates (12) demonstrated bone resorption and fibrous-membrane formation at the cement-bone interface, induced by intra-articular injections of polyethylene particles in a rat model. We found polyethylene wear debris in 92% of the 12 cases with FE (13). Recently, Schmalzried and associates (29) demonstrated that one possible initiating mechanism in the loosening of cemented cups was a biologically active resorptive membrane advancing from the cup periphery toward the dome. Histologically, polyethylene debris was found within the cytoplasm of the macrophages in this membrane.

In addition to the articulating surface, polyethylene debris can be generated from the outer surface of the cup abrading against the cement or bone in loose cemented THRs. Furthermore, the polyethylene liner may abrade against the metal shell due to micromotion or against the screws in the newer modular cementless cups. Creep and wear can deform a thin polyethylene liner sufficiently to result in mechanical failure. Brien and associates (6) reported dissociation of the polyethylene liner in four cases of preassembled PCA cementless acetabular components. Dissociation of cementless acetabular components assembled at surgery can also occur. Significant variability exists in the locking mechanisms of the polyethylene liner with the metal shell. In some designs, micromotion can be observed at the time of implantation, despite the best efforts of the surgeon. The observation of micromotion and in some cases macromotion is more frequent at the time of revision surgery.

IMPROVEMENTS IN PROGRESS

Improvements in minimizing polyethylene wear have been undertaken in two directions. Extended-chain polyethylene has been developed and its use in THR is being investigated clinically. This material has been demonstrated to have three times less creep and a twofold increase in tensile and flexural strength, with no change in the coefficient of friction as compared to regular UHMWP. It is hoped that with comparable thickness, this material will wear less, thus providing longer *in situ* service.

Aluminum oxide ceramic is highly biocompatible and provides greater wettability and lower coefficient of friction than metal. The flexural fatigue and impact strengths appear to be adequate for the mechanical requirements of THR. However, rare fractures of ceramic heads have been reported (24). The size of the femoral head must not be small, and the surgeon should not hammer the ceramic head onto the neck of the femoral stem, to prevent stress risers leading to breakage. The acetabular component must not be implanted in a vertical position, as it may cause point contact between the head and cup, leading to increased wear and breakage (31).

It is hypothesized that the lower friction in the ceramic-polyethylene articulation will generate less wear. Schuller and Marti (30) recently reported a significant reduction of linear polyethylene wear in hips with ceramic heads as compared to those with metallic heads at 9 to 10 years of follow-up. All heads were 32 mm in size, and all reconstructions were cemented. The average total wear in the ceramic group was 0.26 mm as compared to 0.96 mm for the metal group. The mean annual wear rate was 0.03 mm for the ceramic group and 0.10 mm for the metal group ($P<0.001$).

Oonishi and associates (23) reported on a series of 88 cemented THRs with SS and ceramic heads at a minimum 6-year follow-up. All heads were 28 mm in size. The radiographic linear polyethylene wear rate was estimated to be 0.1 mm per year for the ceramic group, and 0.25 mm per year for the metal group ($P<0.01$). Cups with greater lateral opening and poor coverage resulted in 1.3-fold greater wear than better positioned cups in both groups. Cups with smaller outer diameters (thinner plastic) had significantly greater wear rates than the cups with larger outer diameters.

These data clearly support the superior wear characteristics of ceramic heads, although both of these studies only assessed the wear rate, and no information was given on the incidence of loosening and osteolysis. The high cost of ceramic components is of concern in this time of cost containment. Ion impregnation of Co-Cr heads, a less expensive process, has produced a similar reduction of friction at the articulating surface in laboratory testing. Improvements in the sphericity of the prosthetic head and tolerance (conformity) of the head and cup with better manufacturing techniques, such as prematching the cup and head in the factory, may also decrease wear at the articulation.

Preliminary clinical data support adequate cementless cup fixation without supplemental screws. This will eliminate metal debris at the screw-cup junction. Continuing efforts to improve manufacturing techniques to assure stability at modular junctions to minimize fretting are being made. This is important because increasing numbers of modular systems, which maximize fit and fill of the femoral canal, are being developed and marketed. Improved methods of cement preparation and delivery will minimize crack initiation and propagation in the cement, thus providing longer fixation. Current data clearly demonstrate that accelerated debris generation occurs once prosthetic fixation has been compromised.

Above all, investigators must continue to better define the activation and acceleration mechanisms of the biologic response of the host to wear debris. It is hoped that in the future, biochemical or physical modalities can be applied to the patient to arrest or reverse this deleterious biologic process. Until such advances are available and clinically proven, we recommend routine radiographic follow-up of all THRs to detect early signs of osteolysis. If progressive, we recommend revision surgery, even if the patient remains asymptomatic, to prevent serious and irreversible bone loss. Preservation of existing bone stock remains one of the most crucial factors in ensuring the clinical success of revision THR.

ACKNOWLEDGMENT

Part of this research was funded by the generous support of Ms. Emma A. Daniels, President of The May Ellen and Gerald Ritter Foundation.

REFERENCES

1. Agins HJ, Alcock NW, Bansal M, et al. Metallic wear in failed titanium-alloy total hip replacements. *J Bone Joint Surg [Am]* 1988;70:347–356.
2. Agins HJ, Salvati EA, Ranawat CS, et al. The nine- to fifteen-year follow-up of one-stage bilateral total hip arthroplasty. *Orthop Clin North Am* 1988;19:517–530.
3. Bartel DL, Bicknell VA, Wright TM. The effect of conformity, thickness, and material on stresses in ultra-high molecular weight components for total joint replacement. *J Bone Joint Surg [Am]* 1986;68:1041–1051.
4. Blumenthal NC, Cosma V. In vitro model of aluminum induced osteomalacia: inhibition of hydroxyapatite formation and growth. *Calif Tissue Int* 1984;36:439–441.
5. Brien WW, Salvati EA, Betts F, et al. Metal levels in cemented total hip arthroplasty, a comparison of well-fixed and loose implants. *Clin Orthop* 1992;276:66–74.
6. Brien WW, Salvati EA, Wright TM, et al. Dissociation of acetabular components after total hip arthroplasty, report of four cases. *J Bone Joint Surg [Am]* 1990;72:1548–1550.
7. Buly RL, Huo MH, Salvati EA, et al. Titanium wear debris in failed cemented total hip replacement: analysis of 71 cases. *J Arthroplasty* 1992;7:307–316.
8. Collier JP, Surprenant VA, Jensen RE, et al. Corrosion between the components of modular femoral hip prostheses. *J Bone Joint Surg [Br]* 1992;74:511–517.
9. Draenert K. Histomorphology of the bone-to-cement interface: remodeling of the cortex and revascularization of the medullary canal in animal experiments. *The Hip* 1981;9:71–110.
10. Goldring SR, Schiller AL, Roelke M, et al. The synovial-like membrane at the bone-cement interface in loose total hip replacements and proposed role in bone lysis. *J Bone Joint Surg [Am]* 1984;65:575–584.
11. Horowitz SM, Frondoza CG, Lennox DW. Effects of polymethylmethacrylate exposure upon macrophages. *J Orthop Res* 1988;6:827–832.
12. Howie DW, Vernon-Roberts B, Oakshott R, Manthey B. A rat model of resorption of bone at the cement-bone interface in the presence of polyethylene wear particles. *J Bone Joint Surg [Am]* 1988;70:257–263.
13. Huo MH, Salvati EA, Lieberman JR, et al. Metallic debris in femoral endosteolysis in failed cemented total hip arthroplasties. *Clin Orthop* 1992;276:157–168.

14. Huo MH, Salvati EA, Patterson BM, et al. Metal-backed and all-polyethylene cups in cemented total hip replacements. A comparative study in consecutive patients. Presented at the 22nd Annual Meeting of the Eastern Orthopaedic Association, Madrid, October 1991.
15. Isaac GH, Wroblewski BM, Atkinson, et al. Source of cement within the Charnley cup. *J Bone Joint Surg [Br]* 1990;72:149–150.
16. Jacobs JJ, Skipor AK, Black J, et al. Release and excretion of metal in patients who have a total hip replacement component made of titanium-based alloy. *J Bone Joint Surg [Am]* 1991;73:1475–1486.
17. Jasty MJ, Maloney WJ, Bragdon CR, et al. Histomorphological studies of the long-term skeletal responses to well fixed cemented femoral components. *J Bone Joint Surg [Am]* 1990;72:1220–1228.
18. Kummer FJ, Rose RM. Corrosion of titanium/cobalt-chromium alloy couples. *J Bone Joint Surg [Am]* 1983;65:1125–1126.
19. Lee JM, Salvati EA, Betts F, et al. Size of metallic and polyethylene debris particles in failed cemented total hip replacements. *J Bone Joint Surg [Br]* 1992;64:380–384.
20. Livermore J, Ilstrup D, Morrey B. Effect of femoral head size on wear of polyethylene acetabular component. *J Bone Joint Surg [Am]* 1990;72:518–528.
21. McCoy TH, Salvati EA, Ranawat CS, Wilson OD Jr. A fifteen-year follow-up study of one hundred Charnley low-friction arthroplasties. *Orthop Clin North Am* 1988;19:467–476.
22. Morrey BF, Ilstrup D. Size of the femoral head and acetabular revision in total hip replacement arthroplasty. *J Bone Joint Surg [Am]* 1989;71:50–55.
23. Oonishi H, Takayaka Y, Clarke IC, Jung H. Comparative wear studies of 28-mm ceramic and stainless steel total hip joint over a 2 to 7 year period. *J Long-Term Med Implant* 1992;2:37–47.
24. Peiro A, Pardo J, Navarrete R, et al. Fracture of the ceramic head in total hip arthroplasty, report of two cases. *J Arthroplasty* 1991;6:371–374.
25. Rae T. The toxicity of metals used in orthopaedic prostheses. *J Bone Joint Surg [Br]* 1981;63:435–440.
26. Rimnac CM, Wilson PD Jr, Fuchs MD, Wright TM. Acetabular cup wear in total hip arthroplasty. *Orthop Clin North Am* 1988;19:631–636.
27. Ritter MA, Keating EM, Faris PM, Brugo G. Metal-backed acetabular cups in total hip arthroplasty. *J Bone Joint Surg [Am]* 1990;72:672–677.
28. Rose RM, Nusbaum HJ, Schneider H, et al. On the true wear rate of ultra high-molecular weight polyethylene in total hip prosthesis. *J Bone Joint Surg [Am]* 1980;62:537–549.
29. Schmalzried TP, Kwong LM, Jasty M, et al. The mechanism of loosening of cemented acetabular components in total hip arthroplasty. Analysis of specimens retrieved at autopsy. *Clin Orthop* 1992;274:60–78.
30. Schuller HM, Marti RK. Ten-year socket wear in 66 hip arthroplasties. Ceramic versus metal heads. *Acta Orthop Scand* 1990;61:240–243.
31. Sedel L. Ceramic hip, editorial. *J Bone Joint Surg [Br]* 1992;72:331–332.
32. Wright TM, Li S. Polyethylene: mechanisms of wear and enhanced forms. Presented at the 20th Open Scientific Meeting of The Hip Society. Washington, DC, February 1992.
33. Wroblewski BM. Direction and rate of socket wear in Charnley low-friction arthroplasty. *J Bone Joint Surg [Br]* 1985;67:757–761.
34. Wroblewski BM. 15–21 year results of the Charnley low-friction arthroplasty. *Clin Orthop* 1986;211:30–35.
35. Wroblewski BM. Wear and loosening of the socket in the Charnley low-friction arthroplasty. *Orthop Clin North Am* 1988;19:627–630.

*Biological, Material, and Mechanical
Considerations of Joint Replacement,*
edited by B. F. Morrey.
Raven Press, Ltd., New York © 1993.

20

Wear in Total Knee Arthroplasty

Leo A. Whiteside

*Department of Orthopaedic Surgery, DePaul Biomechanical Research Laboratory,
DePaul Community Health Center, Missouri Bone and Joint Center,
Bridgeton, Missouri 63044*

WEAR

Function and Design Considerations

Kinematic characteristics of the knee produce interactions at the bearing surface to produce an especially difficult series of flexibility and wear problems. Many articular surface features that improve kinematics have an adverse effect on wear conditions, and the reverse is also true. To accommodate the ligaments and maintain correct tension throughout the range of motion, the ligaments must be tensioned much as they are in the normal knee. This produces a joint with a shifting load-bearing area and a combination of rolling and sliding at the articular surface (11). Although large surface area contact can be designed in a portion of the arc of knee flexion, surface area contact must be much smaller than optimal at other flexion angles. A knee that is highly conforming in full extension develops point contact or line contact as the knee flexes past 20°. The posterior lip that is necessary to maintain a large contact area in full extension impinges on the posterior femoral condyles as the knee flexes and thus restricts the range of motion of the knee. A partially conforming articular surface in full extension severely compromises the load-bearing contact surface area and allows sliding to occur at the interface. This sliding mechanism creates "plowing" as the condylar surface area travels across the soft polyethylene (Fig. 1). High tensile and shear stresses exist in the subsurface portion of the polyethylene and create a severe mechanical environment (3). Pitting and delamination result from coalescence of subsurface cracks. On the other hand, highly conforming articular surfaces force the polyethylene structure to constrain the movement of the femoral component. This leads to failure of the structural integrity of the polyethylene and results in deformation due to cold flow of the polymer material (10).

Wear, deformation, and cold flow of the polyethylene are all closely related to the thickness of the polyethylene implant (12). Axial load bearing creates stresses in the polyethylene that are transmitted through its substance into the material below. Because the polyethylene is thin and the counterstresses from the undersurface are

---

Reprinted with permission from Whiteside LA, Nagamine R. Biomechanical aspects of knee replacement design. In: Scott WN, ed. *The knee*. Chicago: Mosby (*in press*).

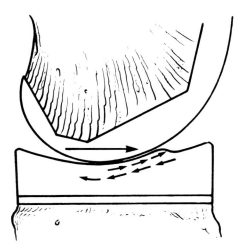

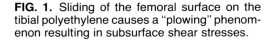

FIG. 1. Sliding of the femoral surface on the tibial polyethylene causes a "plowing" phenomenon resulting in subsurface shear stresses.

concentrated, areas of very high compressive, shear, and tensile stresses exist in the polyethylene between the femoral component and underlying support of the polyethylene. These concentrated stresses increase surface wear and pitting and also magnify the tendency for the polyethylene to cold flow and bend. Metal backing the undersurface of the polyethylene diminishes the tendency to cold flow if the polyethylene is captured peripherally (9). In some knee components linear progression of cold flow with increasing load is found for polyethylene implants thinner than 9 mm if the polyethylene is not backed by a metal shell. As time passes, cold flow and then brittle failure of the polyethylene become an important mechanism for the clinical failure of the implant (9).

Meniscal bearing surfaces that slide with the femoral condylar surface resolve some of the dilemmas created by the kinematic demands and wear problems in the knee. A large surface area can be maintained while knee flexibility is enhanced by allowing the articular surface of the tibia to follow the femoral surface as it is guided by the ligaments (1) (Fig. 2). Very low wear rate and polyethylene deformation have been reported in this mechanical construct (1). However, contact between the undersurface of the polyethylene and edge of the metal tray may damage the polyethylene.

Small areas of contact, combined with complete freedom to rotate and slide from front to back at the articular interface, could be expected to produce especially severe surface wear (8) (Fig. 3). The Ortholoc I total knee replacement is an example of this design configuration. After 5 to 10 years of service, severe surface damage is routinely found when these implants are retrieved during knee revision for unrelated problems such as patellar wear. However, even with Ortholoc I components characterized by linear contact, rotational nonconstraint, and minimal constraint to anteroposterior travel, severe cold flow and catastrophic failure of the polyethylene are rarely seen in this implant. This absence of cold flow and relative durability of the polyethylene-metal construct can be attributed to metal support and peripheral capture of the polyethylene, which prevents cold flow, subsurface wear, and bending of the polyethylene component.

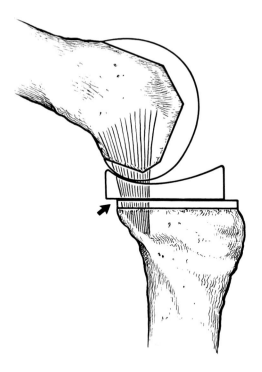

FIG. 2. A meniscal bearing surface helps to prevent stresses on the upper surface, but may increase stresses on the undersurface of the polyethylene by allowing it to slide over the edge of the metal tray.

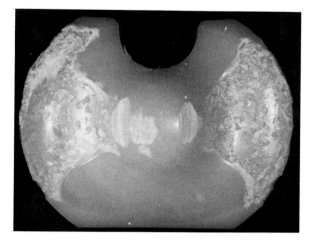

FIG. 3. Wear caused by a femoral condyle with a large radius (flat) distal surface with small radii on each side. Severe wear is present where the medial edge of the femoral component contacted the polyethylene, and cold flow is present where the tibial eminence was impacted.

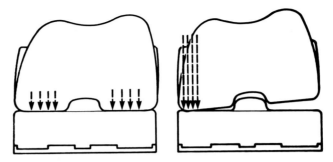

FIG. 4. Flat articular surfaces allow large contact areas, but slight tilt causes edge loading and high contact stress.

Wear along the mediolateral edges of the contact area between the femoral and tibial components is a phenomenon not immediately apparent in design considerations of total knee arthroplasty. Kinematic studies suggest that the lateral side of the knee is often totally unweighted during the stance phase, even in a well-aligned knee, and that the femoral surface can rock into a varus position during the stance phase and load the implant heavily along the medial edge (5). If, on the anteroposterior view, the implant has a single large radius of curvature or other mechanism that prevents smooth tilting of the implant onto one condyle, extreme wear would be expected in the polyethylene under the medial femoral edge (Fig. 4). On the other hand, if the surface were designed with a single radius on the medial femoral condyle and a separate single radius on the lateral femoral condyle with matching radii on the tibial component, then slight tilting could occur without edge loading of the implant (Fig. 5). This should allow smoother functioning of the joint in full extension. Retrieval specimens of the Ortholoc II design have been found to have an improved wear pattern over the Ortholoc I, but also provide an example of edge wear caused by flat contours in the mediolateral plane (Fig. 6). Minimal cold flow is seen over a large surface area, representing the footprint of the femoral component in full extension. However, implants that have been in service for several years in active patients consistently have medial edge wear and cold flow of the intercondylar post—a pattern predicted for flat condylar surfaces. Designs such as the total condylar knee

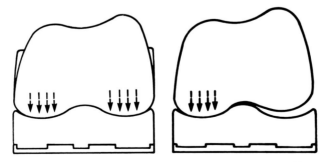

FIG. 5. A single radius of curvature on each femoral condyle also achieves a large contact area, but tilting does not cause edge loading, and contact stresses remain moderate.

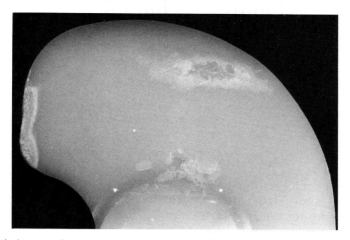

FIG. 6. Polyethylene surface in knee arthroplasty with linear contact and minimal constraint to sliding motions. Pitting and delamination have destroyed the surface, but peripheral capture of the polyethylene has prevented cold flow and destruction of the implant.

replacement, while restricted in some regards, have an advantage in wear because they avoid edge loading (Fig. 7).

The Patella

Patellar wear has been the source of many lessons in implant design. Patellar kinematics dictate a shifting position of load application and an obligatory camming

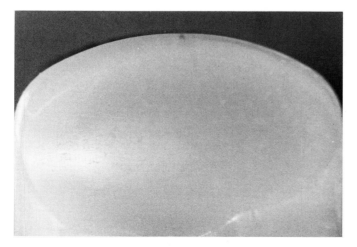

FIG. 7. A total condylar tibial component taken from a patient with persistent valgus deformity. Although lateral condylar cold flow occurred, there was little surface damage because the surface area contact was maintained by a single radius of curvature on the lateral femoral condyle.

action of the anterior femur against the patellar surface. This produces a shifting surface contact area. Despite high loads, the polyethylene must be thin because of anatomical constraints. When enough bone is removed to attach an implant without thickening the articular surface, only 8 to 10 mm of overall thickness of implant can be used to fill the resulting gap. To accommodate the shifting load-bearing surface of the patella, a dome shape appears to be the only design that consistently results in successful patellar tracking. The edges of the dome become dangerously thin, and adding metal backing has produced some disastrous compromises. Metal structures that penetrate the polyethylene surface cause thinning of the polyethylene to a point that yield stress of the polyethylene is exceeded and cold flow and rapid wear cause early failure of the implants (6). However, metal backing of implants that are designed to avoid penetration of the polyethylene by metal have had an excellent track record in total knee arthroplasty (4).

The architecture of the patella makes resurfacing the lateral facet difficult or impossible without changing the thickness and altering the tension of the soft-tissue envelope. A recessed polyethylene dome that leaves the lateral facet to articulate with a smooth femoral condylar surface of the implant has successfully eradicated pain at the patellofemoral joint in total knee arthroplasty and has resulted in very low failure rate. Addition of metal backing to this design has not resulted in an increasing failure rate due to wear (4).

Articular surface materials as well as design are important factors in wear. Increasing surface hardness has consistently increased wear and precipitated disintegration of the polyethylene (2,12). The metal surface also plays an important part in wear at the articular interface. Substituting a titanium component for the standard polished cobalt-chromium surface consistently results in significantly greater wear of both the polyethylene and metal (7) (Figs. 8 and 9), and ion implantation of the

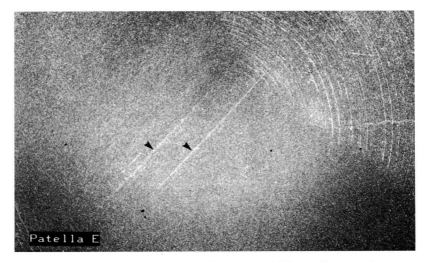

FIG. 8. The top of the dome had mostly polishing and cold flow with only minor scratching in the Co-Cr test group. ×10.62.

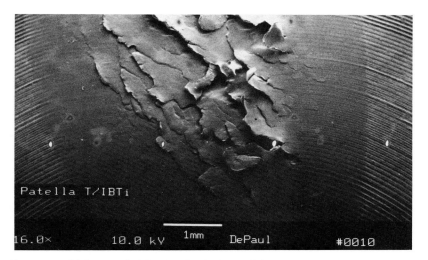

FIG. 9. Extreme cold flow and delamination in four of the six patellae tested against ion implantation of the titanium surface. This form of wear was exclusive to this test group. ×9.6.

titanium surface only marginally improves its wear characteristics (7). Metal surfaces themselves are worn by inclusions in the polyethylene. Even polished cobalt-chromium femoral components are found to have abrasive wear after a few months of active use.

SUMMARY

Kinematic characteristics of the knee create an extreme wear environment, and current materials and designs fall far short of solutions to problems in both wear and flexibility. Achieving a large contact area in full extension and in flexion cannot be achieved by any design. A highly conforming joint surface can achieve excellent surface contact area in full extension, but it blocks knee flexion. On the other hand, a nonconforming articular surface allows the femoral component to roll posteriorly so it does not impinge in flexion, but the nonconforming joint surfaces have such a small contact surface area that wear is unacceptably high. Sliding meniscal bearing surfaces can be made to articulate through a large contact surface area and can also accommodate for impingement that normally occurs with high conformity. However, these surfaces create design dilemmas that have not yet been resolved.

Material considerations are currently a significant factor in clinical performance of total knee arthroplasty, and the metal surface is an important part of this consideration. Polished cobalt-chromium is now the most durable and least damaging of the metal surfaces, but improvement of the metal surface is the next issue to be addressed in the evolutionary improvement of total knee arthroplasty design.

ACKNOWLEDGMENT

The author is grateful for the editorial assistance of D. J. Van Loon, BA, in the preparation of this manuscript.

REFERENCES

1. Argenson JN, O'Connor JJ. Polyethylene wear in meniscal knee replacement. *J Bone Joint Surg [Br]* 1992;74:228–232.
2. Bartel DL, Bicknell V, Wright T. The effect of conformity, thickness, and material on stresses in ultra-high molecular weight components for total joint replacement. *J Bone Joint Surg [Am]* 1986;63:1041–1051.
3. Blunn GW, Hardinge K, Walker PS, Joshi A. The dominance of cyclic sliding in producing wear in total knee replacements. *Clin Orthop* 1991;273:253–260.
4. Cameron H, Cameron G. Stress-relief osteoporosis of the anterior femoral condyles in total knee replacement (a study of 185 patients). *Orthop Rev* 1987;16:22.
5. Harrington IJ. A bioengineering analysis of force actions at the knee in normal and pathological gait. *Biomed Eng* 1976;May:167–172.
6. Lombardi AV, Engh GA, Volz RG, Albrigo JL, Brainard BJ. Fracture dislocation of the polyethylene in metal-backed patellar components in total knee arthroplasty. *J Bone Joint Surg [Am]* 1988;70:675–679.
7. Milliano MT, Whiteside LA. Articular surface material effect on metal-backed patellar components: a microscopic evaluation. *Clin Orthop* 1991;273:204–214.
8. Rose R, Crugnola A, Ries M, Paul I, Ellis E. On the true wear rate of ultra-high molecular weight polyethylene in the total knee prosthesis. *J Biomed Mater Res* 1984;18:207–224.
9. Ryd L, Lindstrand A, Stenstrom A, Selvik G. Cold flow reduced by metal backing. *Acta Orthop Scand* 1990;61:21–25.
10. Walker PS, Hsieh H. Conformity in condylar replacement knee prostheses. *J Bone Joint Surg [Br]* 1977;59:222–228.
11. Wongchaisuwat C, Hemami H, Buchner H. Control of sliding and rolling at natural joints. *J Biomech Eng* 1984;106:368–375.
12. Wright TM, Bartel DL. The problem of surface damage in polyethylene total knee components. *Clin Orthop* 1986;205:67–73.

*Biological, Material, and Mechanical
Considerations of Joint Replacement*,
edited by B. F. Morrey.
Raven Press, Ltd., New York © 1993.

21

Observations of Wear on Retrieved Polyethylene Total Knee Components

Timothy M. Wright and Clare M. Rimnac

*Department of Biomechanics, The Hospital for Special Surgery,
New York, New York 10021*

Observations made from examining retrieved orthopaedic implants can provide evidence of the mechanical performance of the devices. These observations can be used to identify problems in performance and correlate these problems with clinical, design, material, and manufacturing variables. Hypotheses developed from such correlations can then be tested using analytical and experimental techniques. Potential design solutions may result that can be verified through implantation and further retrieval analysis.

An important example of this approach concerns the problem of wear in ultrahigh molecular weight polyethylene total knee components (3). Wear of the polyethylene articulating surface is a significant long-term problem in total knee replacement because of both the osteolysis associated with the release of wear debris (7,11,12) and the tendency for certain total knee replacement designs to fail catastrophically due to excessive wear and fracture of the tibial component (13,24). Finally, failure and dissociation of metal-backed patellar components have been attributed to excessive wear, gross fracture, and permanent deformation of the polyethylene (17,22).

Observations on retrieved components have been used to identify the modes of wear damage and confirm the important clinical and design variables that affect the types and severity of damage (11,13,14,27,28). Analytical and experimental studies have tested hypotheses concerning the influence of these variables on wear behavior (1,6,26) and suggested design solutions aimed at minimizing damage to the articulating surface (1,3). More recently, retrieval analysis has been used to examine the effects of polyethylene material and manufacturing variables (5,16,20,29) on wear damage.

WEAR MECHANISMS

Retrieved polyethylene components examined visually and microscopically have revealed specific damage modes, including burnishing, abrasion, delamination, pitting, surface deformation, scratching, and embedded cement and metallic debris (27,28). The location on the component where damage occurred is a function of component design, but generally damage occurs in high weight-bearing areas, consistent with articulation against the apposing metallic component.

Wear damage to polyethylene is influenced by both clinical and design factors. Observations performed on tibial components of a single design showed statistically significant positive correlations between the amount of polyethylene damage to the articulating surface and both patient weight and the length of time the components had been implanted (27). Other observations on retrieved tibial components of a number of different designs also found a significant positive correlation between the amount of damage and the length of time of implantation (14). Wear damage was also found to be greater in patients who achieved a better ambulatory status postoperatively (10).

The types of damage modes present on polyethylene surfaces are also design dependent. Within polyethylene tibial components for total knee replacement, the appearance of damage modes, such as pitting and delamination, and the occurrence of catastrophic fracture are more associated with designs for which the articulating surfaces are more nonconforming and for which the thickness of the polyethylene layer is small, typically being less than 8 mm (Fig. 1) (27,29).

The fractographic appearance of areas of pitting and delamination is consistent with fracture of the polyethylene material. The surfaces have some of the same features as fractures created experimentally in the laboratory (3,19). Analytical studies have shown that, even for relatively conforming total condylar-type articulating geometries, the stresses occurring on and within polyethylene components are of sufficient magnitude to consider fatigue as a mechanism for these modes of wear. The maximum principal compressive and tensile stresses are high relative to the yield stress of the material, and the movement of the contact area as the knee joint moves through the range of motion assures that portions of the surface will experience cyclic stresses varying from compression to tension. The shear stresses are also significant, with the maximum shear stress occurring below the articulating surface, at about the same depth as the pits and delamination failures observed on retrieved components.

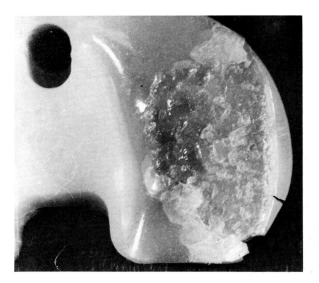

FIG. 1. Retrieved tibial component showing severe delamination of the articulating surface and gross fracture initiating from the periphery.

Recently, experimental evidence has been obtained to further confirm the mechanisms responsible for wear damage. Subsurface crack initiation and propagation were observed to be the dominant mode of failure in cyclic sliding tests of standardized specimens of polyethylene articulating against polished metallic surfaces (6). The geometry mimicked a nonconforming knee replacement in which the polyethylene surface was flat.

More recently, compression fatigue tests were performed on notched polyethylene specimens (18). The applied compressive load ratios (maximum to minimum load) ranged from 16 to 48, as predicted from the results of analyses of total knee components (1). The results demonstrated that crack propagation of as much as 0.15 mm in 100,000 cycles was possible. The mode of crack propagation is consistent with the development of tensile residual stresses at the root of the initial defect upon unloading from compression. These results demonstrate that crack propagation can be expected in the presence of large cyclic compressive loads, consistent with the fracture causing pits and delamination.

DEGRADATION OF POLYETHYLENE

In addition to analysis of surface damage to polyethylene components, the polyethylene can be characterized with respect to changes in density and infrared spectra, using standard methods (9,20). Cylindrical cores, taken perpendicular to the surface, are microtomed into sequential slices (approximately 150 μm thick). Profiles of density and infrared spectra can then be obtained as a function of depth below the articulating surface. These measurements reflect changes in the chemical and physical properties of the polyethylene due to gamma radiation sterilization (21) and oxidative degradation (9). Such changes will result in alterations of the elastic modulus of the polyethylene, an important material property affecting the stresses associated with articulating surfaces (1,26).

The measured changes in polyethylene properties as a result of degradation are nonuniform and are greatest near the surface. The variation in properties caused by degradation as a function of depth from the articulating surface was found to be similar among components in a series of retrieved tibial implants of a single design (29), although the factors influencing these variations are not well understood. In most retrieval studies, the state of the polyethylene prior to implantation is unknown, making it difficult to assess the extent of oxidative degradation that occurred due to *in vivo* exposure. However, comparison of the properties measured from retrieved tibial knee components with typical properties for bulk polyethylene has revealed differences significant enough to predict an increase in the stresses associated with wear damage (8).

To establish the effects of degradation requires comparison of retrieved components to the original stock material from which they were fabricated. To collect such data, a study has been initiated in which the material properties of retrieved polyethylene tibial inserts are being measured and compared to the initial stock properties in the as-received and as-sterilized conditions (20). Preliminary results demonstrate that significant changes occurred to the polyethylene properties beyond those caused by the sterilization process (Fig. 2).

Other confounding, although poorly understood, variables affecting initial mechanical properties of polyethylene, and quite possibly its resistance to degradation,

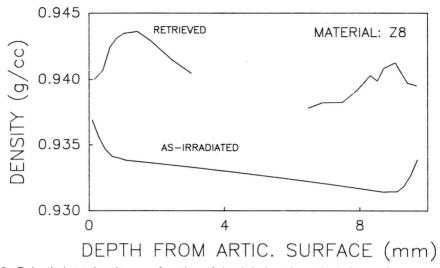

FIG. 2. Polyethylene density as a function of depth below the articulating surface and above the bottom surface of an as-irradiated bulk specimen (Z8 is an internal material code) and a retrieved Insall/Burstein posterior stabilized tibial component. The component was retrieved after 3.5 months of implantation.

are the types of resin used to manufacture the material and the manner in which these resins are fabricated into bulk shapes. Several types of resins have been commonly used to manufacture polyethylene joint components, including RCH 1000 (Ruhrchemie, Oberhausen, Germany), GUR 412 and GUR 415 (Hoechst Celanese, Houston, TX), and Hifax 1900cm (Himont USA, Inc., Wilmington, DE). The differences in physical properties (molecular weight, density, crystallinity) and mechanical properties (elastic modulus, strength, creep resistance) between these resins are significant (16) and probably affect the performance of polyethylene implants (Table 1). Unfortunately, a controlled retrieval study comparing the performance of implants made from the different resins has been difficult to perform, so that no data demonstrating differences in performance exist. Implant manufacturers are aware of the potential problem, however, and most have recently chosen to manufacture implants from a single resin source.

TABLE 1. *Summary of data from 10 lots of ultrahigh molecular weight polyethylene made from 415 GUR resin*

Property	Certification value	Measured value	ASTM F648 guideline
Density (g/cm³)	0.930–0.944	0.930–0.935	0.930–0.945
Yield strength (MPa)	22.3–24.7	21.9–24.7	19.3
Ultimate tensile strength (MPa)	41.0–50.3	30.5–38.5	27.6
Elongation (%)	339–368	260–370	>200
Creep @ 6.9 MPa (%)	1–2	1.6–2.5	<2
Elastic modulus (GPa)	Not reported	1.17–1.59	Not specified

Courtesy of Stephen Li.

The manner in which the resin is fabricated into a bulk shape may also be important to the wear resistance of the resulting component. Implant components have been machined from both extruded rods and compression-molded sheets of polyethylene. In addition, implant components have also been molded directly into final form. These fabrication techniques are known to influence the properties of the polyethylene (16). No significant difference was found, however, in the amount of surface damage between machined and molded tibial components of a single design (28).

METAL BACKING OF POLYETHYLENE COMPONENTS

Metal backing of a polyethylene total knee component has been shown analytically to reduce the stresses in the bone by more evenly distributing the loads transferred to the bone from the component (2). Added advantages of a metal backing include the ability to attach metallic porous structures for fixation by tissue ingrowth and the ability to design modular systems with stem, wedge, and polyethylene insert options.

The wear behavior of the polyethylene inserts in metal-backed total knee components has been demonstrated from observations of retrieved components. For example, the addition of the metal backing requires a reduction in the thickness of the polyethylene to maintain the overall thickness of the implant within anatomical constraints. The severe wear observed on metal-backed tibial components has been attributed, in part, to the thickness (usually <6 mm) of the polyethylene inserts (13,29), with the associated increase in the stresses controlling the damage to the articulating surface.

The method of fixation between the polyethylene insert and the metallic tray can also influence the performance of metal-backed knee components. Analytical studies have shown that when the polyethylene is not rigidly fixed to the metal backing, the stresses associated with surface damage increase (4). In addition, the lack of rigid fixation can allow significant motion at the interface between the polyethylene insert and the metal backing, creating another wear surface from which debris can be released.

The problems with metal backing have been highlighted by the performance of metal-backed patellar components. The addition of a metal backing reduces even further an already thin polyethylene component, leading to increased wear, deformation, and fracture. The gross deformation that occurs in the polyethylene portion of the component makes fixation to the metal backing difficult to design (25). A solution involving any form of interference fit must rely on the polyethylene maintaining its shape throughout the life of the component. Similarly, plastic tabs extending through the metal backing must resist cyclic loading and gross deformation. Consequently, dissociation of the polyethylene from the metal backing is a common failure mode (17,22,23). Dissociation is a serious complication requiring revision and resulting in the generation of considerable metallic debris in addition to polyethylene debris.

FUTURE DIRECTIONS

Methods have been employed to modify polyethylene components in hopes of improving performance. Attempts to improve the mechanical and wear properties of polyethylene through fiber reinforcement have not proved successful. Another method used to modify polyethylene components was heat polishing. Heat polishing involved localized heating, resulting in a smooth, close-tolerance articulating surface. At the same time, however, the heat-polishing process resulted in a thin surface layer (approximately 1 mm thick) of polyethylene with altered physical properties from those of the underlying polyethylene substrate. It has been suggested that the interface between the heat-polished polyethylene and substrate is partly responsible for the significant delamination observed in retrieved heat polished components (5,29).

Perhaps the most reasonable approach to pursue in improving wear performance is to alter the properties of the polyethylene itself. Application of heat and pressure to polyethylene has been shown to have a profound effect on the physical, chemical, and mechanical properties (15). Clinical experience with such an "enhanced" material has been restricted to conforming total hip joint geometries. It remains to be seen, however, what the design considerations must be to apply this technology to develop appropriate "enhanced" polyethylenes for use in more nonconforming total knee joint replacements.

ACKNOWLEDGMENTS

The contributions of Donald Bartel, Stephen Li, Robert Klein, and Lisa Pruitt are gratefully acknowledged as is the support of the National Institutes of Health (grants AR40191, AR38905, and AR01737) and the Clark Foundation.

REFERENCES

1. Bartel DL, Bicknell VL, Wright TM. The effect of conformity, thickness, and material on stresses in UHMWPE components for total joint replacement. *J Bone Joint Surg [Am]* 1986;68:1041–1051.
2. Bartel DL, Burstein AH, Santavicca EA, Insall JN. Performance of the tibial component in total knee replacement. *J Bone Joint Surg [Am]* 1982;64:1026–1033.
3. Bartel DL, Rimnac CM, Wright TM. Evaluation and design of the articular surface. In: Goldberg V, ed. *Controversies of total knee arthroplasty.* New York: Raven Press, 1991:61–73.
4. Bartel DL, Wright TM, Edwards D. The effect of metal-backing on stresses in polyethylene acetabular components. In: Hungerford DS, ed. *The hip, proceedings of the eleventh meeting of The Hip Society.* St. Louis: CV Mosby, 1983:229–239.
5. Bloebaum RD, Nelson K, Dorr LD, Hoffman AA, Lyman DJ. Investigation of early surface delamination observed in retrieved heat-pressed tibial inserts. *Clin Orthop* 1991;269:120–127.
6. Blunn GW, Walker PS, Joshi A, Hardinge K. The dominance of cyclic sliding in producing wear in total knee replacements. *Clin Orthop* 1991;273:253–260.
7. Dannenmaier WC, Haynes DW, Nelson CL. Granulomatous reaction and cystic boney destruction associated with high wear rate in a total knee prosthesis. *Clin Orthop* 1985;198:224–230.
8. Elbert KE, Kurt M, Bartel DL, Eyerer P, Rimnac CM, Wright TM. *In vivo* changes in material properties of polyethylene and their effects on stresses associated with surface damage of polyethylene components. *Trans Orthop Res Soc* 1988;13:53.
9. Eyerer P, Ke Y-C. Property changes of UHMW polyethylene hip cup endoprostheses during implantation. *J Biomed Mater Res* 1984;18:1137–1151.
10. Figgie MP, Wright TM, Santner T, Fisher D, Forbes A. Performance of dome-shaped patellar components in total knee arthroplasty. *Trans Orthop Res Soc* 1989;14:531.
11. Galante JO, Lemons J, Spector M, Wilson PD Jr, Wright TM. The biologic effects of implant materials. A review presented at the plenary session of the 1990 annual meeting of the Orthopaedic Research Society. *J Orthop Res* 1991;9:760–775.
12. Kilgus DJ, Funahashi TT, Campbell PA. Massive femoral osteolysis and early disintegration of a polyethylene-bearing surface of a total knee replacement. A case report. *J Bone Joint Surg [Am]* 1992;74:770–773.

13. Kilgus DJ, Moreland JR, Finerman GAM, Funahashi TT, Tipton JS. Catastrophic wear of tibial polyethylene inserts. *Clin Orthop* 1991;273:223–231.
14. Landy MM, Walker PS. Wear of ultra-high-molecular-weight polyethylene components of 90 retrieved knee prostheses. *J Arthroplasty* 1988(suppl):S73-S85.
15. Li S, Howard EG. Process of manufacturing ultra high molecular weight polyethylene shaped articles. U.S. patent no. 5,037,928, issued 1991.
16. Li S, Nagy EV, Wood BA. Chemical degradation in hip and knee replacements. *Trans Orthop Res Soc* 1992;17:41.
17. Lombardi AV, Engh GA, Voltz RG, Albrigo JL, Brainard BJ. Fracture/dissociation of the polyethylene in metal-backed patellar components in total knee arthroplasty. *J Bone Joint Surg [Am]* 1988;70:675–679.
18. Pruitt L, Koo J, Rimnac C, Suresh S, Wright T. Compression fatigue of ultra high molecular weight polyethylene and its implications for total joint replacements. *Trans Orthop Res Soc* 1993;18:498.
19. Rimnac CM, Wright TM. The fracture behavior of UHMWPE. In: Willert H-G, Buchhorn GH, Eyerer P, eds. *Ultra-high molecular weight polyethylene as biomaterial in orthopaedic surgery.* Toronto: Hogrefe & Huber, 1991:28–31.
20. Rimnac CM, Wright TM, Klein RW, Betts F, Schapiro E. Characterization of material properties of ultra high molecular weight polyethylene before and after implantation. *Soc Biomater Implant Retrieval Symp* 1992;15:16.
21. Roe RJ, Grood ES, Shastri R, Gosselin CA, Noyes FR. Effect of radiation sterilization and aging on ultra high molecular weight polyethylene. *J Biomed Mater Res* 1981;15:209–230.
22. Stulberg SD, Stulberg BN, Hamati Y, Tsao AK. Failure mechanisms of metal-backed patellar components. *Clin Orthop* 1988;236:88–104.
23. Sutherland CJ. Patellar component dissociation in total knee arthroplasty. *Clin Orthop* 1988;228:178–181.
24. Tsao A, Mintz L, McCrae CR, Stulberg SD, Wright TM. Severe polyethylene failure in PCA total knee arthroplasties. *J Bone Joint Surg [Am]* 1993;75:19–26.
25. Wright TM. Design considerations in patellar replacement. In: Goldberg V, ed. *Controversies of total knee arthroplasty.* New York: Raven Press, 1991:145–154.
26. Wright TM, Bartel DL. The problem of surface damage in polyethylene total knee components. *Clin Orthop* 1986;205:67–74.
27. Wright TM, Hood RW, Burstein AH. Analysis of material failures. *Orthop Clin North Am* 1982;13:33–44.
28. Wright TM, Rimnac CM, Faris PM, Bansal M. Analysis of surface damage in retrieved carbon fiber-reinforced and plain polyethylene tibial components from posterior stabilized total knee replacements. *J Bone Joint Surg [Am]* 1988;70:1312–1319.
29. Wright TM, Rimnac CM, Stulberg SD, et al. Wear of polyethylene in total joint replacements: observations from retrieved PCA knee implants. *Clin Orthop* 1992;276:126–134.

Biological, Material, and Mechanical
Considerations of Joint Replacement,
edited by B. F. Morrey.
Raven Press, Ltd., New York © 1993.

22

Design of the Articulation in Total Knee Replacement

Peter S. Walker and Gordon Blunn

*Department of Biomedical Engineering, University College London, Royal National
Orthopaedic Hospital, Stanmore, Middlesex HA 74LP, United Kingdom*

FUNCTIONAL BEHAVIOR OF PARTIALLY CONFORMING ARTICULATIONS

Since the metal-on-plastic surface replacement of Gunston, designed in the late 1960s, the majority of total knee designs, and those used in patients, have been of the partially conforming geometry type. The characteristic of these designs is that the femoral and tibial surfaces generally resemble the surfaces of the articular cartilage. The femoral condyles are usually convex when seen in frontal views, whereas in the sagittal plane, the distal radius is larger than the posterior radius. There have been numerous variations in the geometry of the tibial surfaces, ranging from being in close conformity with the femoral condyles in extension giving maximal conformity, to being flat and thus providing the least conformity without actually being convex. Some designs have allowed unrestrained anteroposterior translation but restrained rotation, whereas other designs, with curved tracks, have provided the opposite effect. Surfaces of high conformity have been found to be incompatible with preservation of one or both cruciate ligaments. On the other hand, designs with flat tibial surfaces have preferably required preservation of both of the cruciates to provide sufficient stability, a scheme that seems to have provided the best function in terms of range of flexion, natural gait patterns, and proprioception. In the middle range, designs of moderate conformity have been found to be best applied to preservation of the posterior cruciate only, the most popular scheme in practice today for reasons of wide application, ease of surgery, reliable fixation, acceptable function, and durability.

Various designs of mobile bearing knee have been in use for a number of years, including the completely conforming Oxford (2) and the variably conforming designs such as the New Jersey LCS (5). A design based on a rolling action has even been proposed (7).

The design parameters of condylar replacements can be examined initially for their effect on clinical performance. If the knee score, using any of a number of methods, is taken as a measure, it is found that many designs of differing articular geometry give similar results. For example, in a recent study (15) comparing a bicompartmental meniscal bearing preserving both cruciates (Oxford), a condylar replacement preserving the posterior cruciate (Kinemax), a condylar replacement with cruciate sacrifice (Insall-Burstein), and a fixed axis hinge (Stanmore), the knee scores and the ranges of flexion were very similar (Fig. 1).

In several studies, flat plastic components used in unicompartmental replacements have given a clinical performance equal to or better than condylar replacements (8) when used as bicompartmentals. The results have been similar to condylar replacements, although there has been a percentage of failures due to instability. The fact that flat surfaces might be susceptible to instability was supported by retrieval data from Blunn et al. (3). From 108 unicompartmental components, used in a uni- or bicompartmental mode, the mean anteroposterior length of the wear tracks was 24 mm, an excursion in excess of that measured for normal knees.

Variations in condylar geometry and preservation or sacrifice of cruciate ligaments may have an effect on long-term loosening due to the differences in the shear forces and "rocking moments" transmitted to the implant-bone interface. Constraint clearly does have an effect, as evidenced by the high loosening rates of partially

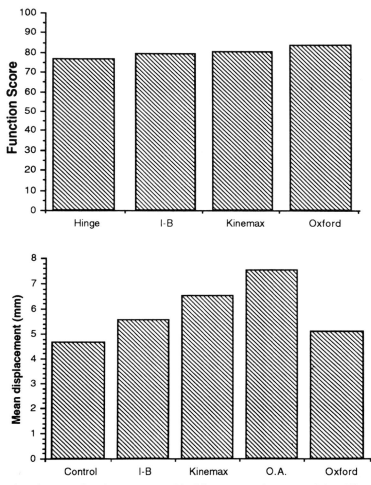

FIG. 1. Functional score of patient groups with different prostheses and the differences in total anteroposterior laxity (Lachman test) at ± 100 N.

constrained linked designs with short intramedullary fixation (Attenborough, Spherocentric), whereas some series of fixed hinges have had very low loosening rates due to the extensive intramedullary fixation (Stanmore, St. Georg, Blauth). However, in the context of conventional condylar designs, differences in fixation performance are difficult to discern from follow-up studies, because of the low loosening rates and variations in design other than those of the articular surfaces themselves, leading to the conclusion that the differences in the interface stresses can be countered by relatively modest and acceptable differences in the means of fixation, such as pegs and so on.

Force Moments and Design Variations

Biomechanical studies have shown certain differences between designs, such as measured differences in the external moments across the knee for different prosthetic designs while walking and ascending and descending stairs (1). Differences were attributed to loss of cruciates, possibly resulting in reduced proprioception, and the reduced quadriceps efficiency due to more anterior contact points than normal. In the studies by Warren et al. (15) noted above, the passive anteroposterior laxity was measured at 20° of flexion (Lachman test) for all designs and found to depend on design type, as well as having a considerable variation within one design type, presumably reflecting the variation in the surgical technique (Fig. 1). However, the variations did not correlate with clinical score, except to the extent that laxity below 5 mm led to a reduced score due to reduced range of flexion and lack of full extension.

Joint Laxity

Laxity under compressive force is more relevant to functional considerations. Thatcher et al. (12) tested a range of condylar total knees by applying a compressive force of 1,000 N, shear forces of up to 350 N, and torques up to 23 Nm, and then measuring the displacements. There was a wide variation in results depending on the femoral-tibial geometry and the presence of stops. Anteroposterior excursions were small in extension, usually 2 to 4 mm in each direction, but in flexion the values were greater and some designs dislocated. In rotation the laxity was between 8° and 15° in each direction for the condylar designs. From a literature review of normal knees, the anteroposterior laxity was 4 to 8 mm in extension, increasing to 6 to 10 mm in flexion, but reducing by 30% to 50% when a compressive force was applied. Warren et al. (15) measured the rotational laxities of the knee while the subjects twisted to the left and then to the right. For normal subjects the mean values were 12° internal rotation and 9° external. For ranges of condylar knees (Oxford, Kinemax, Insall-Burstein), the mean values were 8° to 10° internal and 6° to 7° external. There was little correspondence with the degree of conformity, including the unconstrained Oxford meniscal design, which showed a laxity similar to that of other designs. The conclusion was that the laxity was determined by a combination of the articular surfaces and soft tissues, as well as the function being performed. Augmentations of stability have been provided to substitute for the posterior cruciate, as in the Kinematic/Kinemax Stabilizer and I-B Posterior Stabilized designs. Although these designs have avoided the problem of posterior tibial subluxation, which might otherwise have occurred, there is no evidence of any differences in clinical behavior compared with conventional condylar replacements.

From data such as those above, it is concluded that from a functional point of view, there should be an amount of femoral-tibial conformity, such as to confer similar anteroposterior and rotational laxity characteristics to that of the normal knee. For cruciate-preserving designs, low to moderate conformity is appropriate; for sacrifice of the anterior cruciate ligament, increased posterior tibial curvature is indicated, whereas for sacrifice of both cruciates, increased anterior and posterior curvature, with the option of stabilizing posts, is required. Several designs in these categories have given impressive results at 5- to 10-year follow-up times and even longer. An important question is whether such designs, using currently available materials, are adequate for general use when the life expectancy of many of the patients is 10 to 20 years or longer.

WEAR OF THE POLYETHYLENE

In the present context, the term wear is used to describe the different types of material removal and material damage, consistent with observations from retrievals. First, there is fine particulate wear occurring at the surface with particle size in the range 0.1 to 10 μm. This type of wear, noted in total hips, occurs due to adhesive and three-body abrasive mechanisms occurring at the surface itself. The volumetric wear is proportional to the force acting times the sliding distance. For a constant activity level over the years, the wear rate will be closely constant. (It is difficult to distinguish fine particulate wear from deformation, and the two are likely to occur in unison.) Second, there is abrasive wear due to the action of foreign particles such as cement and bone fragments. This will produce larger polyethylene particles and cutting of the polyethylene surface, as well as particles of the third-body material itself. Third, there is delamination wear, which occurs due to the gradual build-up of subsurface cracks, eventually coalescing to release large fragments from approximately 100 μm and larger. This type of wear may not be evidenced for many years of use, but once it begins, its progress can be rapid, leading to total destruction of the bearing surface. The theory of delamination wear was initially explained for acrylic by Wannop and Archard (14) and for metals by Suh (11). For a sphere loaded against a flat plane, the surface pressure distribution is hemispherical with the maximal pressure (p_{max}) being 1.5 times the mean. There is a radial tensile stress with a maximum around the boundary of $0.13 \times p_{max}$ (assuming a Poisson's ratio of 0.3). The maximal shear stress of $0.31 \times p_{max}$ occurs at the center of the contact at a depth of 0.25 × contact diameter. For a total knee with a typical contact area radius of 4 mm, this depth is 2 mm. When surface sliding occurs with friction, the stress distribution changes. The peripheral tensile stress increases at the trailing edge by a factor of almost 2 for a friction coefficient of 0.1, typical of metal on polyethylene, but by a factor of 5 for a friction coefficient of 0.3, typical of metal on acrylic, which can occur if acrylic particles become embedded in the polyethylene. This tensile stress decays rapidly below the surface, however, and cracks that develop at the surface would cease to propagate. However, they can account for the surface pitting frequently observed on retrievals. The magnitude of the maximum shear stress below the surface changes little with friction, but the depth moves toward the surface with increasing friction, reaching the surface at a friction coefficient of 0.11.

In recent years a great deal of information has been obtained about the factors that contribute to wear, from retrieval, experimental, and theoretical studies. It is difficult to reach firm conclusions about wear mechanisms from retrieval studies because of the large number of variables involved, the incomplete information, and the fact that most retrievals are from failures where other circumstances such as wear or instability may have led to additional wear. However, if enough data can be obtained, hypotheses can be advanced, which can then be tested under controlled conditions. Furthermore, any laboratory study must be able to reproduce the results seen in retrievals to determine validity. Retrieval studies in the past have often concluded that the wear was only slight or only occurred in adverse clinical situations. However, it has not been until recently that retrievals in sufficient numbers and with sufficient follow-up have been possible. The conclusions now are that in certain conditions, severe wear can occur, although considering the large "denominator" from which the retrieval samples have been obtained, it is still not clear whether there will be a major problem after 10 to 15 years and longer.

Delamination wear of PCA knees occurred due to the hot pressing causing a line of weakness in a region approximately 1 mm below the plastic surface, which is a region of high shear stresses. In several designs, thin components have suffered the most severe wear because the stresses are increased due to the underlying metal backing. Wear of all types has been observed in all types of designs with a range of geometries (9). The properties of the plastic material have been implicated as affecting the wear. Higher molecular weight has been considered to be an advantage. Defects in the material such as fusion defects between polyethylene granules have been implicated in providing the initiation sites for cracks and accelerating the delamination type of wear. Components with highly dished tibial surfaces, such as the Total Condylar and Attenborough, have shown a tendency for the entrapment of acrylic particles, which has led to three-body abrasive wear.

Articular Conformity and Debris

It is generally assumed that components with low conformity, and thus high contact stresses, will undergo the highest amount of wear, and vice versa. However, this hypothesis has so far not been consistently supported by the retrieval data. In a current study in our laboratory, more than 200 retrieved knees of several design types have been obtained. Of these, 106 flat unicondylar components were retrieved at follow-up times of up to 19 years. The three types were the Marmor, St. Georg Sledge, and PCA. The wear tracks were typically elongated in the anteroposterior direction with an average length of 24 mm. The Marmor design showed shiny elongated depressions with some surface pitting, but no subsurface defects or cracks were detected from studying sections with scanning electron microscopy. Most of the St. Georg's showed some regions of delamination on the surface to approximately 1 mm in depth. Subsurface cracks were observed, which had evidently initiated around small fusion defects in the polyethylene measuring approximately 150 μm in diameter. The PCA components showed similar wear to that described above for the condylar type. It is noted that the Marmor and Sledge designs did not have metal backing, with the exception of a small number of the Sledges. In the condylar replacement retrievals, delamination wear was observed in components of moderate to high conformity, including the Kinematic 1 and Total Condylar designs. This could be partly explained by high stresses in the plastic being generated by the forces restraining anteroposterior and rotational laxity. Hence, a hypothesis of knee wear based on conformity or contact stresses cannot be supported by the retrieval data so far.

A possible exception was in a study of the Oxford meniscal bearing knee, which is completely conforming at all angles of flexion (2). Twenty-three plastic bearings were retrieved at 10 to 112 months, with all but two being 65 months or less. Depending on the measurement method, the mean penetration rate was 0.026 or 0.043 mm per year. These data were compared with a mean penetration rate in Charnley total hips of 0.19 mm per year. The difference was ascribed to the greater area of contact in the meniscal knees (5.7 cm^2 for each meniscal bearing) than in the hips (3.8 cm^2) leading to lower contact stresses. However, surface pitting was observed, and the follow-up times were relatively short.

Laboratory studies were conducted in an attempt to simulate the sliding conditions of condylar knees occurring *in vivo* (4). The evidence from various studies of knee kinematics was that there was a variety of conditions at the tibial-femoral articulation, including cyclic force at a single point, rolling, and pure sliding. A test machine was constructed to simulate these kinematic conditions. Spherical-ended metal indenters of 25 and 75 mm radii were loaded onto flat polyethylene surfaces under a cyclic force of 2.2 kN at 10 Hz. The plastic specimens were oscillated along a track of 10 mm at 1 Hz. After 10 million cycles the damage to the plastic was examined using scanning electron microscopy. Cyclic forces with no motion resulted in surface indentation only with no subsurface damage. Rolling produced both surface indentation and some surface fine particulate wear but minimal subsurface damage. Sliding resulted in surface wear and subsurface damage consisting of cracks. These cracks were similar to those seen in retrieved specimens as the precursor of delamination wear (Fig. 2A). However, delamination resulting in gross disruption of the surface was not observed. A phenomenon observed on most samples was a layer on the surface ranging in thickness from 10 to 100 μm showing severe disruption, apparently due to the cyclic shear stresses across the surface. The same appearance was noted on many of the retrieval specimens. Thin sections were studied with polarized light microscopy, which revealed stresses due to the photoelastic effect. Surface wear was characterized by local high stresses on surface asperities, a phenomenon that has been noted by Dowson et al. (*personal communication*) (Leeds-Lyon Tribology Symposium). Around the periphery of subsurface intergranular fusion defects, local stress concentrations were observed. This explained the cracks that were seen to emanate from the corners of such defects and would lead to crack propagation, eventually producing delamination wear (Fig. 2B).

The significance of subsurface defects and cracks was indicated in a study by Connelly et al. (6). Polyethylene specimens with an initial v-shaped crack were tested in fatigue at different levels of stress and the crack growth rates studied. There was a steep slope to the curve of the rate of crack propagation against stress intensity, such that a 10% increase in the stress intensity resulted in an order of magnitude increase in crack growth rate. The authors pointed out that fatigue testing of a smooth specimen combines the entire process through crack initiation, crack growth, and catastrophic failure. Preexisting flaws such as fusion defects in the polyethylene would result in a rapid initiation phase, reducing the time for the complete process to occur. Further wear studies were carried out (4) to determine whether

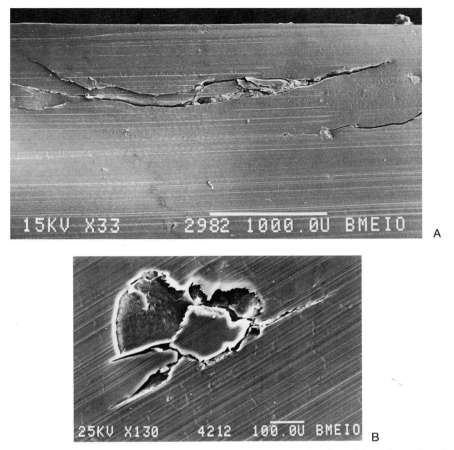

FIG. 2. A: A section through the plastic component of a retrieved unicondylar. The subsurface cracks appear to initiate from and traverse through defects in the plastic. **B:** Cracks propagating from a defect in the plastic.

polyethylene with subsurface fusion defects would lead to extensive delamination compared with material with no microscopically discernible defects. Samples were obtained of "good" polyethylene from unused Marmor unicondylar components, and "bad" polyethylene from unused St. Georg components. The test conditions were as described above, with one test being in serum and the other in distilled water, run for 20 and 10 million cycles. In all tests, there was surface wear of the fine particulate type. In scanning electron micrographs, numerous fine particles were visible on and adjacent to the wear tracks. The depth of the wear tracks was less for the serum lubrication, compared with the distilled water. No subsurface cracks were observed in the scanning electron micrographs on sections of the good material, whereas on the bad material, cracks were observed to emanate from the fusion defects. However, the cracks were not extensive and had not resulted in breakdown of the material.

A THEORY OF WEAR IN CONDYLAR KNEES

The reasons why extensive surface wear and delamination wear have not been observed in a large proportion of retrieval samples and why severe delamination did not occur in the above laboratory wear tests may be due to the different factors leading to the two types of wear (Fig. 3). If it is assumed that the surface wear follows the classical rule of volume = force × sliding distance, then the volume would depend on the articular geometry to the extent that the surfaces controlled the sliding distance. At present, there have been no direct measurements of surface sliding of prosthetic knees in normal activities (with the exception of sequential radiographic studies in mounting a step). However, gait studies have shown that in the stance phase of walking, the angular motion is small. Hence, surface sliding is likely to depend on the conformity of the surfaces in the sagittal view, the least conforming allowing the greatest excursions in response to the shear forces. In such designs, one that was closely conforming in the frontal plane would show a low rate of surface penetration, and one that had low conformity in the frontal plane would show a higher rate of surface penetration. For this type of wear, it is not necessary to introduce contact stress as a variable to explain the different penetration rates.

Delamination wear on the other hand is a fatigue phenomenon, depending on the number of loading cycles and the magnitude of the load and the internal stresses in the material. As noted above, a certain number of cycles will be necessary for the crack initiation and propagation phases. Defects in the material, such as intergran-

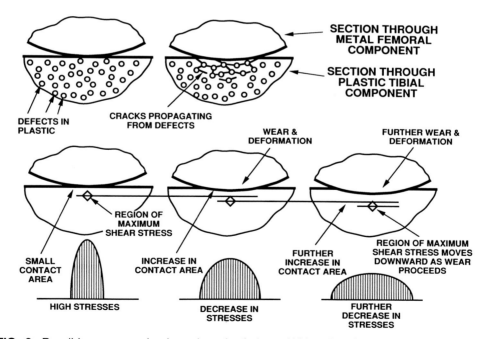

FIG. 3. Possible wear mechanisms in polyethylene. With subsurface defects (*top*) cracks propagate from the defects leading to delamination wear. With no defects (*bottom*) surface wear proceeds but subsurface cracks do not initiate. The changing level of maximal shear stresses helps to prevent (or delay) crack initiation.

ular fusion defects, will effectively eliminate the initiation phase. Some indications of the number of cycles needed for each phase can be obtained from the retrieval and laboratory wear data. In the Marmor prostheses, subsurface cracks were not observed, even in specimens of 10-year follow-up and more. In contrast, delamination wear was seen on most of the St. Georg prostheses at 5 to 10 years. Seedhom and Wallbridge (10) made measurements of the number of gait steps per year in 243 individuals in four different occupations across a wide age span. The average steps per day for men and women were 9,537 and 9,839, respectively. If the load cycle per step is considered to have two force peaks, the average number of force peaks per year for each knee is approximately 3.5 million. Hence, to simulate 10 years of use, 35 million load cycles are needed. Most of our laboratory tests were only up to 10 million (most other tests reported in the literature are also 10 million or less). Hence, delamination wear would not be expected to have occurred. The above suggests that the crack initiation phase, even at high stress, takes at least 10 years to occur, but that the crack propagation phase may take a much shorter time.

The delamination wear may, however, be affected by the surface wear. Delamination depends on a particular location in the material experiencing high stresses for the required number of load cycles. If the relevant type of stress is shear or Von Mises, the location of maximum stress is directly under the center of the contact area at approximately 1 mm below the surface. If the depth of surface wear proceeds at a significant rate, as in the low-conformity Marmor prostheses, then the level of subsurface maximum stress will similarly move downward with time. Thus, a particular level may not experience a sufficient number of load cycles at the required stress level for severe crack initiation and propagation to occur. Under this theory, for polyethylene with few initial subsurface defects, durability may be longer for prostheses of low conformity. For polyethylene with a significant number of subsurface defects, the durability may be more or less independent of conformity. However, more detailed experimentation and theoretical treatment will be needed to quantify the above theory.

ACKNOWLEDGMENTS

The authors are grateful to the Department of Health (UK), and to Howmedica, Pfizer Health Care Products, for support of this work.

REFERENCES

1. Andriacchi TP, Stanwyck S, Galante JO. Knee biomechanics and total knee replacement. *J Arthroplasty* 1986;1:211–219.
2. Argenson JN, O'Connor JJ. Polyethylene wear in meniscal knee replacement. *J Bone Joint Surg [Br]* 1992;74:228–232.
3. Blunn GW, Joshi A, Lilley PA, et al. Polyethylene wear in unicondylar knee prostheses. *Acta Orthop Scand* 1992;63:247–255.
4. Blunn GW, Walker PS, Joshi A, Hardinge K. The dominance of cyclic sliding in producing wear in total knee replacements. *Clin Orthop* 1991;273:253–260.
5. Buechel FF, Pappas MJ. New Jersey low contact stress knee replacement system. *Orthop Clin North Am.* 1989;20:147–177.
6. Connelly GM, Rimnac CM, Wright TM, Hertzberg RW, Manson JA. Fatigue crack propagation behaviour of ultrahigh molecular weight polyethylene. *J Orthop Res* 1984;2:119–125.
7. Elad D, Seliktar R, Mendes D. Synthesis of a knee joint endoprosthesis is based on pure rolling. *Eng Med* 1981;10:97–105.

8. Jensen RE, Collier JP, Mayor MB, Surprenant VA. The role of polyethylene uniformity and patient characteristics in the wear of tibial knee components. *Proc Orthop Res Soc* 1992;17:328.

9. Knutson K, Lewold S, Lidgren L. Outcome of revision for failed unicompartmental knee arthroplasty for arthrosis. American Academy of Orthopaedic Surgeons, poster exhibit, Washington, DC, February 1992.

10. Seedhom BB, Wallbridge NC. Walking activity and wear on prostheses. *Ann Rheum Dis* 1985; 44:838–843.

11. Suh NP. *Tribophysics*. Englewood Cliffs, NJ: Prentice-Hall, 1986.

12. Thatcher JC, Zhou XM, Walker PS. Inherent laxity in total knee prostheses. *J Arthroplasty* 1987;2:199–207.

13. Walker PS. Bearing surface design in total knee replacement. *Eng Med* 1988;17:149–156.

14. Wannop GL, Archard JF. Elastic hysteresis and a catastrophic wear mechanism for polymers. *Proc Inst Mech Eng* 1973;187:615–623.

15. Warren PJ, Olanlokun KF, Cobb AG, Walker PS. The relationship between antero-posterior laxity and function in knee replacements *(submitted)*.

Biological, Material, and Mechanical Considerations of Joint Replacement, edited by B. F. Morrey. Raven Press, Ltd., New York © 1993.

23

The Articulation

Material Considerations

Donald L. Bartel

Department of Mechanical and Aerospace Engineering, Cornell University, Ithaca, New York 14853

The longevity of contemporary total joint replacements is limited because of debris that can accumulate in the tissue surrounding the implant and can subsequently lead to late loosening of the prosthesis and late infection. Much of this debris is generated because of damage that occurs to the articulating surfaces. The minimization or elimination of this problem is one of our most important tasks.

Most total joint replacements involve contact between convex and concave surfaces where the convex component is made from a stiff material such as metal or ceramic and the concave component is made from a much less stiff material such as polyethylene. Convex-convex contact does occur between the patellar and femoral components of some contemporary total knee replacements. However, in this chapter the focus will be on damage due to contact between convex metal and concave polyethylene components because this is the combination with which we have the most experience.

Damage to articulating surfaces may be caused by three-body wear in which foreign bodies, such as polymethylmethacrylate particles, are caught between the surfaces. As the joint moves, these bits of foreign material gouge and scratch the components, releasing particles from the surfaces into the joint space. This, however, is not the only mechanism for generating wear debris. Retrieval analyses show that surfaces can be damaged in the absence of three-body wear. Contact between the metal and polyethylene components produces high stresses on and within the polyethylene. These stresses, along with the relative motion of the contacting surfaces, are sufficient to cause localized failure of the materials, which has been observed as abrasion, pitting, and delamination in retrieved components.

Both the metal and polyethylene surfaces can become damaged; both metal and polyethylene debris have been found in tissue around joint components. However, it is the polyethylene debris that has generally caused the greatest concern. In most cases there is more of it, and the tissue reactions to polyethylene are more severe than to metal debris. Therefore, in recent years most of the research and design efforts that have addressed the minimization of surface damage have been directed toward polyethylene components. These have included retrieval analysis to determine the extent and magnitude of *in vivo* damage; materials testing to determine the strength, stiffness, and fracture characteristics of polyethylene; stress analysis to determine the stresses on and within the polyethylene components due to contact; and design modifications that minimize the stresses associated with damage to the articular surface.

Debris is liberated from polyethylene components by abrasion, pitting, and delamination of the surface (5). Retrieval studies have established that in knees and hips these damage modes increase with time of implantation and with patient weight (7). The forces transmitted across a joint increase with increasing body weight and the number of cycles of loading increases with time of implantation. Therefore, strong evidence exists that damage to artificial joint surfaces involves fatigue processes due to the cyclic loading of the joint.

The stresses acting on and within the polyethylene components for various loading conditions must be determined to understand the mechanisms by which these damage modes occur. These stresses are a function of the magnitude of the contact forces, conformity of the contacting surfaces, kinematic characteristics of the joint, thickness of the polyethylene components, and material properties of the polyethylene. The material properties play a very important role. As will be described, the stresses associated with surface damage are sensitive to the stiffness of the material. As the stiffness of the material increases, the stresses due to contact also increase. Consequently, stronger materials are desirable if surface damage is to be minimized. However, an increase in strength is usually accompanied by an increase in stiffness, which results in an increase in stress. Therefore, benefit is only achieved if the strength is increased to a greater extent than the stresses.

The stresses on and within polyethylene components are also increased as the material degrades in vivo. Retrieval analyses show that the density of the polyethylene increases with time of implantation. Because the stiffness of polyethylene is proportional to the density of the material, increases in density are accompanied by increases in the stresses that cause damage to the articulating surfaces.

Whatever the source of the high stresses, design or degradation, their effect is exacerbated by defects on the surface or within the polyethylene. Consequently, the production of the material itself, the manufacturing processes used to obtain prosthetic components from the material, and the treatments, if any, of the surfaces play major roles in minimizing the damage modes that are responsible for generating debris.

The purposes of this chapter are to review the mechanics of contact in total joint replacements, show the dependence of stresses on material properties of polyethylene, discuss the effects of degradation of polyethylene on stresses associated with damage, and relate these to issues concerning the design of total joint replacements.

DEFORMATION AND STRESS IN POLYETHYLENE COMPONENTS

The elastic modulus of metal components is so much greater than the elastic modulus of polyethylene that any deformation of the metal component may be neglected in comparison to the deformation of the polyethylene component. Consequently, the metal component may be considered to act as a rigid indenter, which under contact, deforms an elastic layer, the polyethylene component. Three types of deformation are important.

First, the polyethylene is squeezed between the metal indenter and supporting bone or metal backing, producing compressive stresses perpendicular to the contact surface. These compressive stresses increase with decreasing thickness of the material, decreasing conformity between the components, and increasing elastic modulus of the polyethylene (3). In each case the penetration of the indenter decreases, resulting in a decrease in contact area and a subsequent increase in contact stress.

Second, the surface of the polyethylene component is stretched as the indenter penetrates the material. The stretching takes place near the edge of the contact area causing tensile stresses at the articulating surface that act tangentially to the surface of the implant. In the center of the contact area, the opposite occurs. The material is subjected to compressive stresses tangential to the surface. As the material is squeezed in a direction normal to the surface, it tries to expand but cannot do so because of the resistance to radial deformation (compressive stresses tangential to the surface) provided by the surrounding material.

These tensile and compressive stresses are important when considered in conjunction with the kinematics of the knee joint. Most total knee replacements are designed to provide motion that causes the contact area to move with respect to the polyethylene. Consequently, a point on the articulating surface will be subjected to compressive stresses when the contact area is centered over the point, tensile stresses when the edge of the contact area has moved to the point, and zero stress when the contact area has moved so the point is outside the contact area. Thus, during flexion and extension of the knee joint, the material at a point on the surface of the polyethylene will be subjected to tensile and compressive stresses that act tangentially to the surface. Such stresses would cause cracks at the surface to propagate perpendicular to the surface of the polyethylene component. The tensile stresses at the edge of contact decrease rapidly with increasing depth, becoming zero less than half a millimeter beneath the surface and reaching their largest compressive value at a depth of approximately 1 mm. The shear stresses at the surface at this location are zero if friction is neglected and increase rapidly with depth. A crack initially propagating perpendicular to the articulating surface would be caused to turn because of the changing stress field. This provides a possible explanation for the formation of the pits that are observed in retrieval studies.

Third, the polyethylene is distorted (subjected to shear stress) as the indenter deforms the surface of the polyethylene. The maximum shear stress occurs beneath the surface at a depth of approximately 1 mm for the nonconforming contact that occurs in total knee replacements and at the surface of the joint for the conforming contact that occurs in total hip replacements. Retrieval analyses have shown that the bottoms of the pits and the zone of delamination both occur at a depth of approximately 1 mm. The maximum shear stresses may be responsible for the initiation and propagation of subsurface cracks, which either extend parallel to the surface of the component (delamination) or turn and propagate toward the surface (pits) (4).

The propagation of cracks normal to the surface is probably associated with the range (algebraic difference) of the maximum principal stresses that cause stretching and compression of the surface. The range of the maximum principal stress and the magnitude of the maximum shear stress both increase when the contact stress increases. Therefore, the stresses associated with pits and delamination increase as the thickness of the component decreases, as the conformity of the articulating surfaces decreases, and as the elastic modulus of the polyethylene increases.

DEPENDENCE OF STRESS AND DEFORMATION ON MATERIAL PROPERTIES

Because the contact stress increases as the stiffness of the material increases, it is important to quantify the contact stress in terms of the elastic properties of polyethylene. Hertzian contact theory is commonly used to determine the contact stresses between elastic components. Unfortunately, it cannot be used to analyze the contact stress in total joint replacements because metal and polyethylene components have such dissimilar elastic moduli and the contact area is not small compared to the size of the implants, particularly in conforming joints such as total hip replacements. The contact stresses can be approximated using the theory of elasticity (2). This approach assumes that the material is linearly elastic. However, polyethylene exhibits a non-linear stress-strain behavior in which the stiffness (elastic modulus) of the material decreases with increasing strain. When the initial elastic modulus (maximum value) is used in a theory of elasticity solution for the stresses, the contact stress will be overestimated. Analyses of component behavior based on elasticity theory, therefore, provide an upper limit on the effects of changes in the elastic properties of the material.

Figure 1 shows the results, obtained using the theory of elasticity, for three implants: a 28-mm total hip replacement, total condylar type knee prosthesis, and prosthesis with a tibial component that is flatter than the total condylar design (the least conforming of the three). Several things should be noted. First, the stresses in all three cases increase as the thickness is decreased. In fact, the stresses are increasingly sensitive to changes in thickness when the thickness of the component is small. Second, the stresses increase with decreasing conformity. The stresses on the acetabular component are much less than the stresses for either knee design and the stresses on the flatter tibial component are the greatest of all. Third, in each case the stresses increase when the elastic modulus is increased from 1,000 to 2,000 MPa.

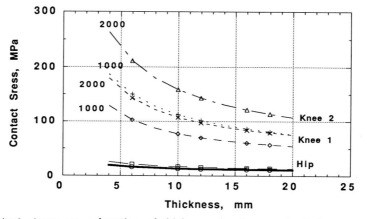

FIG. 1. Contact stress as a function of thickness for three polyethylene components: a 28-mm acetabular cup (Hip), a total condylar type knee (Knee 1), and a less conforming knee component (Knee 2). Results are shown for two values of elastic modulus, 1,000 and 2,000 MPa.

In addition to the general increase in stress with increasing modulus, it should also be noted that the magnitude of the increase is dependent on the conformity of the joint replacement. For the acetabular component, the stresses are small and the increase in stress is also small when the elastic modulus is increased. The increase in stress is much larger for the less conforming knee joints and the largest increment in stress occurs for the least conforming contact. Finite element analyses confirm these observations (1).

The increase in stress due to change in modulus is also dependent on the thickness of the components. As the thickness decreases, the increment in stress due to a change in thickness also decreases. Therefore, a change in the elastic modulus of a thin component produces a greater increase in stress than the same change produced in a thicker component.

Because surface damage is the result of material failure due to cyclic loading, it is natural to attempt to strengthen the material to minimize the possibility of failure. Methods have been developed that enhance the material properties of polyethylene. However, as mentioned previously, when polyethylene is strengthened, the modulus is also increased, resulting in an increase in the stresses associated with damage to the articular surfaces. What Fig. 1 underlines is that the increased potential for damage due to increased stiffness of the material is design dependent. Therefore, an increase in stress due to increased modulus, which is safe for a thick, conforming design, may not be safe for a thin, nonconforming design.

DEGRADATION OF POLYETHYLENE

It has been observed from retrieval studies that the density of polyethylene increases during the time of implantation. Experiments have also shown that the modulus of polyethylene increases linearly with density. Therefore, it is clear that the modulus of the polyethylene generally increases with passage of time after implantation. Furthermore, the increase is not uniform throughout the thickness, but is

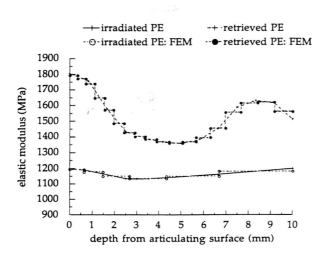

FIG. 2. Elastic modulus as a function of depth from the articulating surface of the acetabular components. Distribution of experimentally determined modulus (irradiated PE and retrieved PE) and the discretization of the modulus used for the numerical analyses (irradiated PE: FEM and retrieved PE: FEM) are shown.

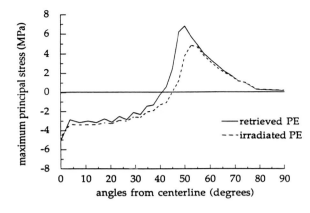

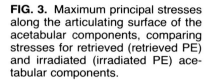

FIG. 3. Maximum principal stresses along the articulating surface of the acetabular components, comparing stresses for retrieved (retrieved PE) and irradiated (irradiated PE) acetabular components.

more pronounced near the superior and inferior surfaces of the implant. Generally, it is greatest near the articulating surface of a polyethylene component.

In some components the peak density (modulus) has been observed at the articulating surface; in others the maximum value has occurred approximately 1 mm beneath the surface (6). This suggests that the change in material properties may be a function of loading since the maximum shear stresses also occur at this depth and the general variation of density with depth is similar to the variation of maximum shear stress with depth.

Because stresses causing surface damage increase with increasing modulus, these *in vivo* changes in material properties due to degradation of the polyethylene increase the risk of debris generation. Figure 2 shows the distribution of elastic modulus through the thickness of a retrieved component. When this distribution was used in a finite-element analysis of the component, it was found that the magnitudes of the maximum principal stresses, which act tangentially to the articulating surface of the component, increased in magnitude (Fig. 3).

Loading, of course, is not the only factor that can cause changes in density. Nonuniform increases in density also occur due to sterilization and oxidative degradation from exposure to the body environment (8). Major research efforts are currently underway to determine the contributions each of these factors makes to the observed changes in material properties.

METAL AND CERAMIC COMPONENTS

As stated previously, the convex surface of a total joint replacement is generally made from either a metal alloy or ceramic material. In nonconforming joints, such as total knee replacements, where pitting and delamination on the scale of a millimeter occur, the stiffness and surface characteristics of the material probably play minor roles, if any, in the stresses associated with these damage modes. Of course, grossly rough surfaces will abrade the polyethylene and much debris will be generated in the process. However, the differences in surface characteristics between various metal alloys, coated or not, and ceramics have probably a second order effect, at most, on the stresses causing macro pitting and delamination.

Contact between conforming surfaces is an entirely different situation. The mechanism by which damage occurs in conforming contact such as total hip replacements is not well understood. It may be that damage here is also due to fatigue processes but that these occur on a micrometer scale. Such a view is not inconsistent with retrieval studies and the amount and type of debris observed in periprosthetic tissues retrieved at revision surgery. Although this picture of damage processes in conforming joints is somewhat speculative, it does suggest that surface characteristics such as roughness, chemistry, and strength may be important factors in minimizing damage.

Changes in surface characteristics may be achieved in several ways. Ceramics may be used instead of metals or the surfaces of metal components may be modified using ion implantation, nitride coating, ceramic coating, or other procedures. The basic assumption in these approaches is that wear occurs primarily by direct contact between the components. Consequently, the goal is to make the surface of the stiffer component of an articulating pair stronger, smoother, and stiffer by choice of material, coating, manufacturing process, or a combination of these. Such improvements are not without disadvantages. For example, a ceramic head for a total hip replacement provides improved surface characteristics compared to a metal head but at an increased risk of fracture compared to a similar metal component.

An alternative approach is to avoid direct contact between the components by designing them to enhance fluid film lubrication. This has been attempted in the past by the use of metal on metal bearing surfaces. Retrieval analyses have shown that some of these devices performed well for many years. Consequently, this concept has been revisited in recent years. When fluid films are achieved in these bearings, the film is likely to be quite thin and the elastic deformations of the articulating surfaces may have to be included in the analysis and design of such components. An alternative approach on this theme is to enhance the possibility of fluid film lubrication by increasing the compliance of the polymeric component. One concept involves the use of a polyethylene substrate with a less stiff layer of material at the articulating surface.

CLOSURE

The generation of debris due to damage of the articular surfaces in total joint replacements is clearly one of the most important problems to be addressed in joint replacement surgery. Modifications of the materials used for bearing surfaces in artificial joints and new materials have great potential for improving the long-term performance of prosthetic joints. In a market-driven environment, it is tempting to produce or try something new before it has been thoroughly tested. Recent history has provided a number of examples of the consequences of such an approach. The patients whom we serve deserve our best efforts to understand the performance and characteristics of existing materials and the consequences of proposed processes, new materials, and material and surface modifications.

Finally, we have ample theoretical, experimental, and clinical evidence that the material choices cannot be isolated from design. A major part of our efforts in this regard must be to document the effects of design variables on surface damage and quantify the relationships between stresses and damage mechanisms.

REFERENCES

1. Bartel DL, Burstein AH, Santavicca EA, Insall JN. Performance of the tibial component in total knee replacement. *J Bone Joint Surg [Am]* 1982;64:1026–1033.
2. Bartel DL, Burstein AH, Toda MD, Edwards DL. The effect of conformity and plastic thickness on contact stress in metal-backed plastic implants. *J Biomech Eng* 1985;107:193–199.
3. Bartel DL, Rimnac CM, Wright TM. Evaluation and design of the articular surface. In: Goldberg VM, ed. *Controversies of total knee arthroplasty*. New York: Raven Press, 1991:61–73.
4. Blunn GW, Joshi A, Hardinge K, Engelbrecht E, Walker PS. The effect of bearing conformity on the wear of polyethylene tibial components. *Trans Orthop Res Soc* 1992;17:357.
5. Hood RW, Wright TM, Burstein AH. Retrieval analysis of total knee prosthesis. A method and its application to forty-eight total condylar prostheses. *J Biomed Mater Res* 1983;17:829–842.
6. Rimnac CM, Wright TM, Klein RW, Betts F, Schapiro E. Characterization of material properties of ultra high molecular weight polyethylene before and after implantation. *Soc Biomater Retrieval Symp* 1992;15:16.
7. Wright TM, Burstein AH, Bartel DL. Retrieval analysis of total joint replacement components: a six-year experience. In: Fraker A, Griffin C, eds. *Corrosion and degradation of implant materials: second symposium*. ASTM STP 859. Philadelphia: American Society for Testing and Materials, 1985:415–428.
8. Wright TM, Rimnac CM, Stulberg SD, et al. Wear of polyethylene: observations of retrieved PCA knee implants. *Trans Soc Biomater* 1991;14:241.

Biological, Material, and Mechanical Considerations of Joint Replacement,
edited by B. F. Morrey.
Raven Press, Ltd., New York © 1993.

24

Surface Analysis of the Taper Junctions of Retrieved and *In Vitro* Tested Modular Hip Prostheses

J. D. Bobyn, A. R. Dujovne, J. J. Krygier, and D. L. Young

Jo Miller Orthopaedic Research Laboratory, Montreal General Hospital, McGill University, Montreal, Quebec, Canada H3G 1A4

Modular connections are being increasingly diversified in both total hip and total knee prostheses to give the surgeon more choice in implant fit and more latitude in design features. This can provide the advantages offered by custom prostheses in optimizing the total joint arthroplasty, particularly in revision surgery, while avoiding the higher costs typically associated with customizing. From a mechanical standpoint, modularity should permit a stable connection of implant components. Often the individual components differ in material properties so that the assembled implant can function to the best advantage. In the hip, for example, apart from allowing adjustment of leg length and offset and easing surgical technique, the coupling of a cobalt-chromium (Co-Cr) or ceramic head with a titanium- (Ti) alloy stem combines the improved wear characteristics of the bearing materials with the superior biomechanical compatibility of the lower stiffness stem material.

The wisdom and safety of utilizing certain modular connections have recently been questioned because of findings of corrosion at the Morse taper head/neck surfaces of hip prostheses (7,14). Of additional concern is the potential for fretting motion at all modular junctions and the release of particulate material that, in a manner similar to that proposed for polyethylene or ceramic particulate debris, may elicit a macrophage-mediated inflammatory response leading to osteolysis (2,4,16,17,19). Fretting between modular parts may also be a trigger mechanism for corrosion through galvanic or crevice mechanisms, as discussed recently in the literature (1,5,9,10,13). Fretting fatigue is another potential problem, and implant fractures, albeit rare, have been reported to occur at modular connection sites.

The purpose of this study was to elucidate the potential for and extent of fretting damage with two types of Morse taper modular connections on hip prostheses. Information was gathered from both retrieved implants that had functioned *in vivo* and implants that were tested *in vitro* in simulated fatigue environments.

MATERIALS AND METHODS

Implants

All observations were obtained from the study of the S-ROM femoral hip prosthesis (Joint Medical Products Corporation, Stamford, CT), a modular design that consists of a proximal sleeve that connects with the stem via a Morse taper (Fig. 1) (6,11). Both the sleeve and stem were machined from Ti-6A1-4V alloy and the implant was combined with a standard Morse taper fitting femoral head manufactured from forged Co-Cr alloy. The tapered male neck was provided with either a polished or as-machined finish and the female taper of the Co-Cr head was left with an as-machined finish. The sleeve that connected with the proximal stem body was provided with an as-machined surface finish that was subjected to a sintering heat treatment used for bonding of the porous coating. The portion of the stem body that interfaced with the sleeve was provided with a light grit-blasted surface finish. The sleeve-stem Morse taper had a nominal contact area of approximately 2,000 mm^2 for the medium-size stem and sleeve; this varied somewhat for smaller and larger implants. The head-neck Morse taper for all specimens studied had a nominal contact area of 560 mm^2. A Morse taper is defined as consisting of a nominal taper of ap-

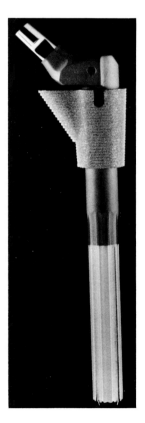

FIG. 1. S-ROM hip prosthesis with modular head-neck and sleeve-stem segments.

proximately 0.625 in. per foot, providing for an included taper angle of approximately 6°.

Twenty-eight S-ROM prostheses were included in this study, 17 of which were retrieved at revision surgery and 11 of which were tested *in vitro*. Details such as period of implantation, stem size, and testing parameters for the *in vivo* and *in vitro* implants are provided in Tables 1 and 2. The *in vitro* implants were used as controls to elucidate the origin of the surface modifications observed *in vivo* and, if possible, validate the use of *in vitro* testing to forecast the performance of modular connections.

The retrieved prostheses had implantation times ranging from 7 months to 6 years. The reasons for removal included loosening, pain, and late infection. Twelve implants were used in primary cases, the remaining five in revisions. The implant size ranged from 11 to 19 mm in diameter.

In Vitro Fatigue Testing

All *in vitro* tested implants were 11 mm in diameter and 150 mm long with a 36-mm neck length and a 32-mm head. Since the purpose of the fatigue testing was to establish a worst-case loading condition, a novel test set-up was implemented following the guidelines of Postak et al. (15). This involved potting the proximal sleeve within a trunnion hub using polymethylmethacrylate (PMMA). Extending from the hub and mounted to a frame was a transverse axis about which the device could pivot upon loading (Fig. 2). The distal lateral aspect of the stem was supported by a reaction transducer. Displacement monitoring using a low-voltage displacement transducer with a sensitivity of 100 μm was active throughout testing to detect relative rotatory motion between the stem and sleeve. The entire frame was supported

TABLE 1. *Description of the* in vivo *specimens and results of surface analysis*

Specimen	Implantation period	Stem size (mm)	% Damaged area		Severity of wear	
			Head-neck	Sleeve-stem	Head-neck	Sleeve-stem
1	7 months	15	10	15	B	B
2	9 months	15	—	35	—	C
3	9 months	17	<5	15	A	B
4	1 year	13	10	<5	B	A
5	1 year	19	<5	25	B	B
6	14 months	15	<5	<5	A	A
7	15 months	17	<5	<5	A	A
8	15 months	17	<5	<5	A	A
9	19 months	11	<5	<5	A	A
10	2 years	13	10	30	B	C
11	2 years	13	<5	<5	B	A
12	2 years	17	<5	10	A	B
13	4 years	14	10	20	B	B
14	4 years	11	25	a	C	C
15	5 years	11	<5	<5	C	B
16	5 years	13	—	10	—	C
17	6 years	13	<5	15	A	B

A, none or negligible; B, burnishing; C, delamination.
aMeasurement not valid because of three-body wear with PMMA.

TABLE 2. *Description of the in vitro specimens and results of surface analysis*

Specimen	Cycles (N)	Load (BW)	Frequency (Hz)	Stem size (mm)	Severity of wear		% Damaged area	
					Head-neck	Sleeve-stem	Head-neck	Sleeve-stem
18	2.0E07	2.5	20	11	B	A	18	5
19	2.0E07	2.5	20	11	B	B	4	8
20	2.0E07	2.5	20	11	B	B	15	8
21	2.0E07	2.5	20	11	B	B	15	5
22	1.0E07	5	10	11	C	B	33	19
23	1.0E07	5	10	11	B	C	15	35
24	1.0E07	5.5	10	11	B	B	14	10
25	1.0E07	5.5	10	11	B	C	11	15
26	1.0E07	6	10	11	C	C	4	12
27	1.0E07	7.5	10	11	C	C	5	20
28	8.3E06	8	10	11	B	C	11	35

A, none or negligible; B, burnishing; C, delamination; BW, body weight.

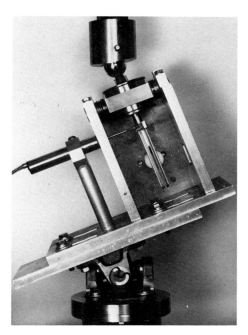

FIG. 2. *In vitro* test arrangement. This is a side view showing the 20° out-of-plane alignment. The coronal slot is visible in the distal stem region, which abuts against a reaction transducer.

by a universal joint attached to the base of an Instron servo-hydraulic testing apparatus. The test set-up was designed to simulate proximal fixation of the device at the sleeve-bone interface only with distal support against the lateral endosteal cortex. Guided by the telemetric data on hip loading published by Davey et al. (8), the stem was angled vertically within the coronal plane and 20° out of the sagittal plane so as to apply an appropriate bending moment and rotatory moment during loading.

The stems were tested at room temperature under head loads ranging from 2.5 to 8 times body weight (1 body weight = 73 kg) at a frequency of 10 or 20 Hertz. Both the head and sleeve were assembled to the stem with a force roughly equivalent to that generated by a standard surgical mallet (three impacts of a 0.5-kg dead weight dropped from a 40-cm height). Loading was applied for 10 or 20 million cycles unless the implant fractured earlier.

Analysis of Taper Surfaces

When possible, the taper surfaces were prepared for analysis by sectioning the taper junction with a high-speed borazone blade and carefully separating the male and female halves to avoid extraneous damage. This was performed with all head-neck and sleeve-stem tapers of the *in vitro* tested stems and approximately one-third of the tapers of the retrieved *in vivo* stems, most of which were received with the head and/or sleeve already disimpacted from the stem. After gross inspection and photography of the male and female taper surfaces, they were lightly cleaned ultrasonically in tetrachloroethylene prior to detailed examination.

First, high-powered stereomicroscopy was used for an overall identification of the severity and extent of fretting wear. The severity of wear was arbitrarily divided into three qualitative classes: A, no or slight wear; B, mild wear (burnishing or slight roughening); and C, extensive wear (delamination, pitting). This classification was performed by two independent observers. Second, computer image analysis was used to quantify the percentage of the nominal area of the taper that showed surface modification or damage from fretting. This was accomplished by analyzing sequential high-power video images of the entire taper surface, manually digitizing the areas of the affected regions, and expressing the total affected area as a percentage of the nominal contact area. The severity of wear did not necessarily correlate with the measurements of the total area showing surface modification. For instance, an implant could have a very small focal area of marked wear and be graded class C severity. Finally, scanning electron microscopy (SEM) and energy dispersive analysis by x-ray (EDAX) were used to determine the detailed characteristics of the fretting scars and products.

The retrieved *in vivo* implants that were disassembled at surgery were carefully examined to distinguish the surface damage that occurred in service from that caused by surgical manipulation.

RESULTS

Head-Neck Junction

In Vivo *Specimens*

Evidence of fretting was observed at the head-neck tapers in all of the retrieved *in vivo* specimens; it differed in extent and severity and was generally quite slight.

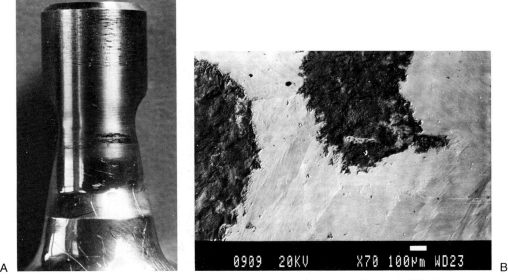

FIG. 3. A: Neck of specimen 14 illustrating obvious regions of surface modification and discoloration. Most of the *in vivo* retrieved specimens showed much less damage. **B:** SEM illustrating the appearance of typical fretting scars.

To the naked eye the fretting typically appeared as surface modification in small, patchy regions or scars that were colored dark gray or black (Fig. 3). At higher magnification, the scars were variously characterized by burnishing, roughening, micropitting, or delamination.

In terms of severity, two implants could not be properly assessed because of excessive damage during retrieval (Table 1). Of the remaining 15 specimens, seven (47%) showed class A damage (none or negligible), six (40%) were in class B (mild burnishing), and two (13%) showed class C damage (delamination, pitting, and material removal). One of the class C implants revealed additional corrosion attack of fretting scars at two sites on the surface of the Co-Cr head (Fig. 4). Corrosion products were detected by EDAX within the affected regions, which at high magnification displayed the characteristic worm-like and pitted appearance of corrosion. This was the only instance of corrosion associated with the mixed-metal head-neck taper connections.

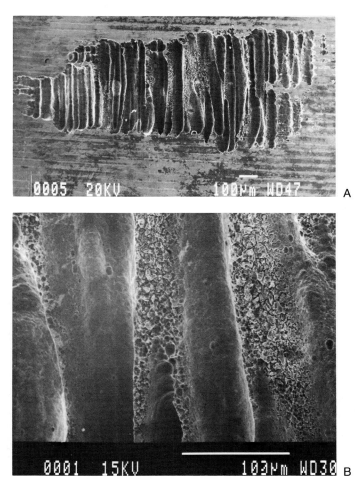

FIG. 4. A: SEM illustrating a small region of corrosive attack on an *in vivo* retrieved Co-Cr head. **B:** Higher magnification showing the pitted character of the corroded region.

In 10 specimens (67%) there was surface modification on less than 5% of the nominal taper area, and it was only detectable at high magnification. In four specimens (27%) the damage was found on approximately 10% of the available surface. Specimen 14 was the most extensively affected, showing damage on approximately 25% of the available surface (Fig. 3). In general, the damaged contact areas were quite randomly distributed over the taper surfaces. Occasionally, circumferential fretting scars were present; these occurred on the most proximal and distal aspects of the taper on either the lateral or medial surfaces of the head and neck. In most cases the scars observed on the mating male and female surfaces were a mirror image of each other.

In all four specimens (100%) in which the retrieved implant was received with the head intact on the neck, there were traces of dried biological fluid on most of the taper surface. This indicates that fluid was either present on the tapers at the time of assembly or infiltrated the junction during *in vivo* service.

In Vitro *Specimens*

In general, the head-neck taper surfaces tested *in vitro* showed greater evidence of surface modification and fretting than *in vivo*. None was classified as class A severity (Table 2). Eight of 11 specimens (73%) showed severity class B changes involving mild burnishing or a slight roughened appearance (Fig. 5). In some instances, the fretting scar was so compacted as to form a glaze. The remaining three specimens (27%) were ranked with class-C damage, where shallow defects, micropits, and highly deformed layers were created by removal and transfer of wear debris from matching male and female surfaces (Figs. 6 and 7). Highly adherent flakes of Ti fretting debris were detected by EDAX on both Co-Cr and Ti alloy surfaces. In specimens 27 and 28 (18%) the initiation of fatigue cracks was observed at fretting

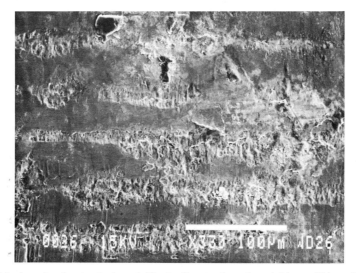

FIG. 5. SEM of an *in vitro* tested neck illustrating surface burnishing within a fretting scar.

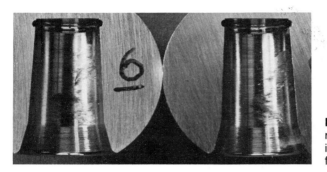

FIG. 6. *In vitro* tested Co-Cr head ranked with class-C fretting severity and the greatest extent of surface change.

scar sites (Fig. 7C). Specimen 28, tested at the highest load of eight times body weight, failed at less than 1 million cycles due to a fracture of the neck through a crack initiated at the fretting scar on the lateral aspect. For the entire group, the damaged contact areas were quite randomly situated and ranged between 4% and 33% of the nominal taper area.

Sleeve-Stem Junction

In Vivo *Specimens*

The sleeve-stem junctions of the retrieved *in vivo* implants all showed some evidence of surface modification or fretting wear (Fig. 8). Six (35%) implants were ranked as class A severity, seven (41%) as class B, and four (24%) as class C (Table 1). Small discolored regions indicative of contact and fretting typically measured only a few square millimeters. These totaled less than 5% of the nominal taper contact area in seven implants (41%), between 5% and 20% in six implants (35%), and greater than 20% in four implants (24%). There was no evidence of gross motion, gross removal of material, or appreciable loss of taper dimensions or tolerances. In some specimens there was an obvious circumferential focus of surface modification at the distal lateral aspect of the taper, whereas the majority displayed a more random appearance of fretting scars, some appearing highly polished and others rougher and darker. A notable exception to these findings was a 4-year retrieval that showed a very large amount of wear (specimen 14, class C wear) and removal of material on the entire medial side of the sleeve-stem taper. Close examination revealed, however, that this was due to a layer of bone cement that had been left inadvertently within the taper at the time of surgery and caused exaggerated three-body wear.

All six (100%) of the *in vivo* specimens received with the sleeve intact on the stem showed evidence of dried biological deposits over most of the taper surfaces once disassembled (Fig. 8B).

In Vitro *Specimens*

As with the head-neck junctions, the *in vitro* tested sleeve-stem junctions showed more surface modification than *in vivo* (Fig. 9). One (9%) was ranked in class A and five each (45%) in class B and class C severity (Table 2). The damaged contact area

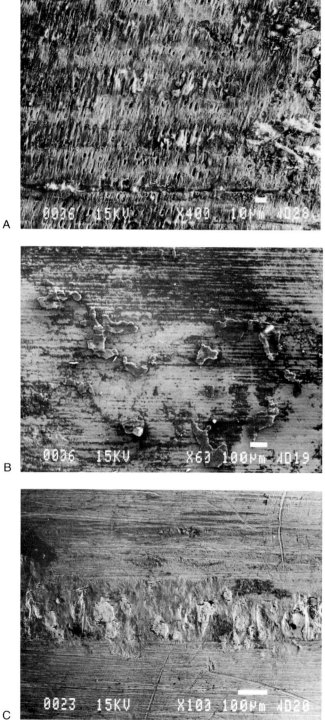

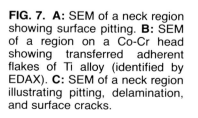

FIG. 7. A: SEM of a neck region showing surface pitting. **B:** SEM of a region on a Co-Cr head showing transferred adherent flakes of Ti alloy (identified by EDAX). **C:** SEM of a neck region illustrating pitting, delamination, and surface cracks.

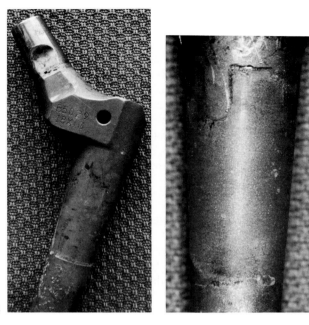

A, B

FIG. 8. A: Stem taper region of specimen 16 retrieved 5 years after surgery. There are several small randomly distributed fretting scars. **B:** Stem taper region of specimen 17 retrieved 6 years after surgery. Distinct fretting scars are less apparent, but the outline of the sleeve on the stem is identified by dried biological deposits.

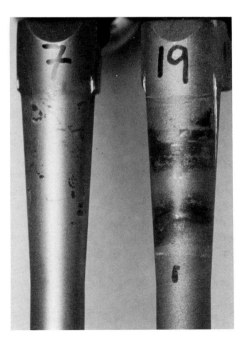

FIG. 9. Two *in vitro* tested stems, the one on the left tested at five times body weight and the one on the right tested at seven times body weight, both for 10 million cycles. The more pronounced surface discoloration and burnishing at the higher load was far more severe than observed with the *in vivo* retrieved specimens.

ranged from 5% to 35% of the nominal taper area. The areas of highest contact (pressure) were most evident at the distal lateral aspect of the sleeve. In general, however, the fretting scars were quite randomly distributed. SEM examination revealed surface roughening at the contact sites in most cases. In a few cases there were apparent delamination and transfer of small amounts of material between stem and sleeve. For all but two specimens the delaminated material was quite firmly adherent; there was no gross evidence of loose wear debris. For specimens 27 and 28 (highest load levels), detectable traces of fine metallic powder could be removed from the male and female taper surfaces with manual pressure. In none of the cases tested *in vitro* was any evidence of gross motion between stem and sleeve detected by the displacement transducer. Furthermore, there was no measurable change in taper dimensions or tolerances, even in implants tested at the highest loads.

Correlation of Fretting with Variables

When the retrieved *in vivo* specimens were divided into subgroups according to duration of implantation, patient weight and age, reason for removal, and implant size, no obvious correlation could be discerned between the extent of fretting wear and these variables.

For the *in vitro* tested implants, visual examination of the taper surfaces showed an apparent influence of load level on the extent of surface modification and fretting damage (Fig. 9). For loads greater than six times body weight there were consistently more discolored contact area, more evidence of surface delamination and material transfer between male and female surfaces, and, in the case of the head-neck junction, evidence of fatigue cracks within fretting scars that did not appear at lower loads.

DISCUSSION

Fretting is defined as a wear mechanism that occurs at low-amplitude, oscillating, sliding movement between two mechanically joined parts under load. There are varying descriptions of the magnitude of motion associated with fretting, but it may generally be defined as less than 20 μm. In the context of modular junctions of total hip prostheses, it would appear inevitable, given the magnitude of loading, that they would be susceptible to fretting wear.

This study has confirmed the occurrence of fretting at the Morse taper junctions of one type of hip stem using both *in vivo* and *in vitro* analysis. Findings of fretting have also been reported for head-neck modular tapers of other prosthetic designs as well (5,10). On Ti-alloy surfaces, the fretting appears as small, distinct, darkly colored patches or scars. The dark color is indicative of Ti-alloy oxidation. The mechanical damage within the fretting scars varied in extent from site to site and implant to implant and overall displayed the entire spectrum of surface modification that has been described for fretting in industrial equipment (3,20). This includes minor damage such as burnishing, moderate damage such as roughening, and the most severe damage of delamination, pitting, and fatigue cracking. The loosening and transfer of flakes of titanium material, as observed at both head-neck and sleeve-stem junctions, have been described by the theories of Waterhouse (20) and Halliday and Hirst (12) as depending partially on the amplitude of the relative micromotion between the involved surfaces.

The extent and severity of fretting were generally more severe in the *in vitro* tested implants. This may have been due to test conditions such as frequency, load level, and number of cycles. It is universally accepted that fretting wear is directly related to both the load level and number of fretting cycles (18). The maximum duration of implantation for the *in vivo* implants was 6 years, whereas most of the *in vitro* implants were tested for 10 or 20 million cycles, equivalent to 10 or more years of function. Despite these differences, the overall similarity between *in vivo* and *in vitro* groups in appearance, severity, location, and size of the fretting scars strongly supports the concept of using *in vitro* testing to assess the stability and wear characteristics of modular connections.

Fretting wear and fatigue are known to be highly dependent on a variety of factors such as slip amplitude, contact stress distribution, contact materials, friction coefficients, contact pressure, surface finish, and environment. All other factors being equal, the design characteristics and fabrication tolerances of the joined parts are particularly important. Looser manufacturing tolerances would lead to smaller contact area (line contact or individual point contact at asperities), higher stress concentration, and higher interfacial motion, all key factors in the development of fretting wear (18). If the location and areas of the fretting scars are valid indicators of quality of fit and contact, it is clear from all the implants studied that the Morse taper connection cannot be made perfectly. The finding of dried biological fluid on the intact retrieved *in vivo* taper surfaces further indicates the absence of male-female contact in some regions and the possibility of fluid ingress during *in vivo* function. Krygier et al. (13) also described fluid ingress during *in vitro* testing of Morse taper junctions in wet environments.

In view of the recent publications and concern about corrosion at head-neck Morse taper junctions, particular interest was paid to identifying sites of corrosion in the 17 retrieved *in vivo* implants. In only one case, a 5-year retrieval, was corrosion detected and this was only in two small focal regions on the Co-Cr taper. Collier et al. (7) reported that significant corrosion was found in 100% of all mixed-metal head-neck tapers retrieved beyond 30 months of service. In our series, with five implants retrieved at 4 years and beyond, there was just the one finding of corrosion and to a vastly smaller extent than that reported by Collier et al. This clearly contradicts the conclusion of Collier et al. that galvanic-induced corrosion is an inevitable consequence of mixed-metal tapers and means that other factors probably influence the chemical stability of Morse taper junctions. Mathiesen et al. (14) demonstrated corrosion at Co-Cr alloy head-neck tapers and referred to the known susceptibility of Co-Cr alloy to crevice corrosion. We have learned from the present study that gaps (crevices) are definitely present at Morse taper connections, and thus a crevice cell could be established the moment the taper is immersed in body fluids (5). Based on the findings of this study, we postulate furthermore that fretting wear could both initiate and propagate depassivation of the taper surfaces while creating additional micropits for crevice corrosion. As stated earlier, it is well-known that machining tolerances play a strong role in governing fretting, fretting wear, and fretting corrosion. It cannot be discounted that in the series of implants studied by Collier et al. the difference in corrosion findings between the group of similar metal tapers and mixed-metal tapers was influenced by differences in machining tolerances and hence propensities for fretting—not simply by the mixed metals themselves. This clearly is a critical subject that requires further research and clarification.

It is important to mention that despite the ubiquitous finding of fretting at Morse taper modular junctions, in no instance was there any evidence of gross wear, loss of material, or appreciable change in nominal dimensions or tolerances of the tapers. It is also important to distinguish between gross implant stability and the small magnitude of motion characteristic of fretting. None of the retrieved *in vivo* implants was removed because of loosening or fracture of modular components. None of the sleeve-stem junctions of the *in vitro* tested implants showed any evidence of gross motion or instability. Yet all of the implants showed some evidence of fretting motion and wear. Fretting at modular connections is absolutely inevitable given sufficient load and loading cycles, and this must be accepted if we wish to gain the advantages offered by modularity.

As a final note, this does not mean that we should accept any serious consequences of modularity. Apart from gross loosening or fracture of modular components, one of the current concerns relates to the generation of particulate debris and corrosion products, macrophage activation, eventual osteoclast stimulation, bony lysis, and implant loosening. Related to this biological cascade of events, the debris released at modular junctions is largely a speculative issue and there are no clear data on what level of debris generation may be acceptable or unacceptable. What is certain is that current manufacturing practice calls for substantially looser tolerances for medical tapers than for tapers in the automotive and machine tool industry (up to eightfold higher). It could only be prudent, given the close relationship between tolerances and fretting, to minimize the possibility of mechanical failure and adverse biological response by using medical device tapers (and other modular connection designs) of the highest possible quality.

ACKNOWLEDGMENTS

The authors are grateful for financial support from the Medical Research Council of Canada and for donation of the implants by the Joint Medical Products Corporation. The authors also thank Drs. Cameron, Engh, Eschenroeder, Moore, Thomkins, Niebaum, Turner, Trick, Christie, and Stein for sending the retrieved prostheses, and Heather Murphy for valuable technical assistance.

REFERENCES

1. Bauer TW, Brown SA, Jiang M, Panigutti MA, Flemming CAC. Corrosion in modular hip stems. Transactions of the 38th Annual Meeting of the Orthopaedic Research Society, 1992:354.
2. Bobyn JD. Polyethylene wear debris. *Can J Surg* 1991;34:531–532.
3. Borai YE. A critical review of the process of fretting fatigue. M.S. Thesis, Concordia University, Montreal, Quebec, 1986.
4. Borssen B, Karrholm J, Snorrason F. Osteolysis after ceramic-on-ceramic hip arthroplasty. *Acta Orthop Scand* 1992;62:73–75.
5. Brown SA, Flemming CAC, Merrit K, Payer JH: Fretting corrosion testing of modular hip designs. Transactions of the 4th World Biomaterials Congress, Berlin, 1992:268.
6. Cameron HU. Recent advances in artificial hip-joint replacement. *Can Fam Phys* 1987;33:649–653.
7. Collier JP, Surprenant VA, Jensen RE, Mayor MB. Corrosion at the interface of cobalt-alloy heads on titanium-alloy stems. *Clin Orthop* 1991;271:305–312.

8. Davey DT, Kotzar GM, Brown RH, et al. Telemetric force measurement across the hip after total hip arthroplasty. *J Bone Joint Surg [Am]* 1988;70:45.

9. Dujovne AR, Bobyn JD, Krygier JJ, Wilson DR, Brooks CE. Fretting at the head/neck taper of modular hip prostheses. Transactions of the 4th World Biomaterials Congress, Berlin, 1992:264.

10. Gilbert JL, Buckley CA, Jacobs JJ, Urban RM, Lautenschlager EP, Galante JO. Mechanically assisted corrosive attack in the Morse taper of modular hip prostheses. Transactions of the 4th World Biomaterials Congress, Berlin, 1992:267.

11. Gorski JM. Modular noncemented total hip arthroplasty for congenital dislocation of the hip. Case report and design rationale. *Clin Orthop* 1987;225:22.

12. Halliday JS, Hirst W. The fretting corrosion of mild steel. *Proc Soc Lond* 1956;236:411–425.

13. Krygier JJ, Bobyn JD, Dujovne AR, Young DL, Brooks CE. Strength, stability and wear analysis of titanium femoral hip prostheses tested in fatigue. Transactions of the 4th World Biomaterials Congress, Berlin, 1992:626.

14. Mathiesen EB, Lindgren JU, Blomgren GGA, Reinholt FP. Corrosion of modular hip prostheses. *J Bone Joint Surg [Br]* 1991;73:259.

15. Postak PD, Polando G, Pugh JW, Greenwald AS. A new method of fatigue testing for proximally supported femoral stems. *Trans AAOS* 1990;320.

16. Santavirta S, Hoikka V, Eskola A, Konttinen YT, Paavilainen T, Tallroth K. Aggressive granulomatous lesions in cementless total hip arthroplasty. *J Bone Joint Surg [Br]* 1990;72:980–984.

17. Schmalzried TP, Kwong LM, Jasty M, et al. The mechanism of loosening of cemented acetabular components in total hip arthroplasty: analysis of specimens retrieved at autopsy. *Clin Orthop* 1992;274.

18. Suh NP. *Tribophysics*. Englewood Cliffs, NJ: Prentice-Hall, 1986.

19. Tanzer M, Maloney WJ, Jasty M, Harris WH. The progression of femoral cortical osteolysis in association with total hip arthroplasty without cement. *J Bone Joint Surg [Am]* 1992;74:404–410.

20. Waterhouse RB. *Fretting fatigue*. London: Applied Science Publishers, 1981.

Biological, Material, and Mechanical Considerations of Joint Replacement, edited by B. F. Morrey. Raven Press, Ltd., New York © 1993.

25

Ceramics for Joint Replacement

Pascal Christel

Department of Orthopaedic Surgery, Lariboisière Saint-Louis Medical School, University Paris 7, F-75010 Paris, France

In the early 1970s, Boutin (1,2), who was already concerned by the wear properties of polyethylene (PE), was the first to introduce alumina ceramics for total hip replacement (THR). Initially, alumina was chosen because of its hardness, which is second only to that of diamond, and resistance to abrasion, which makes this material useful as a cutting tool in the heavy machining industry. From the beginning of his experience, Boutin used the combination of alumina against alumina as a bearing component in THR. Since then, alumina has been also widely used in combination with PE. New ceramics have been recently proposed either as bulk material (e.g., zirconium) or coatings (e.g., titanium nitride [TiN] or diamond-like carbon [DLC]) for femoral heads. All of these ceramic materials belong to a class of biomaterials termed *bioinert ceramics*.

The use of ceramic materials in humans was proposed as early as 1933 (23). However, at that time, the purity and strength of the available Al_2O_3 ceramics did not permit their use as implant materials. It was not until 1965 that Sandhaus (24) proposed alumina type Degussit A1 23 for clinical application. This was the beginning of intensive European studies performed by Hentrich et al. (17), Boutin (2), Heimke et al. (16), and Griss et al. (15).

BIOINERT CERAMICS: BIOLOGICAL CONSIDERATIONS

The early results of biocompatibility evaluation of alumina have led many investigators to consider this ceramic material as bioinert and recommend it as a reference material when performing biocompatibility studies (6). A bioinert material is a material that should induce no tissue response after surgical implantation. The receiving host should ignore the material, and the tissue surrounding the implant material should exhibit both normal structure and activity (6). However, after implantation of alumina in soft tissue, a connective capsule is formed at the ceramic-tissue interface that remains even after a long period of time. Although the morphological characteristics of the encapsulating membrane demonstrate a very low grade tissue response, this shows that alumina-ceramic implants elicit and maintain a foreign-body tissue response. In fact, so-called bioinert materials do not exist. Any surgically implanted biomaterial induces a tissue response with intensity and features that rank the material into either the toxic or biocompatible category.

Alumina was initially proposed and remains in use for cementless orthopaedic and dental implants. In order to characterize its biocompatibility in these specific applications, the study of the bone-ceramic interface appears of primary importance. According to Osborn and Newesely (21), bioceramics may be put into three categories: (i) biotolerant, (ii) bioinert, and (iii) bioactive. The distinction between the three types is based on the characteristics of osteogenesis.

(i) With biotolerant ceramics, *distance osteogenesis* is observed, meaning that there is no direct bone-material contact. This is the case with the bovine-derived bone called Kiel bone.

(ii) Bioinert ceramics show direct bone contact. In this case, sequential fluorochrome labeling demonstrates that bone starts to grow in a centripetal manner at some distance from the ceramic to finally reach its surface, but without chemical bonding. Alumina, zirconium, and carbon belong to this category.

(iii) Bioactive ceramics also show direct bone contact. However, contrary to the previous category, labeling starts at the ceramic surface, demonstrating actual bonding osteogenesis. Hydroxyapatite, β-tricalcium phosphate, natural coral, and sintered bovine bone belong to this third category.

The low-grade tissue response to bulk bioinert ceramics may be related to the fact that these materials are already in their highest possible state of oxidation. They are thermodynamically stable and their ionic structure creates a hydrophilic surface. Accordingly, the wettability of bioinert ceramics, in relation to their surface energy, is higher than that for polymers and metals available in orthopaedics. With alumina, it has been demonstrated *in vitro* that water is adsorbed with high bond strength and that proteins, even at low concentrations, completely cover ceramic surfaces with a monolayer (10).

Ceramics exhibit a high compressive strength; they have been used in heavily loaded environments either for implant fixation (acetabular cup, roots of dental implant) or as friction components. When using alumina-alumina combination in THR, wear debris may be generated. As for any particulate material, the tissue response to ceramic debris depends on its size, shape, and amount. However, compared to polymers, the level of cytokines induced by alumina particles in the tissue surrounding aseptically loosened total hip prostheses has been reported to be lower (27).

DENSE POLYCRYSTALLINE ALUMINA

Manufacturing

The raw powder (99.9% Al_2O_3 + 0.05% MgO) is subjected either to isopressing or injection molding. The obtained green form is machined to the appropriate size and sintered in an oxidizing atmosphere at 1,500 to 1,600°C. Optional hot isostatic pressing (HIP) can be used to further reduce pore size and volume (1,400°C, 1,000 bar), as each pore acts as a notch reducing both static and fatigue strengths. Grinding and polishing constitute the last manufacturing step. High purity and high density of alumina are the factors that ensure a high reliability and long life expectancy of implants. The absence of a glassy phase at the grain boundaries and of pores permitting infiltration of an aqueous medium in the ceramic reduces the stress corrosion effect that can develop at a crack tip or in a flaw. The strength requirements can only be met by a process that yields a practically pore-free material, while maintaining a very low rate of grain growth.

Close control of flaw size and grain size distribution (avoiding large grains) is essential in the manufacturing process. Alumina with a density of greater than 3.95 can be diamond-ground and polished to obtain a surface roughness R_a (average surface roughness) of 0.002 μm, and an R_t (maximum value of surface roughness) of 0.5 μm.

Mechanical Properties

The impact fatigue strength has been measured by using a pendulum test machine, varying the height of the weight (22). With this method a threshold value (10E3 Nm) corresponding to the appearance of the first crack in the surface has been determined.

The dynamic fatigue strength has also been determined in the tensile and compressive zones with a 10-Hz frequency (13). The results have shown that hip joints that are exposed to up to $4 \times 10E6$ cycles a year can withstand these dynamic stresses.

The subcritical crack growth, which is an essential parameter in the estimate of the life expectancy of alumina implants, has been investigated by lifetime measurements in static bending tests in concentrated salt solutions. For crack growth velocities under 10E8 m per second, the results obtained through the crack growth velocity-stress intensity factor relationship have indicated that a material with reduced porosity and flaw size, owing to postcompaction, has an advantage over non-HIP material, with respect to long-term life expectancy. However, from the viewpoint of subcritical crack growth, both HIP and non-HIP aluminas would qualify for load-bearing situations in an aqueous salt solution for a lifetime of 50 years. They demonstrated a 99.9% survival probability of the implant, with maximum tolerable stresses of 115 MPa (14). Similar results have been obtained by Dalgleish and Rawlings (9) when performing investigations in water, bovine serum, Ringer's solution, human plasma, and albumin-salt solutions. It was concluded that aluminas with purities below 99% were unacceptable.

Standards

Several standards list the requirements, specifications, and test procedures for surgical-grade alumina (e.g., ISO 6474, ASTM F 603-78, and AFNOR NF S90-408) (see elsewhere in this volume). Table 1 summarizes the alumina specifications according to the ISO standard.

Friction and Wear

In a hip-joint simulator, friction and wear of alumina-alumina and alumina-PE combinations decreased with time, whereas with metal-PE friction and wear increased with time (13). The wear of alumina-alumina and alumina-PE was 20 and 10 times less, respectively, compared to metal-PE. These observations may be explained by several factors: (i) changes in surface roughness, (ii) sphericity, and (iii) surface physicochemistry.

TABLE 1. *Specifications for surgical-grade dense polycrystalline alumina, according to ISO 6474 standard*

General properties	
Density	3.90 g/cmE3
Chemical composition	
Al_2O_3	99.5%
$SiO_2 + Na_2O$	0.1%
Microstructure (average grain size)	7 μm
Mechanical properties	
Microhardness (2 N) at room temperature	2,300 HV
Compressive strength at room temperature	4,000 MPa
Flexural strength at room temperature	400 MPa
Young's modulus	380,000 MPa
Impact strength	40 cmN/cm²
Wear resistance (ring on disk)	0.01 mmE3/h
Chemical properties	
Corrosion resistance in Ringer's solution	0.1 mg/mE3/day

(i) Secondary to corrosive attack in Ringer's solution, surface roughness of metal increases, whereas surface roughness of ceramic decreases. These observations, made with simulator tests, have been confirmed by the analysis of ceramic-ceramic prostheses retrieved from patients (12).

(ii) Dörre and Hübner (13) have shown that a sphericity deviation as high as 18 μm did not affect the frictional torque, as the lubricating film would not collapse up to this value of sphericity deviation. With a sphericity deviation lower than 5 μm, which is currently obtained, the frictional torque will remain constant during the lifetime of the implant.

(iii) It has also been shown that a water film is strongly adsorbed onto the surface of alumina (10). This wettability may account for the favorable wear performance of alumina.

Alumina Head-Metal Stem Fixation

Before 1977 different means of head fixation were tested, among them, gluing and screw fixation; both failed. In 1977 a self-locking cone was proposed to secure the head to the stem. The taper linearity of the cone must be between 0.5 and 0.75 μm. Considerations relating to the wedge stress as a function of the cone angle led to an optimized angle of approximately 6° (Fig. 1). Small cone angles and low friction are not desirable nor are large angles, such as 10°, which exhibit insufficient rotational stability. Surgeons must be aware that cone angles may differ significantly from one manufacturer to another. In this respect any ceramic head cannot fit any femoral stem. If there is a mismatch between head and neck angles, stress peaks will result, leading to an early fracture of the ceramic head.

The surface finish of the metal cone should be roughened by applying a fine-thread structure (Fig. 2). This spreads the ceramic-metal stress over a large area. The inner surface of the ceramic cone has to be machined in a manner that ensures a large contact resulting in high friction and rotational stability. The grooves on the surface of the metal neck have to be kept small enough to exclude subcritical crack growth. The optimum surface roughness (R_a) is between 0.5 and 1 μm (22).

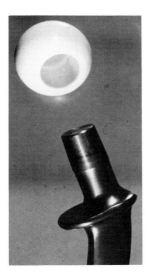

FIG. 1. Alumina-ceramic head–titanium-alloy stem assembly. The cone angle value is between 5° and 6° (Ceraver-Osteal design).

Contamination between both neck and head cones during surgery (blood, cement, tissues) must be avoided. This may be responsible for stress concentration leading to head fracture.

Clinical Considerations

Used clinically since the early 1970s, alumina has by far the longest medical history and has been implanted in several hundred thousands of patients, either in the form of dental implants or bearing components for THR. For the latter, alumina-PE or alumina-alumina combinations are available. Alumina-PE shows five times less wear than metal-PE (8). However, PE remains the weak link and its creep behavior does not differ whether metal or alumina is used. The alumina-alumina combination

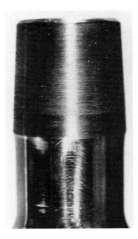

FIG. 2. Detail of the surface finish of the metal cone of the prosthesis in Fig. 1. The micro-threaded surface spreads the ceramic-metal stress transfer over a large area.

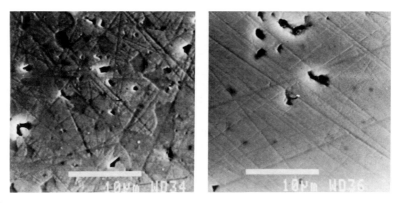

FIG. 3. Scanning electron micrograph view of the weight-bearing surface of an alumina femoral ball retrieved after 2 years (*left*) compared to a nonimplanted head (*right*). There is relief polishing caused by running-in with polishing marks still visible on the surface.

shows negligible wear (Fig. 3) and low friction provided the ceramic has both appropriate properties and clearance between the friction components (12). However, alumina is a very rigid material. The mismatch between bone and ceramic compliances may explain the incidence of alumina cup loosening that has been reported in the literature (20,30). Interestingly, in terms of loosening, results obtained in patients under the age of 50 are much better than in older patients and far superior to metal-PE THR (26). This could be related to a better quality of bone stock in younger patients. In addition to plain cementless and cemented alumina sockets, other methods of fixation have been developed, e.g., metal-backed threaded cups and metal-backed fiber mesh cups fitted with an alumina insert (Fig. 4).

Alumina has a high compressive strength and a low bending strength that limit the diameter of the femoral ball. This characteristic has led to the research and devel-

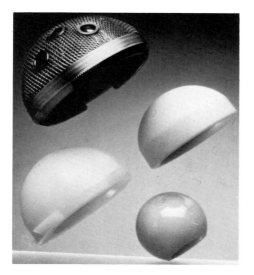

FIG. 4. A metal shell made of titanium alloy covered with a commercially pure titanium fiber mesh can be fitted either with a PE or alumina insert (Cerafit design from Ceraver-Osteal).

opment of new tougher ceramics with improved mechanical properties, such as alumina-zirconium blends or stabilized zirconium.

YTTRIUM PARTIALLY STABILIZED ZIRCONIUM

Material Properties

Zirconium oxide ceramics have three phases: monoclinic, tetragonal, and cubic. The cubic phase is stable but brittle; the tetragonal phase is tough but unstable and may transform into the monoclinic phase. In the presence of a small amount of stabilizing additives (MgO, CaO, and Y_2O_3), tetragonal particles, provided they are small enough, can be maintained in a metastable state at temperatures below the tetragonal-to-monoclinic transformation temperature. The transformation of small tetragonal grains, which should result in a volume increase, is prevented by the compressive stresses applied on these grains by their neighbors. The corresponding class of ceramics is named partially stabilized zirconium (PSZ), the final microstructure of which consists of 0.5-μm diameter grains on average.

The volume change related to the tetragonal to monoclinic phase transformation results in a prestressed material. Thus, a propagating crack can release the stresses in the neighboring grains, which then transform from the metastable state into the monoclinic phase. Because the monoclinic grain volume is larger than the tetragonal one, the associated volume expansion results in compressive stresses at the edge of the crack front and extra energy is required for the crack to propagate further.

The process of producing sintered PSZ is similar to that of alumina. The raw material is made of 0.02 μm particles. Sintering is performed at a temperature below 1,500°C and HIP can be added. When comparing the material properties of Y_2O_3-ZrO_2 ceramics to surgical-grade Al_2O_3, it appears that bending strength and toughness of transformation-toughened zirconium are three times higher than those of alumina. In addition, the ZrO_2-based materials exhibit a lower Young's modulus pointing to an interesting elastic deformation capability when compared to alumina (4). On the other hand, zirconium is less hard than alumina (1,250 vs 2,300 HV). Mechanical properties of Y-PSZ are listed in Table 2.

Friction and Wear

The tribological behavior of PSZ has been investigated by several authors (25,28,29). Using a ring-on-disk test with a ceramic-ceramic combination, Sudanese et al. (29) found that the wear rate of such a combination was unacceptable for zir-

TABLE 2. *Main properties of sintered +*
HIP yttrium-PSZ (Prozyr)

Density	6.1 g/cmE3
Grain size	<0.5 μm
Microhardness (Vickers)	1,000–1,300 HV
Young's modulus	200,000 MPa
Bending strength	1,200 MPa
Fracture toughness	9–10 MPa mE½

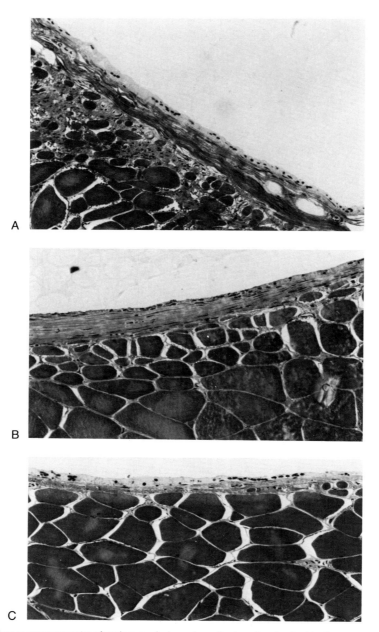

FIG. 5. Tissue response to alumina and zirconia cylinders implanted in the paravertebral muscles of the rabbit (haematoxylin-eosin, original magnification ×400). The features of the encapsulating membrane are identical for both materials. Histomorphometric analysis does not show significant differences between the two materials with time. **A**, alumina at 12 weeks; **B**, zirconia at 12 weeks; **C**, alumina at 26 weeks. (*Figure continues.*)

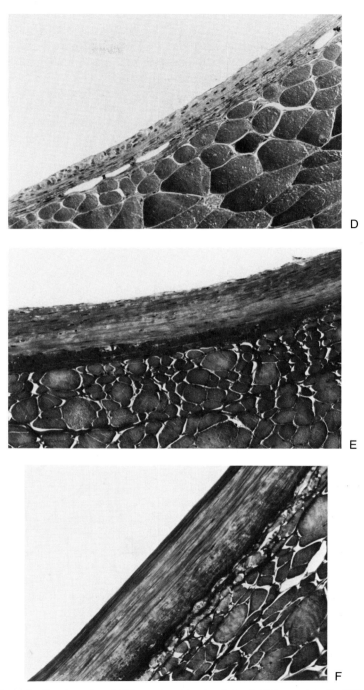

FIG. 5 *(Continued).* **D**, zirconia at 26 weeks; **E**, alumina at 104 weeks; **F**, zirconia at 104 weeks.

conia as compared to alumina (16 mmE3/h vs 0.0033 mmE3/h). When looking at the ceramic-PE combination in comparison with Ti6Al4V- and CoCrMo- (F75) PE, using also an oscillating ring-on-disk tester (25), it was shown that the average wear rate of PE was one order of magnitude higher with metal counterfaces. Also, the wear rate with alumina was five times higher than with zirconia. This was attributed to the finer grain size of zirconia. With a pin-on-disk test, Streicher et al. (28) compared the tribological properties of alumina-, zirconia-, and silicon nitride-PE combinations. The PE wear rate was the lowest for alumina. However, the surface roughness of the ceramic disks, used in this experiment, were twice the values of ball heads made from the same ceramics.

Biological Properties

Long-term implantation, up to 2 years in rabbit and sheep of bulk PSZ cylindrical implants, in either soft tissues or bone, has demonstrated no adverse effect. Histomorphometric analysis of the tissue response was similar for Y-PSZ when compared to alumina (Fig. 5). However, several points still need to be clarified: (i) biocompatibility of zirconium particles, (ii) phase transformation, and (iii) radioactivity.

(i) *In vitro* studies of submicrometer-size PSZ particles using cell cultures have demonstrated a significant cytotoxicity (18). Although no zirconium ion was detectable in the cell culture medium, the formation of an amorphous zirconium gel in the medium as well as the release of yttrium (19) might be responsible for this cytotoxic effect.

(ii) The transformation of the small tetragonal grains into the monoclinic form is triggered by external stresses when overstressed. Also the existence of impurities, like SiO_2, responsible for the formation of a glassy phase at the grain boundaries, can also lead to tetragonal to monoclinic transformation (22). Aging has been studied *in vitro,* through accelerated procedures combining various degrees of heat, humidity, and pressure for different lengths of time or *in vivo,* after implantation in animals. Contradictory results have been published describing a phase transformation rate from tetragonal to monoclinic ranging from a few percent to more than 50%. However, the materials have not always been fully described and characterized, making the comparison and relevance of the different results difficult to establish. Theoretically a transformation as high as 60% from the tetragonal to the monoclinic phase should not give any significant change in toughness of tetragonal zirconium (5).

(iii) Radioactivity emission of zirconium is also an important issue. Zirconium contains traces of thorium, due to the small content of hafnium in the sources of minerals. The emitted radioactivity is very low and often at the detection limit level (3). In addition to the amount of radiation, it is necessary to take into account their nature, alpha or gamma. Most of the alpha particles that are emitted by zirconium are absorbed within the ceramic itself. Those produced at the surface may reach the tissue lying at the interface. The effects on the human body of the delivery of a very low radioactive dose distributed focally over a very long period of time are not well-known. Also, there is no reference on the acceptable parameters of radioactivity for such implant materials.

Although PSZ has been used clinically in Europe for several years for THR, there have been no clinical data reported.

CARBON

Carbon-Carbon Composites

Pyrolytic carbon has been successfully used in cardiovascular devices for many years either as a bulk material or a coating. It is a remarkably biocompatible material; however, its mechanical performance makes it unsuitable for a heavily loaded environment as seen in orthopaedic surgery. Specific biomechanical requirements for orthopaedic applications have led to the development of a new generation of carbon composites with high mechanical strength, low modulus, good toughness, and excellent fatigue behavior. These composites consist of a dense pyrolytic carbon matrix reinforced with carbon fibers (CFRC), the fiber impregnation being achieved either by the liquid impregnation technique (LIT) or Chemical Vapor Infiltration (CVI) at high temperature. The measurements carried out on two- and three-axial CFRC, obtained by LIT using an organic resin as the matrix precursor, have demonstrated similar properties. This may be explained by the material defects related to this particular type of processing. For CVI-CFRC, within a given dimensional arrangement, the fiber type (high modulus or high tensile strength) and, to a lesser extent, the density can influence the composite properties.

It should be pointed out that although the two components of CFRC are intrinsically brittle, it is remarkable that they exhibit a pseudo plastic behavior and do not fail catastrophically in the physiological temperature range. The degree of pseudo plasticity varies according to the type of carbon fibers, the characteristics of the reinforcement, and the manufacturing process (7). CFRC devices are currently at a research stage.

Diamond-like Carbon

Recently, carbon coatings have gained a renewed interest through the diamond-like carbon (DLC) technology. The term diamond-like carbon refers to a variety of amorphous or near-amorphous forms of carbon produced by different means: ion beam deposition, dual ion beam sputtering, laser ablation, ion beam-assisted process, and, most commonly, plasma deposition of methane gas. The material is not like diamond because it is amorphous and contains some residual hydrogen. The physical properties of DLC are somewhere between graphite and diamond. DLC may be deposited both on ion-implanted metallic or polymeric substrates. However, the adhesion of the coating is correlated with the hardness of the substrate. Performance of DLC coatings varies in relation with the production process, and because of their inherent inertness, adhesion remains a major problem in DLC coatings.

The low coefficient of friction and low transfer properties of the ion beam-assisted DLC coating make it a strong potential candidate to improve the friction and wear performance of total joint prostheses (11).

REFERENCES

1. Boutin P. L'alumine et son utilisation en chirurgie de la hanche (étude expérimentale). *Presse Med* 1971;79:639–640.

2. Boutin P. Arthroplastie totale de la hanche par prothèse en alumine frittée. Etude expérimentale et premières applications cliniques. *Rev Chir Orthop* 1972;58:229–246.
3. Cales B, Peille CN. Radioactive properties of ceramic hip joint heads. In: Soltesz U, ed. *Bioceramics, vol 2*. Cologne: German Ceramic Society, 1990:152–159.
4. Christel P, Meunier A, Heller M, Torre JP, Peille CN. Mechanical properties and short-term invivo evaluation of yttrium oxide-partially-stabilized zirconia. *J Biomed Mater Res* 1989;23:45–61.
5. Christel P. Zirconia: the second generation of ceramics for total hip replacement. *Bull Hosp Joint Dis Orthop Inst* 1989;49:170–177.
6. Christel P. Biocompatibility of surgical-grade dense polycrystalline alumina. *Clin Orthop* 1992;282:10–18.
7. Christel P, Claes L, Brown SA. Carbon-reinforced composites in orthopaedic surgery. In: Szycher M, ed. *High performance biomaterials*. Lancaster, PA: Technomic, 1991;499–518.
8. Clarke IC, Dorlot JM, Graham J, et al. Biomechanical stability and design: wear. In: Ducheyne P, Lemons JE, eds. Bioceramics: material characteristics versus in vivo behavior. *Ann NY Acad Sci* 1988;523:292–296.
9. Dalgleish BJ, Rawlings RD. A comparison of the mechanical behavior of aluminas in air and simulated body environments. *J Biomed Mater Res* 1981;15:527–542.
10. Dawihl W, Dörre E. Adsorption behaviour of high-density alumina ceramics exposed to fluids. In: Winter GD, Leray JL, de Groot K, eds. *Evaluation of biomaterials*, London: John Wiley, 1980:239–244.
11. Dearnaley G. Diamond-like carbon: a potential means of reducing wear in total joint replacements. *Clin Mater (in press)*.
12. Dorlot JM, Christel P, Meunier A. Wear analysis of retrieved alumina heads and sockets of hip prostheses. *J Biomed Mater Res* 1989;23:299–310.
13. Dörre E, Hübner H. In: *Alumina, processing, properties and applications*. Berlin: Springer-Verlag, 1984:268–275.
14. Fett T, Hartlieb W, Keller K, Knecht B, Munz D, Rieger W. Subcritical crack growth in high-grade alumina. *J Nucl Mat* 1991;184:39–46.
15. Griss P, Krempien B, von Andrian-Werburg H, Heimke G, Fleiner K. Experimentelle Untersuchungen zur Gewebeverträglichkeit oxidkeramischer Abriebteilchen. *Arch Orthop Unfallchir* 1973;76:270–279.
16. Heimke G, Beisler W, von Andrian-Werburg H, Griss P, Krempien B. Untersuchungen an Implantaten aus Al203-Keramik. *Ber Dtsch Keram Ges* 1973;50:4–8.
17. Hentrich RL, Graves GA, Stein HG, Bajpai PK. An evaluation of inert and resorbable ceramics for future clinical orthopedic applications. *J Biomed Mater Res* 1971;5:25–51.
18. Ito A, Tateishi T, Niwa S, Tange S. In vitro evaluation of the cytocompatibility of wear particles generated by UHMWPE/zirconia friction. *Clin Mater (in press)*.
19. Li J, Liu Y, Hermansson L, Söremark R. Evaluation of biocompatibility of various ceramic powders with human fibroblasts in vitro. *Clin Mater (in press)*.
20. Nizard RS, Sedel L, Christel P, Meunier A, Soudry M, Witvoet J. Ten-year survivorship of cemented ceramic-ceramic total hip prosthesis. *Clin Orthop* 1992;282:53–63.
21. Osborn JF, Newesely H. Bonding osteogenesis induced by calcium phosphate ceramic implants. In: Winter GD, Gibbons DF, Plenk H Jr, eds. *Biomaterials 1980*. London: John Wiley, 1982: 51–58.
22. Rieger W. Medical applications of ceramics. In: *High-tech ceramics: viewpoints and perspectives*. San Diego: Academic Press, 1989:191–238.
23. Rock M. German patent DRP, number 583589, 1933.
24. Sandhaus S. British patent, number 1083 769, 1965.
25. Schwartz GL. Wear and strength of zirconia and alumina ceramic materials. Transactions of the 36th Annual Meeting of the Orthopaedic Research Society. New Orleans, 1990:183.
26. Sedel L, Kerboull L, Christel P, Meunier A, Witvoet J. Alumina-on-alumina hip replacement: results and survivorship in young patients. *J Bone Joint Surg [Br]* 1990;72:658–663.
27. Sedel L, Simeon J, Villette JM, Launay JM. PGE2 level in tissue surrounding failed total hip arthroplasty: effect of materials. Transactions of the 38th Annual Meeting of the Orthopaedic Research Society, 1992:351.
28. Streicher RM, Semlitch M, Schön R. Ceramic surfaces as wear partners for polyethylene. In: Bonfield W, Hastings GW, Tanner KE, eds. *Bioceramics, vol 4*. London: Butterworth-Heinemann, 1991:9–16.
29. Sudanese A, Toni A, Cattaneo GL, et al. Alumina vs zirconium oxide: a comparative wear test. In: Oonishi H, Aoki H, Sawai K, eds. *Bioceramics, vol 1*. Ishiyaku: EuroAmerica, 1989:237–240.
30. Witvoet J, Christel P, Sedel L, Herman S, Blanquaert D. Survivorship analysis of cemented Al203 sockets. In: Oonishi H, Aoki H, Sawai K, eds. *Bioceramics, vol 1*. Ishiyaku: EuroAmerica, 1989:314–319.

*Biological, Material, and Mechanical
Considerations of Joint Replacement,*
edited by B. F. Morrey.
Raven Press, Ltd., New York © 1993.

Discussion of Articulation

Donald L. Bartel

*Department of Mechanical and Aerospace Engineering, Cornell University,
Ithaca, New York 14853*

A panel of 21 surgeons and scientists discussed the current status of research and design efforts relating to the articulating surfaces of total joint replacements. The panel also considered interfaces at junctions and connections between elements of prosthetic components because in contemporary designs relative motion also occurs at these sites. The following conclusions represent broad areas of consensus (there were no major areas of contention) and recommendations.

CONSENSUS

For the majority of low-demand, elderly patients, the materials and material combinations used in properly designed total joint replacements provide excellent performance over a period of one to two decades.

To extend the longevity of total joint replacements we must design implants that minimize surface damage at the articulating surfaces. Such damage produces wear debris that induces adverse tissue reactions in the peri-implant and regenerated joint lining tissues.

The physicochemical properties of the wear debris markedly affect the cellular features and biological behavior of the tissue reaction.

In general, surface damage can be reduced by changing the geometry and material properties to reduce the stresses associated with surface damage, using more wear resistant surfaces, or improving the lubrication of the joint.

The stresses associated with damage to articulating surfaces are a function of the material properties, material combinations, and design. The effects of elastic modulus, thickness, and conformity on stresses associated with surface damage may be calculated and provide a basis for evaluating the design of tibial and acetabular components that is used to advantage in many contemporary designs. Regardless of the adequacy of the design, the quality of the surgical procedure will strongly influence the performance of the device in the patient.

The material, chemical, and physical properties of polyethylene available today vary considerably and have substantial effects on the wear characteristics of total joint components. The damage may be caused in several ways. Adhesive, abrasive, and fatigue mechanisms of surface damage are all known to occur in articulating surfaces. The relative importance and contributions of each of these mechanisms in conforming and nonconforming total joint replacements are yet to be determined.

Data are available describing wear rates in total hip replacements. For example, clinical history suggests that polyethylene wear is less when ceramic rather than metal heads are used. However, it is not yet known how much of this difference is attributable to surface finish, wettability, hardness, or other parameters. It is also generally agreed that the volume of wear debris for ceramic-ceramic and metal-metal bearings in total hip replacement may be less than for metal-polyethylene or ceramic-polyethylene bearings. To be successful, these devices must be manufactured to extremely tight tolerances and three-body abrasive wear must be avoided.

Surface damage may also occur at junctions between elements of modular components. Under load, relative motion may occur at these interfaces that can lead to fretting, corrosion, and generation of debris particles. Because of this, modularity is only justifiable to the extent that the benefits outweigh the risks.

FUTURE RECOMMENDATIONS

Because polyethylene components will continue to be an important element of total joint replacements, the mechanisms by which surface damage occurs must be clarified and the stress distribution and magnitudes that are associated with each of these mechanisms must be determined. The effects of surface roughness, wettability, hardness, and other parameters on the wear of polyethylene in total hip replacements should also be established.

There is a need for more detailed, accurate information on the chemical and physical properties of the polyethylene that is used for acetabular and tibial components from all manufacturers. The data should include such properties as molecular weight, crystallinity, crystal morphology, fabrication methods, degree of fusion, stabilization method, and dose. This information is essential for the interpretation of the varying outcomes that are seen in current clinical data. Furthermore, it is necessary to quantify the effects of these properties on clinical and experimental data.

Modifications in the processing of ultrahigh molecular weight polyethylene can induce significant changes in key physical and chemical properties (e.g., crystallinity, density, modulus, strength, resistance to oxidation). Research is needed to determine the effects of changes in these properties on the wear resistance of prosthetic components, recognizing that the optimum combination of properties may be different for designs in which the articulating surfaces are conforming and designs that employ nonconforming articulations.

Current methods for screening the wear characteristics of material combinations provide useful information on the relationship of specific material properties to wear. However, the issues of design and material cannot be separated and ultimately material combinations must be studied using specimen geometry that simulates their eventual application.

To extend the longevity of total joint replacements it is necessary to understand the ongoing changes in material and physical properties that occur in polyethylene due to sterilization, exposure to the *in vivo* environment, and loading. In particular, in light of current data on postradiation aging, steps are needed to minimize the degradation that can occur to polyethylene components prior to implantation.

Components used at present for total joint replacements are associated with the generation of wear debris. Because it may not be possible to totally eliminate the generation of some wear debris, articular component design, modular junctions, and fixation concepts should be developed that minimize access of wear debris to the peri-implant tissues. When modular components are used, the locking and security of all junctions must be optimized; the relative motion at nonarticular junctions of prostheses should be minimized or eliminated if possible.

Biological, Material, and Mechanical
Considerations of Joint Replacement,
edited by B. F. Morrey.
Raven Press, Ltd., New York © 1993.

26

Prosthesis Wear Particle Effects on Cells and Tissues

Donald W. Howie

Department of Orthopaedic Surgery and Trauma, University of Adelaide,
Department of Orthopaedic Surgery and Trauma, Royal Adelaide Hospital,
Adelaide 5000, South Australia

Prosthetic materials commonly used over the past 20 years have been cobalt-chrome alloys, stainless steel, ultrahigh molecular weight polyethylene (UHMWP), poly-methylmethacrylate (PMMA), and more recently titanium and titanium alloys and aluminum oxide ceramic. Other polymers and materials have been used less commonly.

The use of these materials as the articulating surfaces of prostheses results in liberation of variable numbers of wear particles (20) into the surrounding tissues. The use of cobalt-chrome alloy articulating against itself may result in moderate wear and the accumulation of large numbers of metal wear particles in the tissues (33,34). Initial experience with various types of polymers also resulted in severe wear (22,23), and UHMWP remains prone to wear if used as a convex bearing surface (4,30). Aluminum oxide ceramic may be more resistant to wear. Recently considerable attention has been given to the problem of metal particles, particularly titanium alloy, and generation of wear from the articulating surface of titanium-alloy particles (1).

Wear particles may also be generated from movement that occurs at either the implant-bone interface or implant-implant interface of modular prostheses. It is important to realize that cemented stems are modular and that movement at the interface between stem and cement may cause production of metal and cement debris. Moreover, it is important to realize that implants may be slightly loose yet function well for many years. This may result in production of large numbers of wear particles at the interface where a small amount of micromotion is occurring.

Whereas an adverse tissue response to wear particles has been frequently reported, the mechanism whereby wear particles provoke loosening has remained obscure. Therefore, the role of wear particles in loosening and the possibility of other factors being involved require further investigation. This chapter summarizes human, animal, and *in vitro* studies aimed at providing a better understanding of the relationship between wear particles, bone resorption, and prosthesis loosening. The human studies were performed to determine the types of wear particles and tissue response around failed hip arthroplasties and to relate these findings to the animal studies. The animal studies have concentrated on the tissue response to particles of materials commonly used as the articulating surface of prostheses: cobalt-chrome alloy, UHMWP, and aluminum oxide ceramic. The review of *in vitro* studies has concentrated on toxicity and release of inflammatory mediators.

LOOSENING OF PROSTHESES

Grading Loosening

To better describe the pattern and degree of loosening we have developed an operative grading system (11) and compared this with microscopic findings at the cement-bone interface of revised prostheses. We studied this in resurfacing arthroplasties and what we found applies to the interface between cancellous bone and cement. The grading system will need to be further refined for other implant-bone interfaces but it is a useful guide to the degree of loosening.

The operative grade of loosening was found to correlate reasonably well with the microscopic findings at the interface. The absence of detectable movement at the bone-cement interface (operative loosening grade 0) usually implies the microscopic appearance of either the cement remaining impregnated between surface trabeculae or the cement interdigitating into a thin connective-tissue layer. The presence of fluid ingress and egress at the interface (operative loosening grade 1) implies the presence of connective tissue at the interface. There is likely to be microscopic evidence of loosening, demonstrated by abrasion of the surface of this connective tissue. Slight movement at the bone-cement interface (operative loosening grade 2) implies the presence of a connective-tissue layer or exposed bone at the interface. The presence of gross loosening and the ability to easily remove the prosthesis component (operative loosening grade 3) imply similar appearances at the interface as seen with slight loosening but greater loss of supporting bone.

By comparing the degree of operative loosening with the microscopic findings at the interface, it is possible to classify the implant-bone interface as stable, slightly loose, or grossly loose.

Migration of Particles

We used this classification and histologic examination of the periprosthetic tissues to study stable and loose resurfacing hip arthroplasties. We demonstrated a predominantly macrophage and multinucleate giant-cell response, the presence of large numbers of polyethylene wear particles, and smaller numbers of acrylic, bone, and metal particles (11).

An important finding was the presence of small polyethylene particles in the superior regions of the bone-cement interface of solidly fixed femoral components with stable interfaces. These particles were found within macrophages in the superficial marrow spaces and in a very thin cellular connective-tissue layer separating bone from cement. The particles were found in regions where cement remained impregnated between bone trabeculae or into connective tissue at the interface and where there was no microscopic evidence of loosening. Since these particles were found in areas a considerable distance from the joint cavity, it is proposed that small polyethylene particles migrate along the interface between solidly fixed components. We propose that these particles provoke a macrophage response in the underlying marrow and that this tissue response will contribute to bone resorption at the interface. It may also be possible that macrophages already containing these particles migrate along these interfaces.

Movement of Fluid and Particles Along Interfaces

Ohlin and Lerner (24) concluded that in aseptically loosened total hip replacements, the capsule seems to have a greater production of mediators stimulating bone resorption than bone-cement membranes. The capsule may be exposed to more wear products than are present at the bone-cement interface, but it may also reflect different biologic features of the tissues. The fact that the production of mediators is most often greater in the capsule than in other periprosthetic tissues studied, is hypothetically due to a "prosthetic synovitis" of varying intensity always present in artificial joints and reflects a general foreign-body reaction. The release of mediators capable of inducing bone resorption into the synovial fluid could explain the initiation and maintenance of the loosening process by means of fluid transport. We and others have shown by arthrographic studies that this fluid penetrates the proximal bone-cement interface of femoral stems, invariably is present at the bone-cement interface of cemented sockets, and may reach part of the implant-bone interface around solidly fixed cementless acetabular and femoral components. This may be one explanation of socket loosening in wear-prone prostheses. Additionally, as proposed by Ling *(personal communication),* joint fluid containing wear particles or mediators (24) may move along the space between the stem and its surrounding cement mantle and through defects in the latter to reach the periprosthetic bone. This may be an explanation of the scalloped appearance of bone resorption at a distance from the joint.

TISSUE RESPONSE AROUND FAILED ARTHROPLASTIES IN HUMANS

Factors Influencing Tissue Response

Tissue appearance depends on a number of factors, including the presence or absence of infection (19), degree of loosening, type of prosthesis material, duration of the implant (32), amount and type of wear debris (20,34), and possibly the reactivity of the patient, particularly those with rheumatoid arthritis.

We have studied tissue appearance around a variety of cementless and cemented hip arthroplasties made of the commonly used materials and with articulating surfaces composed of various materials. Of particular interest was the type of cellular response in relation to type and morphology of wear particles.

Noncemented Arthroplasties

Histologic examination of the tissues around cementless metal-on-bone arthroplasties reveals that the capsule around the cementless metal-on-bone arthroplasties and the connective tissue at the implant-bone interface consist mainly of mature fibrous tissue. Occasional macrophages are present in association with small num-

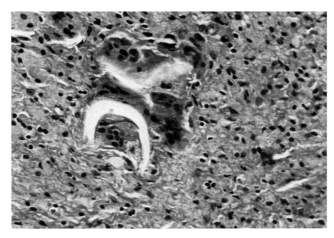

FIG. 1. Photomicrograph of human connective tissue between acetabular cement and bone in a failed Wagner prosthesis taken during joint revision. The tissue is infiltrated by macrophages and multinucleate giant cells. ×260.

bers of metal particles. Multinucleate giant cells are not usually present in significant numbers. Lymphocytes may occasionally be seen.

Around cementless metal-on-metal arthroplasties the capsule and the connective-tissue layer at the prosthesis-bone interface are often stained gray on naked-eye examination of the fresh tissues, but some long-term implants may show little or no staining. Histologic examination reveals that the capsule consisted in most cases of mature fibrous tissues. In some cases a macrophage infiltrate in association with

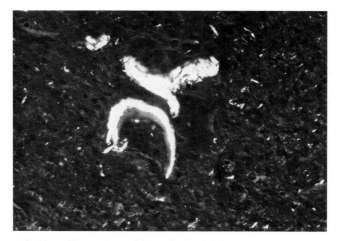

FIG. 2. The same field as Fig. 1 viewed by polarized light showing predominantly small polyethylene particles and measured shards of polyethylene surrounded by multinucleate giant cells. ×260.

metal wear particles is seen. Occasional lymphocytes and lymphocytic aggregates are seen, and there are occasional areas of necrosis.

Electron microscopic examination of the tissue around the cementless metal-on-metal arthroplasties show accumulation of electron-dense particles in macrophages in the capsule and connective tissue at the interface between bone and acetabular and femoral components. Some macrophages that had phagocytosed particles showed extensive accumulation of cytolysosomes. Other macrophages showed total loss of cell membrane and clumping of nuclear chromatin, suggesting degeneration. Other cells retrieved from long-term arthroplasties appear minimally affected by the presence of particles.

Examination of cementless ceramic-on-ceramic arthroplasties reveals that the articulating surfaces of these prostheses usually show little evidence of wear, but occasionally catastrophic wear is present. The capsule and interface tissues are composed of mature connective tissue and a variable but often minimal macrophage response, depending on the number of particles.

Examination of the tissues around cementless metal-on-polyethylene prostheses shows a wide variety of appearances. In some cases there is evidence of significant polyethylene wear-particle accumulation and associated macrophage response. Titanium- or cobalt-chrome-alloy wear particles are present to varying degrees, and this seems to be related to the amount of abrasion of the implant on bone.

Cemented Arthroplasties

A common histologic feature found in the tissues around cemented metal-on-metal arthroplasties is the presence of a macrophage infiltrate in association with very small intracellular metal wear particles. Areas of necrosis are seen occasionally. Multinucleate giant cells are present occasionally in association with cement particles, and lymphocytic aggregates are sometimes seen. Some of our long-term retrievals have shown a surprisingly benign tissue appearance and very few wear particles.

Histologic examination of the tissues around cemented metal-on-polyethylene arthroplasties demonstrates a common pattern; the tissues are infiltrated with varying numbers of macrophages and multinucleate giant cells are common (Fig. 1), lymphocytic aggregates are present occasionally. The tissues contain varying numbers of highly birefringent polyethylene particles (Fig. 2) and voids due to acrylic particles that have dissolved during tissue processing. Metal particles are present around stainless steel, cobalt-chrome, and particularly titanium-alloy components. Small particles of polyethylene are contained within macrophages and larger particles of polyethylene and acrylic are associated with multinucleate giant cells.

Electron microscopy of the connective tissue at the bone-cement interface shows accumulation of particles in macrophages. These particles are assumed to be polyethylene as the particles had not dissolved during tissue processing and metal is not detected on energy dispersive x-ray (EDX) analysis of the particles. Electron microscopy shows macrophages adjacent to cement particles, and, depending on the amount of metal debris, macrophages are seen to contain metal particles and metal particles are also seen extracellularly.

IN VIVO STUDIES

Intra-articular Injection of Wear Particles

The injection of cobalt-chrome particles into rat knee joints causes an initial polymorphonuclear response followed by a macrophage infiltrate and necrosis in the synovium and subsynovium. A lymphocytic response at 7 days is seen but its significance is unclear. At 3 months macrophages and necrosis persist in the tissues. Further studies of the long-term effects of cobalt-chrome particles (14) demonstrate that after 6 months and 1 year necrotic areas persist with particles both intracellularly and lying within an amorphous ground substance. The changes that occur in particle and macrophage scores of the subsynovium over 1 year demonstrate that some particles are cleared from the joint, but many remain within the subsynovium (14). Thus, although some particles are being cleared, one may still expect particles to remain within the joint and to accumulate if there is continued production of wear particles from a joint prosthesis.

One week following injection of aluminum oxide particles and cobalt-chrome particles of similar size, there is a difference in the macrophage-to-particle ratio, suggesting that the response to the cobalt-chrome in terms of the number of macrophages was more severe. At 4 weeks and at 3 months we did not find a difference in the macrophage response. Thus, it appears that the type of wear particle may determine tissue response.

Polyethylene particles were prepared in a wear simulator. Injection of these particles produces the typical appearance seen around prostheses with a polyethylene articulating surface. Large shards of polyethylene and also aggregates of small particles were contained within multinucleate giant cells (Figs. 3 and 4). Examination of tissues revealed that, as a rough guide, particles larger than the size of a nucleus of a macrophage (i.e., approximately 5 μm) produce what under light microscopy appears to be a multinucleate giant-cell response. A mononucleate-cell response is produced by particles smaller than this.

Repeated injections of polyethylene-wear particles were administered in one knee and saline particles in the other knee of rats with acrylic plugs inserted in their distal

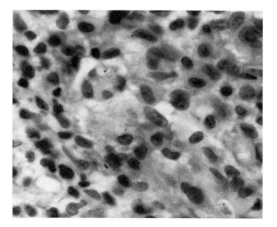

FIG. 3. The rat subsynovium following multiple injections of polyethylene particles. The subsynovium is infiltrated by macrophages and multinucleate giant cells. (Hematoxylin-eosin; original magnification, ×240).

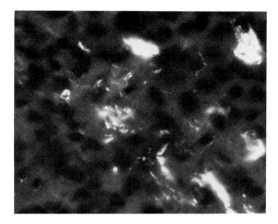

FIG. 4. Same field as in Fig. 3 viewed by polarized light showing small birefringent polyethylene particles contained within macrophages, whereas large particles and aggregates of small particles are contained within multinucleate giant cells. (Hematoxylin-eosin; original magnification, ×240).

femurs (16). The cement plug was adjacent to the joint. If one injects saline there is no change in that appearance, whereas repeated injections of polyethylene particles produce a different appearance. Polyethylene particles were found within the knee joint but also at the interface between the cement plug and bone. Transverse section of the bone near the joint showed that, instead of the plug being encompassed in bone, there was now connective tissue with voids that contained the polyethylene particles. Further studies using this model have not as yet allowed us to quantitate bone resorption because of the large variability in appearance around the plug. However, this model supports our hypothesis that in the absence of infection, loading, or macro-movement at the interface, one sees an adverse response to prosthesis wear particles that are present at the implant-bone interface.

Ultrastructural Appearances of Cellular Response to Prosthesis Wear Particles

The majority of studies of the effects of wear particles in humans and animals have relied largely on the light microscopy appearances of tissue response to wear particles. However, light microscopy alone does not allow a comprehensive assessment of the effects of very small particles of cells because subtle ultrastructural changes are beyond the resolution of the light microscope. Thus, the ultrastructural appearances of rat knee synovium were examined at intervals from 1 day to 4 weeks following the intra-articular injection of cobalt-chrome-alloy, aluminum oxide-ceramic, and polyethylene wear particles in rat knee joints. The appearances were compared with previous light microscopy studies (13,15) and with the appearances in the tissues around failed human arthroplasties (33).

Electron microscopic examination of the synovium of rat knees following the injection of cobalt-chrome-alloy particles demonstrates that these particles cause varying degrees of degeneration and necrosis of synovial and subsynovial macrophages containing endocytosed particles. Appearances similar to the "rounding up" of degenerate macrophages described following the phagocytosis of cobalt-chrome particles *in vitro* (6) also were seen on the surface of the synovium in this study (Fig. 5). These findings confirm the focal ulceration and necrosis observed in light microscopic studies of rat knee synovium following the intra-articular injection of cobalt-

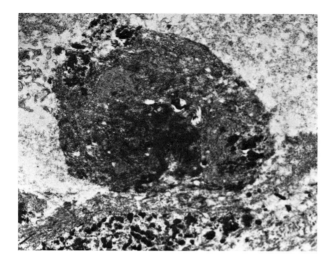

FIG. 5. Electron micrograph of the synovium 1 week following the injection of cobalt-chrome particles. A necrotic cell containing endocytosed particulate material shows a smooth, rounded profile with loss of its ruffled border, loss of nuclear definition, and lack of recognizable cellular organelles (magnification ×17,500).

chrome wear particles (13) and observed in human tissues around cobalt-chrome prostheses.

EDX microanalysis of the intracellular particles confirms the presence of cobalt and chrome in the particles similar to results obtained when the tissues around human prostheses were analyzed.

Four weeks following the injection of cobalt-chrome particles there was proliferation of macrophages and type-B synovitis. Macrophages in the subsynovium showed evidence of increased numbers of cytolysosomes. This finding is consistent with *in vitro* studies that have demonstrated the release of lysosomal enzymes by macrophages in response to various metal particles (27,29). Increased lysosomal enzyme activity, as indicated by positive staining for acid phosphatase and naphthol esterase, also has been described in foci of macrophages and multinucleate giant cells in association with various types of wear particles in the tissues around human prostheses (5).

By contrast with cobalt-chrome particles, synovial ulceration and marked macrophage degeneration did not occur following the injection of aluminum-oxide particles (Fig. 6). This is consistent with light microscopic studies showing the absence of necrosis following the intra-articular injection of aluminum oxide in rats knees (15).

Of interest is the finding of early cytotoxic effects of cobalt-chrome particles on macrophages, followed later by the presence of apparently healthy macrophages containing endocytosed material. It is not yet clear whether the early corrosion of cobalt-chrome particles within cells, possibly liberating toxic cobalt salts within cells, causes the cytopathic effects observed early after exposure *in vitro* (6) and observed *in vivo* in the present studies. Such corrosion could result in a progressive lessening of toxicity of the particles, thereby allowing the accumulation of abundant particles in macrophages that do not exhibit any degenerative features. By contrast, aluminum oxide, which is highly resistant to corrosion, has shown minimal cytopathic effects in this study.

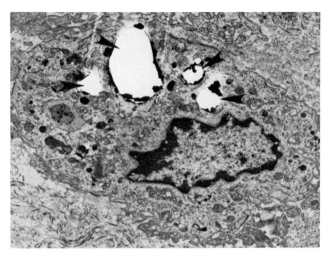

FIG. 6. Electron micrograph of the subsynovium 1 week following the injection of aluminum-oxide particles. A macrophage containing endocytosed particles (*arrows*) shows no evidence of degeneration (magnification ×5,500).

After polyethylene-particle injection, degeneration of lining synoviocytes was occasionally seen. The subsynovium was infiltrated by macrophages and multinucleate giant cells that had phagocytosed particles (Fig. 7). Degeneration of macrophages was not a feature of the subsynovial response. Particles less than approximately 5 μm in maximum dimension, and often less than the resolution of the light microscope, were contained within single macrophages. Although these findings confirm

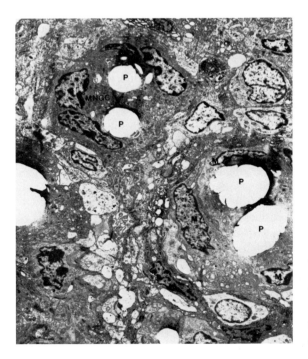

FIG. 7. Low-power electron micrograph of the synovium and subsynovium 4 weeks following the injection of polyethylene particles. Within the subsynovium there are two cellular aggregates surrounding particles (P). One aggregate (MNGC) does not show the presence of cellular membranes separating the nuclei, whereas the other aggregate (M) of nuclei has identifiable cellular membranes and is an aggregate of mononuclear macrophages surrounding particles (magnification × 4,000).

to a large degree the light microscopic appearances, the important findings in the study were the size of particle that is phagocytosed by a single macrophage and that either aggregates of small particles or single large particles may be surrounded by either densely aggregated macrophages or multinucleate giant cells.

IN VITRO STUDIES

The advantage of *in vitro* tissue culture techniques is that they are a quick, sensitive, quantitative test of the response to materials by living cells and, in particular, human cells. The disadvantage with *in vitro* testing is that it precludes complex tissue interactions because the cell culture is stagnant and, therefore, separated from a blood supply and from possible neural, hormonal, and metabolic control mechanisms (28). This makes extrapolation of the results to the clinical situation difficult.

Rae (28) summarized the usual techniques of tissue-culture assessment of biocompatibility of implant materials and emphasized the possible influence of the following factors: the physical form of the material, sizes and shapes of particles, presence of soluble products, method of assessment of toxicity, and choice of cell and tissue type.

In Vitro Studies of Inflammatory Mediators in Periprosthetic Tissues

Goldring et al. (8) first demonstrated the elevated levels of prostaglandin E_2 (PGE$_2$) and collagenase in the tissue they described as a "synovial cell like" lining adjacent to loose cemented femoral stems and in a later paper (17) showed less PGE$_2$ in connective tissue around more rigidly fixed implants. Goldring et al. (8) also suggested differences in the histology of periprosthetic pseudo membranes, rheumatoid patients having more papillary transformation and lymphocytic hyperplasia than osteoarthritic patients.

Thornhill et al. (31) demonstrated elevated levels of PGE$_2$ and interleukin-1 (IL-1) production by the synovium-like cells of the tissue around an animal model. Goldring (7) also showed that PGE$_2$ or PGE$_2$-dependent factors are released by membrane tissues and suggested a role for IL-1. Kim et al. (18) reported equal amounts of PGE$_2$ in membranes around titanium and cobalt-chrome cementless total hip replacements (articulating against polyethylene) and Austin Moore stems, whereas collagenase and IL-1 were lower around the Austin Moore stems. Ohlin et al. (25) confirmed bone resorption *in vitro* by a cell-dependent mechanism that stimulated osteoclasts and suggested the presence of a PG-dependent mechanism and a nonprostanoid, one not affected by cyclooxygenase inhibitor.

Levels of PGE$_2$ in synovial fluid of patients with aseptic loose total hip replacements were compared with solid joints by Horowitz et al. (10) and were much higher. However, Gruen et al. (9) did not believe that osteolysis was initiated by biochemical factors because the levels of inflammatory mediators in the tissues around hips with osteolysis were not different from hips with fixed stems without focal osteolysis. Chiba et al. (3) suggested that tumor necrosis factor, IL-6, and IL-1 were the important mediators of bone resorption as these were higher in membranes from osteolytic foci.

From the above it can be seen that there is considerable support for the role of PGE$_2$ and cytokines in bone resorption. It is important to realize that cytokine production in response to wear particles is likely to be modified by a number of factors, including intracellular effects and the presence of inhibitors (Fig. 8). However, it would seem reasonable that osteoclasts are stimulated by these inflammatory mediators released by macrophages. It may also be that macrophages play a more direct role in bone resorption.

Periprosthetic Bone-Resorbing Cells

The role of inflammatory cells in aseptic loosening has been studied by examining the bone-resorption capacity of these cells. Pazzaglia and Pringle (26) examined macrophages and giant cells from around loose total hip prostheses. The cells had ingested particles and were tested for their ability to resorb bone *in vitro*, using osteoclasts as the control. Macrophages and giant cells did not form pits or resorption lacunae on the bone substrates, and thus the authors believed that the results supported the view that bone resorption around implants is mediated by osteoclasts. A role of macrophages in the attachment phase of bone resorption was suggested.

Athanasou et al. (2) found different results. They examined macrophages and foreign-body macrophage polykaryons from the capsules of failed hip arthroplasties, which they distinguished from osteoclasts by their antigenic phenotype and lack of response to calcitonin. When cultured on cortical bone slices, both macrophages and macrophage polykaryons produced small resorption pits and were associated with areas of superficial resorption of the bone surface. The authors thought that these results indicate that foreign-body-induced macrophages and macrophage polykaryons are capable of a type of low-grade bone resorption that may be of pathogenic significance in the loosening of cemented joint prosthetic components. We have investigated the use of this assay method but found the tests difficult to quantitate when there is low-grade resorption because of the uneven surface of the cut bone and the inherent variability of the bone surface. Suffice it to say that the importance

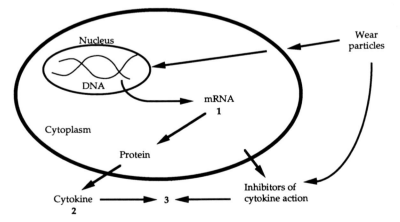

FIG. 8. The possible effects of wear particles on cytokine production. The effects can be assessed by detecting (1) cytokine mRNA using *in situ* or Northern hybridization (1), immunoreactive protein using immunohistology or enzyme-linked immunosorbent assay (2), and (3) biologic activity using specific responder cells *in vitro* (3).

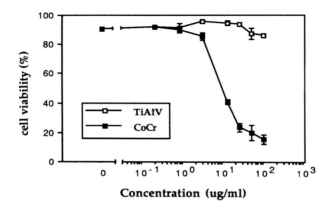

FIG. 9. Preliminary studies of the differences in toxicity pattern of rodent macrophages exposed to particules of titanium-aluminum-vanadium (TiAlV) and cobalt-chrome (CoCr).

of the direct effects of macrophages on periprosthetic bone resorption remain unclear.

Toxicity and Release of Inflammatory Mediators

The degree of particle toxicity is determined by a number of factors that include the inherent toxicity of the material to cells, solubility of the particle in body fluids, size of particles, degree of phagocytosis and particles by different types of cells, and solubility of the particle within cells.

As well as causing cell necrosis, particles adversely affect the functional capability of cells and induce lysosomal enzyme and inflammatory mediator release by phagocytic cells. Murray and Rushton (21) investigated *in vitro* particulate-debris induction of bone resorption. Macrophages that phagocytosed particles became activated and stimulated up to 15 times as much bone resorption as did control macrophages.

Metal particles remain a concern. They may be produced by wear at the articulating surface, abrasion due to micromotion at the prosthesis-bone interface or femoral stem-cement interface, and fretting at metal-metal articulation of modular prostheses.

Our studies suggest differences in the pattern of toxicity and also in the release of inflammatory mediators, particularly PGE_2 but also cytokines, in response to titanium alloy and cobalt-chrome alloy (12) (Fig. 9). We believe that this relationship between toxicity and inflammation is important when defining the relative biocompatibility of prosthetic materials and their wear particles.

SUMMARY

The findings in our studies and those of others have demonstrated that the appearances of the periprosthetic tissues are related to the type, number, and size of particles. However, it must be remembered that the appearances at revision surgery do not tell the full story. It is clear that throughout the life of a prosthesis, there are ongoing production of wear particles and clearance of wear particles from the surrounding joint. Clearly the appearance and tissue response around any given prosthesis will be related to the balance between the rate of production of wear particles, the ability of the tissues to deal with the particles, and the rate of clearance of the particles from the joint.

It is important to appreciate that wear particle-associated inflammation may not be enough in itself to cause progressive loss of bone. It is likely that other factors, which may include continuing production of particles, micromotion at the implant-bone interface, fluid movement, and pressure effects, act in concert with wear particles to induce bone lysis.

As there is no ideal bearing material that currently fulfills all the requirements of arthroplasty design, some degree of wear-particle production and accumulation in the periprosthetic tissues can be expected. The amount and type of wear debris produced will depend on a number of factors, some of which are within the control of prosthesis designers and surgeons. It is important, therefore, that designers and users of prostheses are aware of the inherent wear characteristics of a given implant material and the potential of wear particles of this material to cause an adverse tissue response and thus contribute to bone resorption and prosthesis loosening.

ACKNOWLEDGMENTS

This work was undertaken with the following departments and the author acknowledges the assistance of the staff in the Department of Orthopaedic Surgery and Trauma, Royal Adelaide Hospital; Department of Pathology, University of Adelaide; and Division of Tissue Pathology and Medical Illustration and Electron Microscopy Units of the Institute of Medical and Veterinary Science.

The author acknowledges the assistance of Prof. B. Vernon-Roberts, Dr. R. Garrett, Mr. D. Haynes, Ms. M. McGee, Mrs. J. McLean, Ms. S. Hay, Ms. S. Rogers, Mr. B. Dixon, Dr. T. Mukherjee, Dr. M. Pearcy, and Mrs. E. Patterson.

This research was supported in part by grants from the Daws Research Fellowship and Research Foundation, Royal Adelaide Hospital; Adelaide Bone and Joint Research Foundation; Australian Orthopaedic Association and Royal Australasian College of Surgeons; and National Health and Medical Research Council.

REFERENCES

1. Agins HJ, Alcock NW, Bansal M, Salvati EA, Wilson PD, Pellicci PM. Metallic wear in failed titanium alloy total hip replacements. *J Bone Joint Surg [Am]* 1988;70:347–356.
2. Athanasou NA, Quinn J, Bulstrode CJK. Resorption of bone by inflammatory cells derived from the joint capsule of hip arthroplasties. *J Bone Joint Surg [Br]* 1990;72:988–992.
3. Chiba J, Iwaki Y, Kim KJ, Rubash HE. The role of cytokines in femoral osteolysis after cementless total hip arthroplasty. Transactions of the 38th Annual Meeting of the Orthopaedic Research Society, 1992;17:350.
4. Dahl E, Mikkelsen DA. Wear of the polyethylene head of the Oscobal prosthesis. *Acta Orthop Scand* 1976;47:643.
5. Eftekhar NS, Doty SB, Johnston AD, Parisen MV. Prosthetic synovitis. *Hip* 1985;169.
6. Garrett R, Wilksch J, Vernon-Roberts B. Effects of cobalt-chrome alloy wear particles on the morphology, viability and phagocytic activity of murine macrophages in vitro. *Aust J Exp Biol Med Sci* 1983;61:355–369.
7. Goldring SR, Jasty M, Roelke MS, Rourke CM, Bringhurst FR, Harris WH. Formation of a synovial-like membrane at the bone-cement interface. Its role in bone resorption and implant loosening after total hip replacement. *Arthritis Rheum* 1986;29:836–842.
8. Goldring SR, Schiller AL, Roelke M, Rourke CM, O'Neill DA, Harris WH. The synovial-like membrane at the bone-cement interface in loose total hip replacements and its proposed role in bone lysis. *J Bone Joint Surg [Am]* 1983;65:575–584.

9. Gruen TA, Dorr LD, Bloebaum R, Emmanuel J, Saberi MT. Osteolysis in bone ingrowth total hip arthroplasty. Transactions of the 37th Annual Meeting of the Orthopaedic Research Society, 1991;16:528.

10. Horowitz SM, Salvati E, Glasser DB, Lane JM. Prostaglandin E2 is increased in the synovial fluid of patients with aseptic loosening. Transactions of the 37th Annual Meeting of the Orthopaedic Research Society 1991;16:335.

11. Howie DW, Cornish BL, Vernon-Roberts B. Resurfacing hip arthroplasty: classification of loosening and the role of prosthesis wear particles. *Clin Orthop* 1990;255:144–159.

12. Howie DW, Haynes DR, Hay S, Rogers SD, Pearcy MJ. The effect of titanium alloy and cobalt chrome alloy wear particles on production of inflammatory mediators IL-1, TNF, IL-6 and prostaglandin E2 by rodent macrophages in vitro. Transactions of the 38th Annual Meeting of the Orthopaedic Research Society 1992;17:344.

13. Howie DW, Vernon-Roberts B. The synovial response to intraarticular cobalt-chrome wear particles. *Clin Orthop* 1988;232:244–254.

14. Howie DW, Vernon-Roberts B. Long-term effects of intraarticular cobalt-chrome alloy wear particles in rats. *J Arthroplasty* 1988;3:327–336.

15. Howie DW, Vernon-Roberts B. The synovial macrophage response to aluminum oxide ceramic and cobalt-chrome alloy wear particles in rats. *Biomaterials* 1988;9:442–448.

16. Howie DW, Vernon-Roberts B, Oakeshott R, Manthey B. A rat model of resorption of bone at the cement-bone interface in the presence of polyethylene wear particles. *J Bone Joint Surg [Am]* 1988;70:257.

17. Jasty M, Rubash HE, Paiement G, Bragdon C, Harrigan TP, Harris WH. Distribution of bone ingrowth into proximally coated, femoral porous canine total hip replacements. Transactions of the 32nd Annual Meeting of the Orthopaedic Research Society 1986;11:344.

18. Kim KJ, Greis P, Wilson SC, D'Antonio JA, McClain EJ, Rubash HE. Histological and biochemical comparison of membranes from titanium, cobalt-chromium and non polyethylene hip prostheses. Transactions of the 37th Annual Meeting of the Orthopaedic Research Society 1991; 16:191.

19. Mirra JM, Amstutz HC, Matos M, Gold R. The pathology of the joint tissues and its clinical relevance in prosthetic failure. *Clin Orthop* 1976;117:221.

20. Mirra JM, Marder RA, Amstutz H. The pathology of failed total joint arthroplasty. *Clin Orthop* 1982;170:175.

21. Murray DW, Rushton N. Macrophages stimulate bone resorption when they phagocytose particles. *J Bone Joint Surg [Br]* 1990;72:988–992.

22. Newman PH, Scales JT. The unsuitability of polyethylene for movable weight-bearing prostheses: report of a case of cup arthroplasty of the hip. *J Bone Joint Surg [Br]* 1951;33:392.

23. Ohlin A. Failure of the Christiansen hip: survival analysis of 265 cases. *Acta Orthop Scand* 1990;61:7–11.

24. Ohlin A. Socket wear, loosening and bone resorption after total hip arthroplasty. Doctoral dissertation, Lund University, 1989.

25. Ohlin A, Johnell O, Lerner UH. The pathogenesis of loosening of total hip arthroplasties. *Clin Orthop* 1990;253:287–296.

26. Pazzaglia UE, Pringle JAS. Bone resorption in vitro: macrophages and giant cells from failed total hip replacement versus osteoclasts. *Biomaterials* 1989;10:286–288.

27. Rae T. The haemolytic action of particulate metals (Cd, Cr, Co, Fe, Mo, Ni, Ta, Ti, Zn, Co-Cr alloy). *J Pathol* 1978;125:81–89.

28. Rae T. A review of tissue culture techniques suitable for testing the biocompatibility of implant materials. In: Winter GD, Leray JL, de Groot K, eds. Evaluation of Biomaterials. John Wiley & Sons Ltd. 1980:289–93.

29. Rae T. The biological response to titanium and titanium-aluminium-vanadium alloy particles. Tissue culture studies. *Biomaterials* 1986;7:30–36.

30. Revell PA, Weightman B, Freeman MAR, Vernon-Roberts B. The production and biology of polyethylene wear debris. *Arch Orthop Trauma Surg* 1978;91:167–181.

31. Thornhill TS, Ozuna RM, Shortkroft S, Keller K, Sledge CB, Spector M. Biochemical and histological evaluation of the synovial-like tissue around failed total joint replacement prostheses in human subjects and a canine model. *Biomaterials* 1991;11:69–72.

32. Vernon-Roberts B. The initial state. In: Lewis JL, Galante JL, eds. *The bone-implant interface: workshop report*. Chicago: American Academy of Orthopaedic Surgeons, 1985:8.

33. Vernon-Roberts B, Freeman MAR. The tissue response to total joint replacement prostheses. In: Swanson SAU, Freeman MAR, eds. *The scientific basis of joint replacement*. Kent: Pitman Medical Publishing, 1977:86.

34. Willert HG. Semlitsch M. Reactions of the articular capsule to wear products of artificial joint prostheses. *J Biomed Mater Res* 1977;2:157–164.

Biological, Material, and Mechanical Considerations of Joint Replacement, edited by B. F. Morrey.
Raven Press, Ltd., New York © 1993.

27

Adverse and Toxic Effects of Prosthetic Materials

Jonathan Black

Department of Bioengineering, Clemson University, Clemson, South Carolina 29634-0905

Solid materials are generally classed as metals, polymers, ceramics (including glasses), and composites of two or more different materials. These classes reflect the primary electronic bonding in each general type and the resulting physical and mechanical properties: Metals (metallic bonds) have high melting points and moderate to good corrosion resistance; high elastic modulus, hardness, strength, and toughness. Polymers (covalent and Van der Waals (hydrogen) bonds) have low melting points and moderate solubility; low elastic modulus, hardness, strength, and toughness (but high ductility). Ceramics (ionic bonds) have very high melting points and very low solubility; very high elastic modulus and hardness, moderate strength but low toughness due to extremely low ductility. Composites, or more generally composite materials, embody the designed combination of examples of several of these material types to produce materials with new, more desired combinations of properties, primarily mechanical ones. Thus, a fiber reinforced polymer may gain tensile strength from the fiber and ductility from the matrix and exhibit a modulus somewhere between those of fiber (high) and matrix (low). However, not all properties of such composites are desirable: a fiber-reinforced polymer may be weak in compression and have low fatigue strength due to poor fiber-matrix adhesion.

Prosthetic design for replacement of major joints in the human body is said generally to be *materials limited;* that is, the various requirements imposed on the designer by the desired device function and lifetime, combined with space and biological response constraints, result in a wide variety of designs fabricated from a quite narrow range of materials.

Moreover, all of the many designs available for components for replacement of a particular joint are more alike than they are different. The simplest way to think about a component of a joint replacement is to consider that it has three elements: an articulation element that controls, to a greater or lesser degree, the desired motion with respect to an adjacent bone, a structural element that positions this articulating element with respect to the bone to which it is attached, and a fixation or attachment element that anchors the component, i.e., fixes it, relative to that bone (Fig. 1). The analysis is slightly complicated by the use of four fixation strategies, alone or in combination: press-fit, cementation, interlock (e.g., ingrowth, macro-interlock, screw threads), and adhesion. In actual practice, a component may have more than

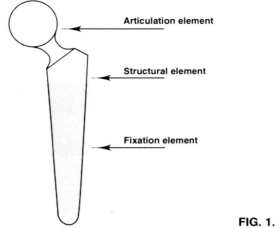

FIG. 1. Elements of THR component.

three physical parts; however, there are only these three functional elements and each part may be identified with one or more of these elements.

This generic similarity of component design makes it possible, among other things, to consider biological response to materials of fabrication in a generic manner. Today the choices of materials for each element are, as noted before, very limited. Table 1 shows the typical materials in use today and candidate materials for use in the near future, with total hip replacement (THR) used as an example.

TABLE 1. *Present and future materials used in the functional elements of THR*

Component	Materials	
	Present	Future
Acetabular		
Functional element		
Articular	UHMWPE	Ceramic (Al_2O_3?)
Structural	Co-base, Ti-base alloy	Polymer matrix composite
Fixation		
Press-fit	Co-base, Ti-base alloy	??
Cementation	PMMA	??
Interlock	Co-base, Ti, Ti-base	??
Adhesion	CaHAP	??
Femoral		
Functional element		
Articular	Co-base alloy	Al_2O_3 (ZrO_2?)
Structural	Co-base, Ti-base alloy	Polymer matrix composite
Fixation		
Press-fit	Co-base, Ti-base alloy	??
Cementation	PMMA	??
Interlock	Co-base, Ti, Ti-base	??
Adhesion	CaHAP	??

UHMWPE, ultrahigh molecular weight polyethylene (ASTM F-648), Co-base, cobalt-base alloys (ASTM F-75, F-562, F-563, F-799); Ti, titanium (ASTM F-67); Ti-base alloys, titanium base alloys (ASTM F-136, F-620); PMMA, polymethylmethacrylate (ASTM F-451); Al_2O_3, aluminum-oxide ceramic; ZrO_2, zirconium-oxide ceramic; CaHAP, calcium hydroxyapatite (ASTM F-1185); ?, possible; ??, unknown. Table reflects current and near-term U.S. practice.

Thus, consideration of adverse effects of biomaterials used in prosthetic joint replacement can be limited to consideration of these few materials and their degradation products.

MECHANISMS FOR IMPLANT BIOMATERIAL-HOST INTERACTIONS[1]

An implant is, by definition, placed in contact with living tissue during a surgical procedure. It can produce an effect (host response) at the tissue-implant interface, either by its physical presence or at local, systemic, or remote sites by consequence of its coupling with the host. This coupling is a consequence of the chemical, electrical, and/or mechanical features of the implant and its interaction with the host environment.

To date, there is no evidence that the electrical properties (e.g., conductivity, permitivity, dielectric constant) of total joint replacement components affect the host adversely, although such an argument has been made concerning the interference of metallic fracture fixation devices with early healing (2).

Mechanical coupling has two aspects: (i) surface morphology (e.g., roughness, porosity), which affects tissue response and sets the stage for later load transfer, and (ii) local relative motion between implant and tissue ("micromotion"), which can both alter tissue repair and produce wear debris.

Chemical coupling also has two aspects: (i) production of denatured host protein and (ii) release of elution or corrosion products. However, the mere chemical analytical demonstration of degradation products, for instance, alloy constituents in the capsular tissues around the hip during THR revision arthroplasty, is not a direct guide to the possibility of an elicited host response. Metal may be present in capsular tissue in the following forms: soluble organometallic complexes, solid (alloy) wear debris, matrix-bound organometallic complexes, intracellular soluble or precipitated metal compounds, and extracellular precipitated compounds. Among soluble forms, atomic valence may have a profound effect on biological activity, as in the case of chromium (17). Each form has different solubility and transport properties and thus presents a different potential hazard to the host at local, systemic, or remote sites. If biomaterial degradation products are significantly transportable (in solid form) or soluble, then systemic and remote-site host responses are also possible.

Current considerations focus on three physical aspects of biomaterials used in prosthetic joint replacement: the bulk material itself, *circum* device wear debris, whether metallic, polymeric, or ceramic, and soluble metal bearing species, found locally or in serum and urine.

In the initial searches for suitable prosthetic biomaterials, emphasis was placed on finding completely inert materials and biocompatibility was defined in terms of absence of host response. All biomaterials, other than viable autologous tissue, elicit a host response, and modern bioengineering attempts to design the material, by selection of composition and structural and processing parameters, to produce either a desirable or, at the very least, a minimal, tolerable response. Such biomaterials are termed *interactive* (4). Modern processing of metallic alloys is designed to minimize hard and soft tissue response, whereas processing of calcium-hydroxyapatite coat-

---

[1]Space does not permit a full discussion of this topic. The reader is referred to Black (3) for further information as it relates to biological performance of materials in orthopaedic applications.

ings is directed toward producing optimum osteoconductive activity while preserving coating integrity. This latter response, as in the case of bone and/or soft-tissue ingrowth into porous surfaces, is viewed as desirable or beneficial and is termed *adaptive*. (See Chapter 10 in ref. 4 for a full discussion of this topic.)

Adverse host responses to implanted materials may be classified as: metabolic, bacteriologic, immunologic, and neoplastic. The latter two topics are addressed elsewhere in this volume by Merritt and Brown (Chapter 12) and Rock (Chapter 28), respectively, and will not be discussed here.

METABOLIC HOST RESPONSE

Metabolic adverse responses may be due to direct chemical interactions of soluble components with host tissue and its enzymatic systems or indirect interactions, mediated by cellular factors produced in response to foreign materials. (See Chapter 26 by Howie for a discussion of adverse secondary response to wear debris.) Table 2 summarizes clinically observed biological effects of excesses of metal constituents of cobalt- and titanium-based alloys.

Consideration of direct effects is complicated by the recognition that many of the metallic species involved have normal metabolic roles (15) and that, in most cases, the exact nature of the metal-containing ion released from implants *in vivo* is not known. Studies of total joint replacement arthroplasties have shown elevated serum and urine levels of cobalt, chromium, and nickel (13,14,16) and titanium (11) in the presence of cobalt- and titanium-based alloy components, respectively, in patients with loose devices exhibiting generally high values. Table 3 provides reference data for normal individuals; patients with joint replacements may show concentrations of from 1.5 to 10 times these values.

TABLE 2. *Biological effects of alloy constituents*

Element	Effect of excess	Observations
Aluminum[a]	Encephalopathy; vitamin D-resistant osteoporosis; microcytic anemia; Alzheimer's disease (?)	Interacts with phosphate; protein cross-linker
Chromium	Toxic as Cr[VI](through reduction to Cr[III]); presumptive carcinogen; hepatotoxicity/ nephrotoxicity; contact dermatitis	Required for glucose tolerance
Cobalt	Toxic primarily as Co[II]; cardiomyopathy; hypothyroidism; possible carcinogen; possible contact dermatitis	Component of vitamin B_{12}
Manganese	Psychiatric disorders; neurotoxicity	Role in chrondroitin sulfate synthesis
Molybdenum	Anemia; dysentery (animals); pseudogout (effect as copper antagonist)	Constituent of several oxidases
Nickel	Presumptive carcinogen; contact dermatitis	Element in systemic response to stress
Titanium[a]	Unknown; some compounds are dermatological irritants	[a]
Vanadium	Carcinogen (?)	Competes with phosphate in Na^+-, K^+-ATPase

Adapted from ref. 6 with additional information from ref. 8.
[a]No known normal biological role.
?, possible.

TABLE 3. *Serum and urine concentration of implant alloy elements (normal individuals)*

Element	Plasma conc. (μg/L = ppb)	Urine conc.[a] (μg/L)
Aluminum	2.2	6.4
Cobalt	0.05	0.33
Chromium	0.06	0.13
Manganese	<1	<0.5
Molybdenum	Unknown	Unknown
Nickel	0.2	1.0
Titanium	3.3	0.41
Vanadium	0.16	0.61

Adapted from ref. 4.
Primary sources: aluminum, titanium, vanadium (11); cobalt, chromium, nickel (it is widely believed that urine collection, especially from female subjects, is subject to contamination[a]) (16); manganese (8); creatinine (9).

However, individuals show variations in normal levels for any one metal of up to one order of magnitude (10-fold). Thus, elevations must be considered relative to what is normal for a particular patient (usually unknown) rather than in relation to nominal normal values and ranges. In addition, it has been shown, in the case of internal fracture fixation hardware, that concentrations of metal near implants may be up to 500 to 1,000 times those in the surrounding normal tissues (12). Limited studies of cadavers also show 10 to 50 times concentrations of some alloy elements in remote site tissues, such as lung, liver, and kidneys (7,14).

It is reasonable to assume that within implant patient populations examples of each of the symptoms in Table 2, referable to excess of alloy constituents or other causes, may be found. However, no clinical link has been demonstrated so far by retrospective or prospective study, since this issue has not been examined except in the case of neoplastic transformation (see Chapter 28) and then without supporting laboratory analyses of metal content to substantiate specific elevations. Furthermore, as previously stated, little is known, even when such data are reported, of the actual chemical form and thus biological availability.

INFECTION

Implant-associated infection is still a clinical problem, although of low frequency. Intraoperative and immediate postoperative infections are now quite rare, typically less than 0.5% in most series, due to better operating room practices and the widespread use of air handling systems such as laminar flow suites. Late infection continues to be a problem and has been associated with hematogenous "seeding" from remote sites, such as dental abscesses or urinary tract infections (5). The implant provides a substrate, which, if not fully integrated with surrounding tissue and colonized by host cells, may provide a preferential site for bacterial growth. Gristina (10) described this process of cellular integration versus bacterial adhesion and colonization in graphic terms as "the race for the surface." However, there is no general evidence that the composition of the prosthetic material or its surface morphology play a role in the incidence of implant site infections, either acutely or chronically. Not withstanding this, it is possible to imagine biomaterials that actively suppress infection by release of antibiotics (5), bactericidal corrosion products (1), or by impeding bacterial adhesion (7), thus interfering with growth of colonies.

CONCLUSION

Material properties are important to both device performance and host response. Modern biomaterials are sufficiently selected by clinical practice that most function well in a majority of applications. The lack of detailed studies of clinical physiology and epidemiology of these biomaterials has deprived scientist and clinician alike of an understanding of the principles that govern both the common success and uncommon failure of biomaterials in prosthetic devices. Until such studies are performed and their results understood at a conceptual level, progress toward new biomaterials for joint replacement prostheses will continue to be largely empirical.

REFERENCES

1. Berger TJ, Spadaro JA, Chapin SE, Becker RO. Electrically generated silver ions: quantitative effects on bacterial and mammalian cells. *Antimicrob Agents Chemother* 1958;9:357–358.
2. Black J. *Electrical stimulation: its role in growth, repair and remodeling in the musculoskeletal system*. New York: Praeger, 1987.
3. Black J. *Orthopaedic biomaterials: biomaterials in orthopaedic research and practice*. New York: Churchill-Livingstone, 1988.
4. Black J. *Biological performance of materials: fundamentals of biocompatibility,* 2nd ed. New York: Marcel Dekker, 1992.
5. Brause BD. Infected orthopedic prostheses. In: Bisno AL, Waldvogel FA, eds. *Infections associated with indwelling medical devices*. American Society for Microbiology, Washington, DC: 1989:111–127.
6. da Silva JJRF, Williams RJP. *The biological chemistry of the elements*. Oxford: Clarendon Press, 1991.
7. Dobbs HS, Minski MJ. Metal ion release after total hip replacement. *Biomaterials* 1980;1: 193–198.
8. Friberg L, Nordberg GF, Vouk VB. *Handbook on the toxicology of metals, 2nd ed. Vol. II: specific metals*. Amsterdam: Elsevier, 1986.
9. Ganong WF. *Review of medical physiology, 14th ed*. Norwalk, CT: Appleton & Lange, 1989:593ff.
10. Gristina AG. Biomaterial-centered infection: microbial adhesion versus tissue integration. *Science* 1987;237:1588–1595.
11. Jacobs JJ, Skipor AK, Black J, Tuttle MC, Urban RM, Galante JO. Metal release and excretion in patients with titanium-base alloy total hip replacement components. *J Bone Joint Surg [AM]* 1991;73:1475–1486.
12. Lux F, Zeisler R. Investigations of the corrosive deposition of components of metal implants and of the behavior of biological trace elements in metallosis tissue by means of instrumental multielement activation analysis. *J Radioanal Chem* 1974;19:289–297.
13. Michel R. Trace metal analysis in biocompatibility testing. *CRC Crit Rev Biocompat* 1987;3: 235–317.
14. Michel R, Nolte M, Reich M, Löer F. Systemic effects of implanted prostheses made of cobalt-chromium alloys. *Arch Orthop Trauma Surg* 1991;110:61–74.
15. National Research Council (US), Subcommittee on the Tenth Edition of the RDAs. *Recommended daily allowances, 10th ed*. Washington, DC: National Academy of Sciences, 1989.
16. Sunderman FW Jr, Hopfer SM, Swift T, et al. Cobalt, chromium and nickel concentrations in body fluids of patients with porous-coated knee or hip prostheses. *J Orthop Res* 1989;7:307–315.
17. Wapner KL, Morris DM, Black J. Release of corrosion products by F-75 cobalt base alloy in the rat. II: Morbidity apparently associated with chromium release *in vivo*. *J Biomed Mater Res* 1986;20:219–233.

Biological, Material, and Mechanical Considerations of Joint Replacement, edited by B. F. Morrey. Raven Press, Ltd., New York © 1993.

28

Toxicity Oncogenesis

Case Reports

Michael G. Rock

Department of Orthopaedics, Mayo Clinic, Rochester, Minnesota 55905

The benefits afforded millions of patients in whom various orthopedic implants have stabilized fractures and replaced diseased arthritic joints cannot be challenged. Early fracture stabilization, which was popularized by the Swiss Association for Osteosynthesis group, has shortened hospital stay, minimized morbidity associated with multiple injury, and allowed for early reconstitution of function. Similarly, partial or total joint replacement for the posttraumatic or arthritic patient has been associated with reproducible and consistent pain relief and return to activities. Total hip arthroplasty could arguably be considered the greatest technical advance in orthopaedics; yet concern with longevity of the reconstruction, continued integrity of the components of the reconstruction, and the body's ability to accept large foreign objects continue to plague the orthopedic community.

Minimal acceptable requisites for an implant include chemical stability, biocompatibility, and appropriate mechanical properties. Additionally, the metals used as implants should exhibit excellent corrosion resistance. This is assisted in part by the development of a passive layer of oxide on its surface that acts as insulation from the surrounding corrosive *in situ* environment. The three metals most commonly used in orthopaedic implants include 316-L stainless steel, vitallium (cobalt-chromium-molybdenum-based alloy), and titanium (titanium-aluminum-vanadium-based alloy). Although they exhibit excellent resistance to corrosion, including galvanic, crevice, fretting, intergranular, and stress, ultimately with sufficient cyclic loading, these implants will experience corrosion fatigue. Oxidation of these large metallic components produce chlorides, oxides, and hydroxides in combination with particulate metal matter. The oxide surface of the implant is continually being shed, due to the nature of the environment in which it is placed, ultimately exposing progressively deeper zones of the implant and demonstrating the phenomenon of corrosion. This is particularly true in lower extremity implants that are subjected to 1 or possibly 2 million cycles per year. Evolving efforts to reduce the possibility of fatigue failure among implants have included forging, isostatic pressing, and ion implantation to produce a superior metal microstructure minimizing surface delamination.

Much of the impetus in developing implants with greater corrosion-resistant tendencies was precipitated by the excessive soft-tissue staining noted by orthopedic surgeons at the time of fixation removal or revision joint arthroplasty. The presence of particulate metal matter in local tissue from such implants has been confirmed (12,23,31). Recent reports suggest that this effect persists despite attempts to increase implant fixation and durability with porous coating (1,9,18,47). Similar experiences have been noted in the animal model (49). The introduction of porous-coated implants has allowed for the possible contribution of wear to local and possibly even systemic concentrations of particulate metal matter. If the porous-coated implant is not secured and translates against the surface of the bone, the surface excrescences that allow bone ingrowth will be shed from the implant, ultimately exposing the host to greater overall surface area and concentration of the constituents of the alloy. Such loosening and shedding of these beads occur at the time of implantation, due at times to the excessive force administered to direct the implant into the bone, as well as with future migration of the implant upon settling. Although no firm figures are available, it is estimated that 2% of patients will experience radiographic evidence of bead shedding and migration (7). Recent analysis of porous-coated total knee arthroplasty patients suggests that this figure may grossly underestimate the incidence (32).

Possibly of greater concern is the detection of these same metal ions in areas remote from the implant, including serum, urine, and regional draining lymph nodes. Elevated serum levels of metal ions consistent with the composition of the implanted alloy have been confirmed in the experimental model (48) and humans after total hip arthroplasty (4,17). Particulate metal matter does not appear to be unique in its ability to accumulate locally at the site of implants or even at distant and remote sites. The same phenomenon has been noted with polyethylene and to a lesser extent, at least locally, with polymethylmethacrylate (28,46).

The body's response to the local presence of debris is contingent on the size and amount, as well as the rate of accumulation. The body attempts to neutralize these foreign particles by precipitating granulomatous foreign-body reactions and/or removal through local lymphatic channels. Preferential binding of principally metallic debris is initiated at the cellular level within local tissue for cobalt and chromate VI, and with extracellular binding to albumin for nickel and chromate III and transferrin binding of chromium, cobalt, and nickel. If the local accumulation of debris exceeds the body's ability to neutralize and/or transport, the debris migrates from the site to remote areas including bone-cement and bone-implant surfaces very possibly contributing to, if not initiating, loosening.

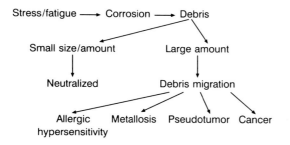

FIG. 1. Local tissue reaction to implant.

Such concentration of debris locally and systematically could theoretically lead to hypersensitivity, metabolic toxicity, or possibly even the induction of carcinogenesis (Fig. 1).

EFFECT OF CORROSION

Hypersensitivity

Hypersensitivity to various metals including cobalt, chromium, and nickel does occur and can generally be determined by appropriate skin testing. Less than 1% of patients subjected to joint arthroplasty show such sensitivity, suggesting that routine skin testing is not cost effective. Furthermore, it is well-known that skin testing does not reflect the sensitivity reaction that occurs in the deep tissue (see Chapter 12). Recent studies suggest that more than half of the patients presenting for removal of fixation or prosthetic components are sensitive on *in vitro* cell migration inhibition tests, with 28% reacting, and thereby may not be skin-test positive due to chemotactic suppression. This implies that patients can not only be sensitized with the implant but may also elicit an immune response in presensitized individuals (27). When it does occur, local metallic debris, to which the patient is hypersensitive, will cause local vascular obliteration, precipitating local bone necrosis, thereby weakening the bone-cement interface and, with time and repetitive challenge, ultimately culminate in implant loosening.

Metal Toxicity

Increasing concern over the biocompatibility of the various implant metals currently in use has precipitated sophisticated analysis of cellular response including histology, scanning electron microscopy, and enzyme histochemical analysis, as well as attempting to determine local and systemic concentrations of the metal ions. It must be stated that all of the released metal from the three conventional alloys currently in orthopedic use have definable biologic roles, with the sole exclusion of titanium. The current accepted normal value range of these elements is extremely wide due in large part to the variations in analytical techniques used by various facilities as well as the methods of specimen preparation apart from obvious anticipated differences due to heredity, diet, occupation, and other extrinsic factors that may contribute indirectly.

Attempts to quantify local concentrations of metallic debris in the vicinity of the implant appear fraught with inaccuracies, mostly due to sampling error and the inability to measure bioavailable or nonbioavailable metal species. This variation even within the same patient was dramatically illustrated by Agins et al. (1). It is generally believed that it is more accurate to determine serum and urine concentrations as a reflection of systemic exposure.

With the advent of atomic absorption spectroscopy, the ability to detect levels of metallic elements has improved tremendously. In studying 15 patients prior to and 6 months after conventional total hip replacement with a cemented vitallium component, Black et al. (6) determined that the mean value of serum chromium is 50% higher relative to preoperative determinations, whereas cobalt remained unchanged in that short postoperative follow-up. Similarly, nickel exhibited a threefold increase in serum concentration during the same timeframe, but all of these figures were within the wide acceptable normal range for these metallic ions in the human. Similar analyses have been performed on patients with titanium ingrowth implants that have revealed that in the presence of a loose, uncemented femoral component, the serum concentration of titanium rose twofold (47). Again, this was within the accepted normal range in humans recommended by the Second Generation of Biological Reference Standard. Furthermore, when analyzing the serum-to-urine concentration in patients subjected to conventional total hip arthroplasty, it became apparent that the urinary concentration of chromate in particular did not rise with the same magnitude as the serum level. This suggests that the rise in serum values that occurs within the first 2 to 3 weeks postoperatively exceeded the urinary ability to excrete or that the chromate was bound to circulating protein, such as transferrin, making it unexcretable.

Chromium is known to have an affinity for the reticuloendothelial system and gains ready access into the erythrocyte. It is therefore distinctly possible that metal ions, although apparently exhibiting normal values in the circulation post-joint replacement, may be accumulating without organs and tissues remote from the implantation site, ultimately reaching concentrations in these target organs and tissues that may precipitate toxic events. Without extension necropsy studies, this obviously remains conjectural and cannot be firmly determined until such studies are performed. Such accumulation of this debris in tissue remote from the implant but similar in concentration to that seen in serum has previously been reported in the animal model (49). Therefore, it is entirely plausible that metallic ions can accumulate in organs and tissues remote from implantation and that these concentrations unlike the systemic circulation could increase due to the unidirectional intracellular ingestion of these particles.

It therefore appears that at present there is no compelling evidence to suggest that toxic levels of the various metallic ions that constitute currently acceptable orthopedic implants exist locally or systemically. With increased man-year exposure, the possibility of deposition and storage of this material in various tissues and organs has to be considered. As suggested by Steinemann (38), the potential release could amount to 0.15 to 0.3 $\mu m/cm^2$ per day, which translates to between 11 and 22 mg per year in patients with total hip replacements. This coincides with the total body burden of such metallic ions in a 70-kg man. If, as is suggested by the above determination that this additional load is not excreted, the possibility of generating toxic levels in certain target organs and tissues could manifest as intracellular toxicity. Under a toxic load of cobalt, nickel, or aluminum, a virtual absence of lactic dehydrogenase and succinate dehydrogenase activity occurs, implying a low level of respiration (30). In addition, glucose-6 phosphate dehydrogenase activity was considerably lower in the cells exposed to the cobalt, nickel, and aluminum as well as cobalt-chromium alloy, indicating decreased cell metabolism. Alternatively the acid phosphatase is markedly elevated, which is more classically seen with macrophage activity. There is also emerging evidence that aluminum competes with magnesium, a normally occurring catalyst in allowing polymerization of tubulin, a primary structural protein found in central and peripheral nerves. Such a reversal of aluminum/magnesium effect on the central nervous system has been found in patients experiencing Alzheimer's dementia. Titanium, once thought to be bioinert, has recently been associated with granulomatous disease of lung, adenocarcinomas of lung, and a distinct antiplatelet effect. What is potentially more disturbing is that these figures for serum concentrations have come from patients who have been subjected to conventional cemented vitallium components. With the advent of uncemented porous-coated implants, these figures are expected to increase, creating the very distinct possibility of toxic levels in the serum and other tissue and organs that will respond with altered cellular dynamics and function, as mentioned above.

Carcinogenesis

Perhaps one of the greatest concerns with metal dissemination locally and within the systemic circulation is the possibility of inducing carcinogenesis. This is thought to be possible by one of two mechanisms: (i) A "solid-state" mechanism has been proposed, whereby a large foreign object implanted *in vivo* possibly stimulates mutagenesis of local cells, thereby creating tumor by its mere presence. Most large foreign objects upon implantation will initiate a very marked fibrous reaction. The cells within this fibrous reaction ultimately mutate and become cancer growths. (ii) The other inescapable possibility is that particulate metal matter has an innate capacity to induce cancer.

Well-documented cases of carcinoma and sarcoma have developed in refinery workers who inhaled nickel and chromium and in miners who were exposed to iron or even at local injection sites of iron dextran (13). Although the results have not been universally accepted, many animal experiments have shown a direct correlation between the initiation of sarcomas and the injection of particulate metal debris. This appears to be related to the concentration, as well as the physical nature, of the metal implanted (40). Metal ions, particularly cobalt, chromium, and nickel, are known to induce infidelity of DNA synthesis by causing the pairing of non-complimentary nucleotides and thereby creating a misinterpretation of the genetic code (37).

Furthermore, it must be remembered that particulate metal matter may not be the only solid-form material that can be, and has been proven to be, carcinogenic in appropriate environments. In 1954 long before the first total hip arthroplasty was performed, Laskin (22) postulated on the carcinogenic capabilities of polymethylmethacrylate after subcutaneous introduction of this material in mice. His conclusions suggested that similar occurrences of tumors may appear in humans that were being treated at that time with methylmethacrylate for dental deficiencies and that this evolution of cancer may take up to 20 years of exposure given the proportional time exposure before tumors were seen in the mice. A similar conclusion was reached by Carter and Roe (10) on the use of polyethylene plastic before it was conventionally used in the management of arthritic joints. Regardless of form, whether powder or large solid segments, polyethylene plastic produced sarcomas in 25% and 35% of rats, respectively. Their conclusions also suggested a latent period of 25 years in humans before such an event could be expected to occur.

It is, therefore, with interest that investigators were forewarning the medical community of the carcinogenic effect of metals and polymers years before the development and introduction of joint replacement using these very same materials. In 1969, Sir John Charnley introduced total hip arthroplasty as an alternative in the management of arthritic hips. No other orthopedic procedure has been adopted with such enthusiasm. Twenty-three years later we are still witnessing an incremental increase in the yearly utilization of this operation, attesting to the obvious success associated with it. According to some investigators, we may be coming into an era of increased tumor activity in the vicinity of or possibly remote from implantation sites of these orthopedic appliances (5).

CASE REPORTS AND ANALYSIS

Osteolysis

In 1976, Harris et al. (16) were the first to describe an aggressive granulomatous lesion around a cemented femoral stem in a total hip replacement. This was a condition of localized tumor-like bone resorption that appeared radiographically as large lytic defects within the femur, approximating the cement mantle of the implant. Initially thought to be neoplastic, these lesions were surgically biopsied and found to be consistent with well-organized connective tissue containing numerous histiocytic, monocytic, and fibroblastic reactive zones. Immunohistologic evaluation revealed multinucleate giant cells and nonspecific esterase-positive monocyte macrophages. These findings suggest a foreign-body type reaction, and with the subsequent isolation of polyethylene, methylmethacrylate, and metal debris, it was theorized that these constituents of the construct likely migrated down around the implant cement mantle in cemented prosthesis and implant bone interface in ingrowth noncircumferentially coated implants. Such a reaction suggests an excessive accumulation of debris at the site of articulation that surpasses the body's ability to neutralize and/ or transport the material resulting in migration of debris to sites remote from the source.

Descriptive analysis of the process has suggested the presence of a brisk immunologic reaction to the foreign matter with rapid accumulation of histiocytes, macrophages, and giant cells at the site of accumulated debris, which in turn precipitate the release of enzymes capable of bone absorption including prostaglandin E_2, tumor necrosis factor, interleukin-1 (20,34). This rapid appearance of bone loss radiographically, which is often associated with a deteriorating clinical course, has been termed type-II aseptic loosening.

Various components of the implant have been implicated in its initiation and continued bone loss, but the prevailing thought is that polyethylene debris is likely the cause. Initially thought to be a rather uncommon phenomenon and generally in the presence of compromised unstable implants, it has now been determined by several authors that the incidence of this phenomenon approximates 5% to 7% and that it is seen as commonly in cemented and uncemented components as well as stable constructs (24,35). The actual chemical factors responsible for the formation of the cell that produces the enzymes that subsequently cause the presumed osteoclastic activity are still unknown. Suffice it to say that it is a condition that we are seeing with increasing frequency, and, as suggested by both Santavirta et al. (34,35) and, more recently, Tanzer et al. (42), this phenomenon seems to be progressive, prompting these authors to recommend early intervention and revision to prevent further bone loss and risk of fracture.

The osteolysis, even in its massive form, that was noted with cement techniques may very well be a prelude to the experience with uncemented porous-coated implants. In the situation of no motion of the bone-implant interface, as mentioned previously, constituents of the alloy are released primarily by surface corrosion. If, on the other hand, the implant is not fixed or becomes loose, the surface particles may become free and generate an extensive local metallosis effect primarily as a result of wear, not corrosion. The full effect of noncemented implants on local tissue has not yet materialized. Given the added surface and tendency for the beads to come loose not only at the time of surgery but also later with cyclic loading, one can only assume that the local concentration of particulate material, not only metal but also polyethylene, will be infinitely increased over the conventional cemented implants and that the reaction noted with the latter of significant bone resorption and lysis may be trivial compared to the noncemented implants.

Oncogenesis

In 1978, clearly 2 years after the introduction of pseudo tumors of bone induced by the presence of large foreign bodies, in this case total hip arthroplasty, Arden and Bywaters (2) reported a case of a 56-year-old patient who developed a high-grade fibrosarcoma of soft tissue 2.5 years after receiving a metal-on-metal McKee-Farrar hip prosthesis. The tumor apparently did not have a direct association with the underlying bone or any components of the total hip arthroplasty. No formal analysis of the tumor for debris products was performed.

This case drew attention to the possibility of tumors being initiated in the presence of large orthopedic appliances. It was not until 1984 when this concept became fashionable in large part due to three articles that appeared simultaneously in the *Journal of Bone and Joint Surgery* recounting two malignant fibrous histiocytomas and one osteosarcoma at the site of a total hip arthroplasty (3,29,39).

This sudden and rather unexpected evolution prompted an editorial in the same journal addressing the issue of sarcoma and total hip arthroplasty and encouraged the orthopedic community worldwide to report such cases to a central registry to obtain more accurate figures on the incidence of such a problem (15). These tumors occurred 2, 4, and 5 years after hip replacement that was performed with various femoral and acetabular components, some with metal-on-metal articulations and others with metal on polyethylene. In two of these cases, the proximal femur was extensively involved with tumor that was in direct contact with the component (3,29). The remaining case was a soft-tissue sarcoma not in direct approximation to the prosthesis (39). Two of these tumors were malignant fibrous histiocytomas (3,39), one of bone and one of soft tissue. The remaining tumor was osteosarcoma (29). In this particular case, there was evidence of gray-brown pigmentation both intra- and extracellularly between the tumor and femoral component. No formal metal analysis was performed. Three additional cases emerged prior to 1988 at 15 months, 4.5 years, and 3.5 years after implantation. These were two malignant fibrous histiocytomas (11,15) and a malignant giant-cell tumor (33).

In 1988, five additional cases were reported occurring at 10 (45), 10 (21), 11 (25), 11 (41), and 12 (45) years after implantation. The sarcomas included two osteosarcomas, two malignant fibrous histiocytomas, and one synovial sarcoma. Two of these were soft tissue in a location with no direct association with the implant (25,45), yet in the case reported by Tait (41) there was evidence of nickel within tumor cells. The remaining three patients all had direct contact with either the cement or implant with the tumor originating in bone.

In 1990, an additional case was reported of an osteosarcoma of bone appearing at the site of a total hip arthroplasty eight years after implantation (8). This had direct contact with the underlying implant and cement with extensive soft tissue involvement. Both Martin et al. (25) and Brien et al. (8) analyzed the tumor for particulate debris and found no evidence of methylmethacrylate or polyethylene did not determine the presence of cobalt and chromium in the case of Martin et al. (25) and the typical constituents of stainless steel, those being chromium, nickel, molybdenum, manganese, and barium in the case of Brien et al. (8). As such, there have been 13 reported cases of tumor in close proximity, if not in direct extension, to an underlying total hip joint replacement (4) or total knee replacement.

MAYO CLINIC EXPERIENCE

Having reviewed the Mayo Clinic pathology registry, we add two additional patients, neither of whom had their joint replacement procedure performed at our institution. The first is that of a 79-year-old man who, 9 months previously, came to total hip cement utilizing Harris-Gallante uncemented femoral and acetabular components and presented with increasing discomfort in his left groin. He was found to have a large (11 × 6 × 3.5 cm) tumor engulfing the proximal femur extending down the canal and out into the soft tissues. Obvious direct contact to implant was noted. There was no evidence of any particulate debris in the tumor excised. The second case was that of a 56-year-old man who developed an osteosarcoma of soft tissue 14 months after left total knee arthroplasty with tumor extending down to both the femoral and patellar components. There was no particulate debris in the resected tumor.

OTHER DATA

Of the 15 reported cases, six tumors were of soft-tissue origin and nine of bone (Table 1). The histogenesis of the soft tissue tumors included three malignant fibrous histiocytomas, one synovial sarcoma, one soft-tissue osteogenic sarcoma, and one fibrosarcoma. The histogenesis of the primary bone tumors included four osteogenic sarcomas, three malignant fibrous histiocytomas, one malignant giant-cell tumor of bone, and one angiosarcoma. Direct contact with the underlying tumor was noted in 11 of the 15 cases. The remaining four were of soft-tissue origin that appeared to be remote from the implant with an obvious interval of normal tissue. In three of the cases, particulate metal matter was determined to be present in the tumor (21,25,43) including one case of a soft tissue sarcoma that appeared on image and exploration to be remote from the implant but had obvious evidence of nickel present within the tumor cells (25). In the series by Brien et al. (8), the concentration of the metal found in the tumor was within 30 percent of what was determined to be the composition of the metal in the stainless steel implant.

Apart from tumors developing at the site of prosthetic replacement, there have been eight known malignant tumors that developed at the site of previous internal fixation (21) (Table 2). To date, there have been no malignancies noted around a titanium implant, with the vast majority of malignancies both in the prosthetic and internal fixation groups being in the vicinity of chrome-cobalt-vitallium implants.

TABLE 1. *Malignancy associated with joint endoprosthesis*

Author	Year	Prosthesis	Time interval (years)	Histiogenesis
Castleman et al.[a]	1965	Austin-Moore	1	Malignant giant-cell tumor
Arden & Bywaters[a]	1978	Mckee-Farrar	2.5	Fibrosarcoma[c]
Bago-Granell et al.[a]	1984	Charnley-Mueller	2	Malignant fibrous histiocytoma
Penman & Ring[a]	1984	Ring	5	Osteosarcoma
Swann	1984	Mckee-Farrar	4	Malignant fibrous histiocytoma[a]
Ryu	1987	Uncemented vitallium	1.4	Malignant fibrous histiocytoma[c]
Vives et al.[a]	1987	Charnley-Mueller	2	Malignant fibrous histiocytoma
Vanderlist[a]	1988	Charnley-Mueller	11	Histiocytoid angiosarcoma
Lamovec et al.	1988	Charnley-Mueller	11	Synovial sarcoma[c]
Lamovec et al.[a]	1988	Charnley-Mueller	10	Osteosarcoma
Tait[b]	1988	Charnley-Mueller	11	Malignant fibrous histiocytoma[c]
Martin et al.[a,b]	1988	Charnley-Mueller	10	Osteosarcoma
Brien et al.[a,b]	1990	Charnley	8	Osteosarcoma
Rock[a]	1992	PCA ingrowth	8	Malignant fibrous histiocytoma
Rock[a]	1992	PCA TKA	1.2	Osteosarcoma[c]

[a]Direct contact to implant and/or cement.
[b]Particulate metal identified within tumor cells.
[c]Soft-tissue sarcoma.
PCA, porous-coated anatomic; TKA, total knee arthroplasty.

This is not to exonerate stainless steel because tumors in proximity to implants made of this alloy have been reported in the animal literature (8). In 1976, other veterinarians were encouraged to report similar experiences, nearly 8 years before such concern was voiced with the application of these implants in humans.

It would appear that the diagnosis of a tumor superimposed or at least in the vicinity of these replacements carries with it a rather dismal prognosis. Figures available suggest that the vast majority of patients succumb within the first year after diagnosis and many within the first several weeks to months from the time of tumor detection.

TABLE 2. *Malignancy associated with internal fixation*

Author	Year	Prosthesis	Time interval (years)	Histiogenesis
McDougall McNally	1956	Stainless steel	30	Ewing's sarcoma
Delgado	1958	—	3	Undifferentiated sarcoma
Dube & Fisher	1972	Stainless steel	36	Hemangioendothelioma
Tayton	1980	Vitallium	7.5	Ewing's sarcoma
McDonald	1981	Vitallium	17	Lymphoma
Dodion et al.	1982	Vitallium	1.2	Lymphoma
Lee et al.	1984	Vitallium	14	Malignant fibrous histiocytoma
Hughes et al.	1987	Vitallium	29	Malignant fibrous histiocytoma

CRITICAL ANALYSIS AND ITS SIGNIFICANCE

As impressive as these cases may be, they must be put into perspective given the global use of internal fixation and prosthetic devices. Approximately 300,000 to 350,000 total hip joint replacements are performed worldwide on a yearly basis. It is assumed that approximately 3 million people will have had total hip arthroplasties performed by the end of this year. To date, there have been 15 reports of malignant tumor arising in close proximity to these implants (13 total hip and two total knee arthroplasties) (see Addendum). No direct contact was noted in four. However, if we determine the frequency of sarcomas in total hip arthroplasties, this incidence in this select patient population would be one case in 230,000. There are approximately 3,000 new primary bone tumors and 5,000 soft-tissue sarcomas in the United States per year. This would give an incidence of approximately 1 in 100,000 for the general population to develop a primary bone sarcoma and 1 in 40,000 to develop a soft tissue sarcoma. This is obviously not stratified for age given that many primary bone tumors develop in the second and third generation of life, yet it does afford the opportunity of putting this rather unusual event in perspective.

The prevalence of osteosarcoma among the osseous malignancies in this series is not entirely unexpected. Of the total osteosarcoma population 15% to 20% occur after the age of 50 years. Most of these cases are superimposed on Paget's disease or in previously irradiated tissue, yet *de novo* cases of osteosarcoma do occur in this age group. Malignant fibrous histiocytoma of bone is somewhat less common. A review of the Mayo Clinic files reveals 71 cases with more than half of these occurring after age 55. Malignant fibrous histiocytoma of soft tissue is the most common soft-tissue sarcoma. It is not surprising, therefore, that four of six soft-tissue tumors in the combined series are of this histogenesis. As such, the distribution of sarcomas in the combined series could have been predicted from general population data given the age of the patients and anatomical distribution.

There have been two separate reports that have critically analyzed the cancer risk after total hip arthroplasty (14,36). The combined person years of exposure after operation between the two series was 20,015. The overall cancer incidence among total hip replacement procedures in both series did not appear to be any different than what was expected or anticipated. The cancer-observed/expected ratio was especially low for the first 2 years following surgery in both series, implying that patients undergoing this procedure are otherwise generally healthy. In both series, the observed/expected ratio of developing lymphoma or leukemia was two to three times higher in patients who had total hip arthroplasty. Additionally, there was a twofold decrease in breast carcinoma among patients who had total hip arthroplasty.

Of interest, Gillespie et al. (14) suggested a similar decrease in the incidence of rectal, colon, and lung cancer among total hip arthroplasty patients. The results suggest or are possibly compatible with the hypothesis of chronic stimulation of the immune system, thereby potentially allowing for malignancies to occur within the lymphoreticular system. We have already determined a predilection for particulate metal matter to accumulate in the reticuloendothelial system. This has been further supported by studies in animals subjected to metal implants, especially those containing nickel, in which there was an increase in malignancies of the lymphoreticular system (44). Additionally, due to the added immune surveillance, tumors of breast, possibly colon, rectal, and lung may be decreased. A hyperimmune state is not unexpected given the dissemination of debris locally at implantation sites as well as the well-recognized and documented capacity of this material to gain access to the systemic circulation and possibly storage sites including the reticuloendothelial system. This trend obviously needs continued surveillance.

SUMMARY

In summary, my interpretation of the literature suggests that implants commonly used for fixation and reconstruction may not be entirely inert. Corrosion is an inevitable byproduct of implanting large foreign metallic devices. Accumulation of particulate debris is to some extent going to occur in all patients who have large metallic prosthetic devices. This necessarily includes the distinct possibility of systemic exposure to these foreign objects that the body attempts to neutralize and excrete. Due to the heightened immunologic surveillance and/or possible storage of particulate metal matter in sites remote from the implantation site, patients with total hip arthroplasty may be at added risk for remote malignancies, particularly of the lymphoreticular system. The incidence of primary mesenchymal tumors in close proximity to implants appears to be coincident with the incidence in the general public. As authors have suggested, however, we may not have yet witnessed the true frequency of these tumors due to the lack of a sufficient time interval to allow the ultimate expression of the host to a large *in situ* foreign object. We have entered the third decade of total joint replacement. Continuous review and reporting of adverse events with implants are obviously necessary. It is incumbent on large institutions performing such replacements with regularity to analyze cancer risk not only at the site of implantation but also at remote sites. We have embarked on such a review at the Mayo Clinic, which offers a unique opportunity to assess such risk factors due in large part to our effective retrieval system through a registry that has closely monitored all 40,000 joint arthroplasty patients.

ADDENDUM

Several recent reports have surfaced since the submission of this chapter, which include unpublished reports sent to the editor of six additional tumors in close proximity to total hip arthroplasties (14a) and an additional case report and review of the literature (19). Upon combining the reviews of available literature, the total number of tumors in close proximity to a joint replacement increases to 27, 19 of which are published. Of these, 20 are primary bone tumors, six are primary soft-tissue sarcomas, and one is a metastatic adenocarcinoma. Fourteen are known to have been in direct contact with the components, seven had no contact with intervening noncancerous tissue, and in six patients the tissue of contact was not known. The histogenesis of malignant fibrous histiocytoma in 11, osteosarcoma in six, other sarcomas in nine, and metastatic adenocarcinoma is an anticipated distribution in this patient population. Given that the interval to tumor induction from bone stimulation should be at least as long as the accepted 5-year interval from irradiation therapy to sarcoma degeneration, 13 patients of the 27 would qualify. Taking this and contact to implant as requisites for possible association of tumor and implant, the incidence of 1 in 230,000 still exists.

The above determinations are at best marginally accurate. The true incidence worldwide is difficult, if not impossible, to assess accurately, due in large part to the lack of a tracking system either in this country or abroad, to determine the rate of which total hip arthroplasty is being performed.

Additionally, we are relying on prompt and accurate reporting of tumors near implants by orthopedic surgeons everywhere, which is rather unlikely. What is needed, therefore, are in-depth review and more accurate prospective tracking of arthroplasty patients by institutions that perform this operation with regularity and have the mechanisms in place to follow those patients carefully.

REFERENCES

1. Agins HJ, et al. Metallic wear in failed titanium alloy total hip replacements. A histological and quantitative analysis. *J Bone Joint Surg [Am]* 1988;70:347–356.
2. Arden GP, Bywaters EGL. Tissue reaction in surgical management of juvenile chronic polyarthritis. In: Ardin GP, Ansell BM, eds. London: Academic Press, 1978:269–270.
3. Bago-Granell J, et al. Malignant fibrous histiocytoma of bone at the site of a total hip arthroplasty. A case report. *J Bone Joint Surg [Br]* 1984;66:38–40.
4. Bartolozzi A, Black J. Chromium concentrations in serum blood clot and urine from patients following total hip arthroplasty. *Biomaterials* 1985;6:2–8.
5. Black J. Does corrosion matter? *J Bone Joint Surg [Br]* 1988;70:517–520.
6. Black J, et al. Serum concentrations of chromium, cobalt, and nickel after total hip replacement. A six-month study. *Biomaterials,* 1983;160–165.
7. Bobyn JD, Engh CA. Biologic fixation of hip prosthesis. Review of the clinical status and current concept. *Adv Orthop Surg* 1983;7:137–150.
8. Brien WW, et al. Osteogenic sarcoma arising in the area of a total hip replacement. A case report. *J Bone Joint Surg [Am]* 1990;72:1097–1099.
9. Buchert BK, et al. Excessive metal release due to loosening and spreading of cintered particles on porous coated hip prosthesis. Report of two cases. *J Bone Joint Surg [Am]* 1986;68:606–609.
10. Carter RL, Roe FJC. Induction of sarcomas in rats by solid and fragmented polyethylene: experimental observations and clinical implications. *Br J Cancer* 1969;23:401–407.
11. Castleman L, et al. Case records of Massachusetts General Hospital. Case 38-1965. *N Engl J Med* 1965;273:494–504.
12. Coleman RF, Herrington J, Scales JT. Concentration of wear products in hair, blood, and urine after total hip replacement. *BMJ* 1973;1527–1529.
12a. Delgado ER. Sarcoma following a surgically treated fractured tibia, a case report. *Clin Orthop* 1958;12:315–318.
12b. Dodion P, Putz P, et al. Immunoblastic lymphoma at the site of an infected vitallium bone plate. *Histopathology* 1982;6:807–813.
13. Doll R. Cancer of lung and the nose. Nickel workers. *Br J Indus Med* 1958;15:217–223.
13a. Dube VE, Fisher DE. Hemangioendothelioma of the leg following metallic fixation of the tibia. *Cancer* 1972:30:1260–1266.
14. Gillespie WJ, et al. The incidence of cancer following total hip replacement. *J Bone Joint Surg [Br]* 1988;70:539–542.
14a. Goodfellow J. *J Bone Joint Surg [Am]* 1992;74:645.
15. Hamblen DL, Carter RL. Sarcoma and joint replacement (editorial). *J Bone Joint Surg [Br]* 1984;66:625–627.
16. Harris WH, et al. Extensive localized bone resorption in the femur following total hip replacement. *J Bone Joint Surg [Am]* 1976;58:612–618.
16a. Hughes AW, et al. Sarcoma at the site of a single hip screw. A case report. *J Bone Joint Surg [Br]* 1987;60:470–472.
17. Jacobs JJ, et al. Metal release and excretion from cementless titanium total knee replacements. *Trans Orthop Res Soc* 1991;16:558.
18. Jacobs JJ, et al. Release and excretion of metal in patients who have a total hip replacement component made of titanium-base alloy. *J Bone Joint Surg [Am]* 1991;73:1475–1486.
19. Jacobs JJ, Rosenbaum DH, Hay RM, Gitelis S, Black J. Early sarcomatous degeneration near a cementless hip replacement: a case report and review. *J Bone Joint Surg [Br]* 1992;5:740–744.
20. Kreicbergs A. Pseudotumor after metal fixation of a fracture. Surgery: a case report. *Acta Orthop Scand* 1983;54:739–742.
21. Lamovec J, et al. Synovial sarcoma associated with total hip replacement. A case report. Addendum: osteosarcoma associated with a Charnley-Mueller hip arthroplasty. *J Bone Joint Surg [Am]* 1988;70:1558–1560.

22. Laskin DM. Experimental production in sarcomas by methyl methacrylate implant. *Proc Soc Exp Biol Med* 1954;87:329–333.

22a. Lee YS, et al. Malignant fibrous histiocytoma at site of metal implant. *Cancer* 1984;54:2286–2289.

23. Lux F, Zeisler R. Investigations of the corrosive deposition of components of metal implants and of the behavior of biological trace elements in metallosis tissue by means of instrumental multi-element activation analysis. *J Radial Anal Chem* 1974;19:289–297.

24. Maloney WJ, et al. Bone lysis in well fixed cemented femoral component. *J Bone Joint Surg [Br]* 1990;72:966–970.

25. Martin A, et al. Osteosarcoma at the site of a total hip replacement. *J Bone Joint Surg [Am]* 1988;70:1561–1567.

25a. McDonald I. Malignant lymphoma associated with internal fixation of a fractured tibia. *Cancer* 1981;48:1009–1011.

25b. McDougall, A. Malignant tumor at site of bone plating. *J Bone Joint Surg [Br]* 1956;38:709–713.

26. Memoli VA, et al. Malignant neoplasms associated with orthopedic implant material. Presented at 28th Annual Orthopaedic Research Society Meeting in New Orleans, LA, January 1982.

27. Merritt K, Brown SA. Biological effects of corrosion products from metals. In: Fracher AC, Griffin CD, eds. *Corrosion and degradation of implant materials, second symposium.* ASTM-STP 859. Philadelphia: American Society for Testing Materials, 1985:195–207.

28. Pazzaglia U, Beyers PD. Fractured femoral shaft through an osteolytic lesion resulting from the reaction to a prosthesis. *J Bone Joint Surg [Br]* 1984;66:337–339.

29. Penman HG, Ring PA. Osteosarcoma in association with total hip replacement. *J Bone Joint Surg [Br]* 1984;66:632–634.

30. Rae T. A study on the effects of particulate metals of orthopaedic interest on murine macrophages in vitro. *J Bone Joint Surg [Br]* 1975;57:444–450.

31. Rock, MG, Hardie R. Analysis of local tissue response in 50 revision total hip arthroplasty patients. Presented at the Symposium on Retrieval and Analysis of Surgical Implants and Biomaterials, Snowbird, UT, August 1988.

32. Rosenquist, et al. Loosening of the porous coating of biocompartmental prostheses in patients with rheumatoid arthritis. *J Bone Joint Surg* 1986;68:538–542.

33. Ryu RKN, et al. Soft tissue sarcoma associated with aluminum oxide ceramic total hip arthroplasty. A case report. *Clin Orthop* 1987;216:207–212.

34. Santavirta F, et al. Aggressive granulomatous lesions associated with hip arthroplasty: immunopathological study. *J Bone Joint Surg [Am]* 1990;72:252–258.

35. Santavirta F, et al. Aggressive granulomatous lesions in cementless total hip arthroplasty. *J Bone Joint Surg [Br]* 1990;72:980–984.

36. Sinibaldi K. Tumors associated with metallic implants in animals. *Clin Orthop* 1976;118:257–266.

37. Sirover MA, Loeb LA. Infidelity of DNA synthesis in vitro: screening for potential metal mutagens or carcinogens. *Science* 1976;194:1434.

38. Steinemann SG. Corrosion of titanium and titanium alloys for surgical implant. In: Lutergering G, Swicker U, Bunk W, eds. *Titanium science and technology,* vol. 2. Berlin, 1985:1373–1379.

39. Swann M. Malignant soft tissue tumor at the site of a total hip replacement. *J Bone Joint Surg [Br]* 1984;66:629–631.

40. Swanson SAV, Freeman MAR, Heath JC. Laboratory tests on total joint replacement prostheses. *J Bone Joint Surg [Br]* 1973;55:759–773.

41. Tait NP. Case reports, malignant fibrous histiocytoma occurring at the site of a previous total hip replacement. *Br J Radiol* 1988;61:73–76.

42. Tanzer M, et al. The progression of femoral cortical osteolysis in association with total hip arthroplasty without cement. *J Bone Joint Surg [Am]* 1992;74:404–410.

42a. Rayton KJJ. Ewing's sarcoma at the site of a metal plate. *Cancer* 1980;45:413–415.

43. Vanderlist JJJ. Malignant epitheloid hemangioendothelioma at the site of a hip prosthesis. *Acta Orthop Scand* 1988;59:328–330.

44. Visuri T. Cancer risk after McKee-Farrar total hip replacement. *Orthopedic* 1992;14:137–142.

45. Vives P, et al. Histiocytome fibreux malin du fémur après prothèses totale de hanche. *Rev Chir Orthop* 1987;73:407–409.

46. Willert HD, et al. Osteolysis in alloy arthroplasty of the hip. The role of ultrahigh molecular weight polyethylene wear particles. *Clin Orthop* 1990;58:95–107.

47. Witt JD, Swann M. Metal wear in tissue response in failed titanium alloy total hip replacements. *J Bone Joint Surg [Br]* 1991;73:559–563.

48. Woodman JL, Black J, Jiminez SA. Isolation of serum protein organometallic corrosion products from 316 LSS and HS-21 in vitro and in vivo. *J Biomed Mater Res* 1984;18:99–114.

49. Woodman JL, Jacobs JJ, Gallante JO, Urban RN. Metal ion release from titanium-based prosthetic segmental replacements of long bones in baboons. A long term study. *J Orthop Res* 1984;1:421–430.

*Biological, Material, and Mechanical
Considerations of Joint Replacement,*
edited by B. F. Morrey.
Raven Press, Ltd., New York © 1993.

29

Allergy and Hypersensitivity

Arne Hensten-Pettersen

NIOM, Scandinavian Institute of Dental Materials, N-1344 Haslum, Norway

Allergy and hypersensitivity reactions to medical materials and devices are of concern to physicians and patients (2,9,15). Compared to the large number of implants inserted per year, there seems to be little published clinical research or animal experimentation that addresses this issue. A MEDLINE search done in connection with this conference indicated that from 1966 to 1992, approximately 14,000 papers were published on artificial implants, 11,000 were on allergy, hypersensitivity, and immunology, whereas only 45 papers combined the topics. The databases reflect the key words in the papers but do not cover all information in the field. Most papers are individual case reports and retrospective studies on limited, select patient groups, usually accompanied by a literature review.

MECHANISMS IN ALLERGY AND HYPERSENSITIVITY

Allergy is a hypersensitive state acquired through exposure to a particular antigen (allergen). Reexposure to the antigen can subsequently alter the capacity of the immune system to react. Originally, the term allergy denoted any altered reactivity, whether decreased or increased, but is now usually restricted to indicate increased reactivity, i.e., immunologic hypersensitivity reactions.

The normal effector mechanisms for humoral immunity depend on the activation of B cells and for cell-mediated immunity on T cells. Excessive stimulation of these effector mechanisms by antigen in a sensitized host can lead to tissue damage. Pathologic processes induced by immunologic responses may be classified as types I to IV (30).

Type I: Anaphylactic Hypersensitivity

The reaction of antigen with specific immunoglobulin E (IgE) antibody bound through its Fc part to the mast cell, leads to the release from the mast cells of granules containing mediators including histamine, leukotrienes, and platelet-activating factor, plus eosinophil and neutrophil chemotactic factors (30).

The offending antigen is identified by intradermal prick tests or provocation testing. The immediate wheal and flare reactions may sometimes last for as long as 24 hr and are characterized by a dense cellular infiltrate and being more edematous than the early reaction. Examples are anaphylactic shock, immunologic urticaria, hay fever, and extrinsic asthma. The antigens capable of raising IgE antibodies are usually complete antigens of high molecular weight. However, IgE antibodies to chromium and nickel compounds have been detected (29).

Relevance to orthopedic biomaterials. Rostoker et al. (33), in an extensive literature review of adverse reactions to osteosynthesis materials, cited three cases of immediate reactions to metals (two to nickel and one to chromium). The diagnosis needs careful documentation, as simultaneous exposure during surgery to other materials capable of eliciting type I reactions may confound the issue. In surgical latex gloves, both the latex per se and the starch powder may contain antigens that can react with specific IgE antibodies (43).

Type II: Antibody-Dependent Cytotoxic Hypersensitivity

This type involves the death of cells bearing antibody attached to a surface antigen. The cells may be taken up by phagocytic cells to which they adhere through their coating for IgG or C3b or lysed by the operation of the full complement system. Cells bearing IgG may also be killed by polymorphs and macrophages or by K cells through an extracellular mechanism (antibody-dependent, cell-mediated cytotoxicity). Examples are transfusion reactions, antibody-mediated graft destruction, and hypersensitivity resulting from the coating of erythrocytes or platelets by a drug (30).

Relevance to orthopedic biomaterials: Unknown.

Type III: Complex-Mediated Hypersensitivity

This results from the effects of antigen-antibody complexes through (i) activation of complement and attraction of polymorphonuclear leukocytes that release tissue-damaging enzymes on contact with the complex and (ii) aggregation of platelets to cause microthrombi and vasoactive amine release. Where circulating antibody levels are high, the antigen is precipitated near the site of entry into the body. The reaction in the skin is characterized by polymorphonuclear infiltration, edema, and erythema. It reaches a maximum at 3 to 8 hr (Arthus reaction). In relative antigen excess, soluble complexes are formed that are removed by binding to the CR1 C3b receptors on red cells. If this system is overloaded or if the classical complement components are deficient, the complexes circulate in the free state and are deposited under circumstances of increased vascular permeability at certain preferred sites; the kidney glomerulus, joints, skin, and choroid plexus. Complexes can be detected in tissue biopsies by immunofluorescence and in serum by assessing C1q or changes in C3 and C3c (30).

Relevance to orthopedic biomaterials: Necrosis of periprosthetic tissues, with histologic appearance and serum complement analyses consistent with type-III hypersensitivity reactions, has been observed in three of 30 cases of atypical loosening of total hip prostheses (20). In a study of methylmethacrylate sensitivity in orthopedic surgery (26), no relationship was found between the cardiovascular reactions observed during cementation of femoral prostheses and the complement system, measuring complement factors C3 and C4.

Type IV: Cell-Mediated or Delayed-Type Hypersensitivity

The interaction of antigen with primed T cells leads to release of soluble mediators, lymphokines, which account for the appearance of an indurated and erythematous reaction that reaches a maximum often at 24 to 48 hr, hence, a delayed reaction. The reaction is characterized histologically by infiltration with mononuclear phagocytes and lymphocytes. Another subpopulation of T cells may be activated by class I major histocompatibility antigens to become directly cytotoxic to target cells bearing the appropriate antigen (30). Examples of delayed-type hypersensitivity reactions are tissue damage occurring in microbial infections, insect bites, and allergic contact dermatitis.

Allergic contact dermatitis is of special interest to the topic of this volume and will be further elaborated. Allergic contact dermatitis is a cell-mediated immunologic response to chemicals with a molecular weight generally less than 1,000. When the foreign chemical contacts and penetrates the skin, it becomes associated with a Langerhans-cell transmembrane glycoprotein, the class-II histocompatibility antigen. T cells only recognize the chemical when it is associated with the class-II determinants. Lymph node T cells with complementary receptors specific for the chemical or antigen recognize the antigen–T-cell complex. Recognition is followed by rapid proliferation of the T cells and the subsequent differentiation and dissemination of effector and memory T cells. These cells circulate throughout the body via the blood and lymphatic systems and retain their specificity for the original chemical. A subsequent cutaneous contact with the original or a cross-reactive chemical may result in the characteristic inflammatory skin reaction. The circulating memory T cells recognize the antigen formed at the application site and undergo rapid activation and secrete lymphokines. Thus, after elicitation, the skin of the sensitized individual is characterized by erythema, edema, vesiculation, and pruritis (38). Continuing provocation of delayed hypersensitivity by persisting antigen leads to formation of chronic granulomata. Some chemicals require, in addition, an exposure to light before they can react. They may elicit photoallergic reactions simulating sunburns, i.e., actinic dermatitis. Most photoallergic reactions have been attributed to organic chemicals and drugs. Cobalt has been observed to be a photosensitizer (31).

In vivo tests for delayed hypersensitivity reactions are skin patch tests and/or *intra*dermal injection of antigens. *In vitro* tests for delayed hypersensitivity include macrophage migration inhibition (6,12,25) and assessment of blast-cell transformation (23). Future test methods will probably more directly measure release of specific lymphokines and other inflammation mediators.

Relevance to orthopedic biomaterials: A high incidence of metal hypersensitivity was found in patients with metal-to-metal hip arthroplasties. Patients with metal-to-plastic prostheses had no greater incidence of metal hypersensitivity than a control group awaiting operation (1). Local and generalized eczematous reactions have been observed following insertion of metal implants in those subsequently shown to be allergic to cobalt, chromium, and nickel (13,42). In a Swedish survey Carlsson and Möller (5) traced 37 subjects with metal allergy who had metallic device implants. The mean observation period was 6.3 years. None of the 19 living at the time of the survey had suffered any dermatologic or orthopedic complications attributable to their contact allergy. Information about the cause of death of the 18 other patients would have been of interest. Metal allergy may be a predisposing factor for infection of periprosthetic tissues (16).

Other Reaction Mechanisms Related to Hypersensitivity

Atopy

The term atopy is inconsistently used in medicine. Immunologists use it to denote IgE-mediated reactions, i.e., atopic allergy, occurring in approximately 10% of the population (30). Dermatologists classify 10% to 20% of the population as atopic (37). Atopic dermatitis is a chronic, pruritic inflammation of the skin, often occurring in association with a personal or familial history of allergic rhinitis, asthma, or hay fever. Its diagnosis and etiopathology are dominated by controversy because of the complex interrelationship between its morphology and genetic, physiologic, and immunologic factors, all of which seem to be involved in the presentation and evolution of the disease. Pruritis, which is elicited by complex etiologic factors, is the cardinal feature of the disease. Three other characteristic lesions accompany the irritation, namely, papules, lichenification, and eczematous lesions. These changes may be present in any combination in an atopic individual and can vary from time to time (10).

In a study of adverse reactions, tentatively diagnosed as nickel allergy associated with orthodontic appliances, nine patients were patch tested with 5 per cent nickel sulfate. One patient with oral aphtous ulcers had a strong reaction to nickel, but the ulcers persisted after removal of the appliances. The other eight had negative patch tests. Six of them were diagnosed as atopic individuals (36).

Relevance to orthopedic biomaterials: Unknown.

Urticaria

Many reports on adverse reactions to orthopedic devices describe patients with urticarial reactions. Contact urticaria is a wheal and flare response elicited by the application of various compounds to intact skin. Immunologic contact urticaria is an IgE-mediated reaction due to histamine release from mast cells, as described above. Nonimmunologic contact urticaria (NICU) is clinically indistinguishable from the other variety and occurs without previous sensitization. The reaction remains localized and does not spread to become generalized urticaria, nor does it cause systemic symptoms. Its pathogenetic mechanisms are not clearly understood. NICU may be elicited by a number of compounds, notably benzoic acid, which is found in many fruits, added as a preservative in salad dressings and other processed foods, and is also a degradation product of benzoylperoxide used in composite dental filling materials, denture base resins, and methylmethacrylate-based bone cements.

Relevance to orthopedic biomaterials: Role of NICU unknown.

Paresthesia

Orthopedic surgeons and dental laboratory technicians may have dermatitis associated with the use of methylmethacrylate monomer, often in the form of marked dryness and fissuring of the skin. A unique feature of allergic contact dermatitis caused by methylmethacrylate monomer is a persistent paresthesia of the fingertips in the form of a burning sensation, tingling, and slight numbness. This type of paresthesia has also been observed in orthodontists who had become sensitized to other monomers in orthodontic bonding materials (9). The paresthesia may be due to a direct neurotoxic effect of the monomer after it penetrates the skin.

Relevance to orthopedic biomaterials: May be associated with occupational problems. Unknown relevance in patients.

Intolerance

Intolerance reactions may clinically mimic the urticaria and edema of type-I hypersensitivity reactions, but are not mediated via the immune system. They are associated with insufficient levels of enzymes that normally metabolize substances such as fructose, lactose, acetylsalicylic acid, ethanol, and benzoic acid.

Relevance to orthopedic biomaterials: Unknown.

Selection of Test Substances

None of the elements or chemical components of orthopedic devices is exclusive to orthopedics. The composition and formulations have usually been adopted from other uses and modified for orthopedic purposes. Most of the metallic elements, monomers, and associated chemicals and their degradation products have been implicated as offending substances in hypersensitivity reactions when used in nonorthopedic situations.

Studies on metal allergy and orthopedic devices have often limited their evaluation to cobalt chloride, nickel sulfate, and hexavalent chromium compounds such as potassium dichromate. In their elemental form these metals are the most abundant in the devices and are also common sensitizers in the population. However, the minor elements of the alloys may also be of importance because allergic reactions are not dose dependent (15). Elves et al. (8) included titanium, molybdenum, and vanadium compounds in their patch-test battery and found one patient with a positive reaction to vanadium. Most studies have accepted that titanium is not a sensitizer. However, Lalor et al. (19) found indications that titanium also may be of considered in this connection.

The selection of relevant test substances is also uncertain when assessing hypersensitivity to resin-based materials. The bone cements, usually based on monomeric and polymeric methylmethacrylate, contain reactive chemicals that initiate and control the polymerization reaction, in addition to stabilizers and antioxidants. The polymerization reactions of this type of material may yield residual monomers and activated end groups, which may react further with tissue proteins. Benzoyl peroxide may degrade to benzoic acid (18), and formaldehyde may be formed as an oxidation product of the monomer (34). A complete test series may need to include these and probably other substances.

CLINICAL IMPLICATIONS OF HYPERSENSITIVITY

Sensitization and Immunologic Tolerance

The issue of prosthetic hip replacement and induction of metal sensitivity remains unsettled (1,3,22). In two studies (7,41) the postoperative group excluded those with preexisting sensitivity, and other studies had different prospective and retrospective groups (1,4). Rooker and Wilkinson (32) patch tested their patients before and after hip replacement with stainless steel/high-density polyethylene prostheses. Of the six patients positive to nickel, chromium, and/or cobalt, five were negative to these metals after the operation. The sixth patient had received a titanium-based prosthesis and remained nickel sensitive. Loss of metal sensitivity was also observed in three of 18 patients who had been exposed to orthopedic implants for several years and who had positive reactions to one or more metals before arthroplasty (5). Induction of immunologic tolerance may thus be a possible additional benefit of orthopedic surgery.

Guinea pigs fed nickel or chromium prior to being sensitized are more difficult to sensitize to these elements (39,40). A lower incidence of nickel allergy in subjects who were exposed to nickel-containing alloys through orthodontic treatment prior to ear piercing has also been demonstrated (2,37). Thus, in nonsensitized individuals, oral antigenic contact to nickel and chromium may induce immunologic tolerance rather than sensitization. One nickel-sensitive subject experienced rapid clinical improvement of a long-standing eczema of her hands and forearms in direct relationship to the insertion of four single nickel-based dental crown restorations (35), but such changes have not been reported in other studies in dentistry.

ANIMAL STUDIES

There are ethical and potential practical problems associated with implanting devices containing materials that one knows for certain that the patient is hypersensitive to. There are surprisingly few animals studies on this subject. Merritt and Brown (25) implanted stainless steel screws in the humeri of nickel-sensitized rabbits and found severe reactions to implants to be associated with metal sensitivity. Gjerdet et al. (11) implanted stainless steel and cobalt-chromium-based wires subcutaneously in nickel-sensitized rabbits and found no difference in tissue reaction between sensitized and nonsensitized animals. There were, however, marked tissue reactions in the sensitized animals to some of the wires that had been treated with silver solder prior to insertion. Niemi et al. (28) implanted palladium-based alloys subcutaneously in palladium-sensitized guinea pigs. There were no marked tissue reactions, except for a moderately increased number of mast cells around the implants in the sensitized animals. Lewin et al. (21) implanted cobalt-chromium and stainless steel screws in guinea pigs sensitized to nickel, cobalt, and chromium and found no significant differences between contact allergic and control animals by qualitative examination. Heggers et al. (14) found a cellular immune response to methylmethacrylate in experimentally sensitized guinea pigs. Different types of methylmethacrylate-based resins were implanted in the subcutaneous tissue of formaldehyde-sensitized and control guinea pigs, and Kallus (17) found an enhanced, transient tissue response in the sensitized animals. The tissue reaction was proportional to the formaldehyde content of the polymers. An orthopedic bone cement evaluated by the same methods elicited comparable tissue reactions in formaldehyde-sensitized animals (T. Kallus, *personal communication*).

REQUIREMENTS FOR CLINICAL DOCUMENTATION

Hypersensitivity reactions following insertion of orthopedic implants are difficult to evaluate. At a workshop on alloy systems in dentistry, it was suggested that good documentation requires an extensive investigation that includes (24):

1. Establishing that the patient's history, signs, and symptoms are consistent with hypersensitivity reactions,
2. Identifying the eliciting substances,
3. Establishing the patient's ability to react,
4. Demonstrating that the patient is symptom free on removal of causative substance(s),
5. Eliciting a reaction by reexposure.

No published case reports satisfy these requirements. Several of the requirements may also come in conflict with practical and ethical considerations and may not be in the patient's own best interest. Agreement on similar guidelines in orthopedics might help to evaluate allergy and hypersensitivity reactions to implanted devices.

GENERAL CONCLUSIONS

Both local and systemic reactions may sometimes occur following implantation of metallic devices (13,33,42). Metal allergy has been suggested as a predisposing factor for infection of periprosthetic tissues (16). However, it looks like the majority of individuals—even the majority of sensitized individuals—will tolerate low levels of allergens in the tissues without adverse effect. Induction of immunologic tolerance may be a potential benefit.

The mechanisms by which local cutaneous and systemic reactions occur as a result of nickel in orthopedic implants remain somewhat obscure and seem unpredictable in the clinic. Some reactions appear to be type I in nature. In others there is good evidence of type-IV hypersensitivity. In some patients, however, type-I, -III (Arthus), and -IV reactions seem to coexist (42). The reaction patterns elicited by other metals seem to be similar to those elicited by nickel.

Information on allergy or hypersensitivity reactions to nonmetallic constituents of orthopedic devices is scarce (27).

REFERENCES

1. Benson MKD, Goodwin PG, Brostoff J. Metal sensitivity in patients with joint replacement arthroplasties. *BMJ* 1975;4:374–375.
2. Burrows D. Mischievous metals—chromate, cobalt, nickel and mercury. *Clin Exp Dermatol* 1989; 14:266–272.
3. Burrows D, Creswell S, Merrett DJ. Nickel, hands and hip prostheses. *Br J Dermatol* 1981; 105:437–444.
4. Carlsson A, Magnusson B, Möller H. Metal sensitivity in patients with metal-to-plastic total hip arthroplasties. *Acta Orthop Scand* 1980;51:57–62.

5. Carlsson Å, Möller H. Implantation of orthopaedic devices in patients with metal allergy. *Acta Dermatol Venereol* 1989;69:62–66.
6. Christiansen K, Holmes K, Zilko PJ. Metal sensitivity causing loosened joint prostheses. *Ann Rheum Dis* 1979;38:476–480.
7. Deutman R, Mulder J, Brian R, Nater JP. Metal sensitivity before and after total hip arthroplasty. *J Bone Joint Surg [Am]* 1977;59:862–865.
8. Elves MW, Wilson JN, Scales JT, Kemp HBS. Incidence of metal sensitivity in patients with total joint replacements. *BMJ* 1975;4:376–378.
9. Fisher AA. Contact dermatitis in medical and surgical personnel. In: Maibach HI, Gellin GA, eds. *Occupational and industrial dermatology.* Chicago: Year Book Publishers, 1982:219.
10. Gigli I, Baer RL. Atopic dermatitis. In: Fitzpatrick TB, Eisen AZ, Wolff K, Freedberg IM, Austen KF, eds. *Dermatology in general medicine.* New York: McGraw-Hill, 1979:520.
11. Gjerdet NR, Kallus T, Hensten-Pettersen A. Tissue reactions to implanted orthodontic wires in rabbits. *Acta Odontol Scand* 1987;45:163–169.
12. Grasshoff H, Schmidt D, Kluge K, Müller WA. Hüftgelenkendo-prothetik und Metallsensibilisierung. Untersuchungen mit dem Leukozytenmigrationstest. *Beitr Orthop Traumatol* 1990;37: 211–215.
13. Guyuron B, Lasa CI. Reaction to stainless steel wire following orthognathic surgery. *Plast Reconstr Surg* 1992;89:540–542.
14. Heggers JP, Talmage JB, Barnes ST. Cellular immune response to methylmethacrylate in experimentally sensitized guinea pigs. *Milit Med* 1978;143:192–195.
15. Hensten-Pettersen A. Casting alloys: side effects. *Adv Dent Res* 1992;6:38–43.
16. Hierholzer S, Hierholzer G. Metallallergie als pathogenetischer Faktor für die Knocheninfektion nach Osteosynthesen. *Unfallheilkunde* 1984;87:1–6.
17. Kallus T. Enhanced tissue response to denture base polymers in formaldehyde-sensitized guinea pigs. *J Prosthet Dent* 1984;52:292–299.
18. Koda T, Tsuchiya H, Yamauchi M, Ohtani S, Takagi N, Kawano J. Leachability of denture-base acrylic resins in artificial saliva. *Dent Mater* 1990;6:13–20.
19. Lalor PA, Revell PA, Gray AB, Wright S, Railton GT, Freeman MAR. Sensitivity to titanium. A cause of implant failure? *J Bone Joint Surg [Br]* 1991;73:25–28.
20. Langlais F, Postel M, Berry JP, Le Charpentier Y, Weill BJ. L'intolérance aux débris d'usure des prothèses. *Int Orthop* 1980;4:145–153.
21. Lewin J, Lindgren JU, Wahlberg JE. Apparent absence of local response to bone screws in guinea pigs with contact sensitivity. *J Orthop Res* 1987;5:604–608.
22. Löer F, Schleupner KH, Zilkins J. Déclenchement d'allergies suite à l'implantation d'endoprothéses totales de hanche? *Chirurgie* 1986;112:462–467.
23. McMillan C, Burrows D. In vitro testing of nickel contact hypersensitivity. In: Maibach HI, Menné T, eds. *Nickel and the skin: immunology and toxicology.* Boca Raton, FL: CRC Press, 1989:79–89.
24. Merritt K. Biochemistry. Hypersensitivity. Clinical reaction. In: Lang BR, Morris HF, Razzoog ME, eds. *International workshop. Biocompatibility, toxicity and hypersensitivity to alloy systems used in dentistry.* Ann Arbor: University of Michigan School of Dentistry, 1986:193.
25. Merritt K, Brown SA. Tissue reaction and metal sensitivity. An animal study. *Acta Orthop Scand* 1980;51:403–411.
26. Monteny E, Delespesse G, Screyen H, Spiette M. Methylmethacrylate hypersensitivity in orthopaedic surgery. *Acta Orthop Scand* 1978;49:186–191.
27. Monteny E, Oleffe J, Donkerwolke M. Methylmethacrylate hypersensitivity in a patient with cemented endoprosthesis. *Acta Orthop Scand* 1978;49:554–556.
28. Niemi L, Syrjänen S, Hensten-Pettersen A. The biocompatibility of a dental Ag-Pd-Cu-Ag-based casting alloy and its structural components. *J Biomed Mater Res* 1985;19:535–548.
29. Novey HS, Habib M, Wells ID. Asthma and IgE antibodies induced by chromium and nickel salts. *J Allergy Clin Immunol* 1983;72:407–412.
30. Roitt IM. *Essential immunology.* Oxford: Blackwell Scientific Publications. 1991:253–275.
31. Romaguera C, Lecha M, Grimalt F, Muniesa AM, Mascaro JM. Photocontact dermatitis to cobalt salts. *Contact Dermatitis* 1982;8:383–388.
32. Rooker GD, Wilkinson JD. Metal sensitivity in patients undergoing hip replacement. *J Bone Joint Surg [Br]* 1980;62:502–505.
33. Rostoker G, Robin J, Binet O, Paupe J. Dermatoses d'intolérance aux métaux des matériaux d'osteosynthèse et des prothèses. *Ann Dermatol Venereol* 1986;113:1097–1108.
34. Ruyter IE. Release of formaldehyde from denture base polymers. *Acta Odontol Scand* 1980; 38:17–27.
35. Spiechowicz E, Glantz PO, Axéll T, Chmielewski W. Oral exposure to a nickel-containing dental alloy of persons with hypersensitive skin reactions to nickel. *Contact Dermatitis* 1984;10: 206–211.

36. Staerkjaer L, Menné T. Nickel allergy and orthodontic treatment. *Eur J Orthodont* 1990;12:284–289.
37. van der Burg CKH, Bruynzeel DP, Vreeburg KJJ, van Blomberg BME, Sheper RJ. Hand eczema in hairdressers and nurses: a prospective study. I: Evaluation of atopy and nickel hypersensitivity at the start of apprenticeship. *Contact Dermatitis* 1986;14:275.
38. von Blomberg BME, Bruynzeel DP, Sheper RJ. Advances in mechanism of allergic contact dermatitis: in vitro and in vivo research. In: Marzulli F, Maibach H, eds. *Dermatoxicology*. Washington, DC: Hemisphere Publishing, 1991:255.
39. Vreeburg KJJ, de Groot K, von Blomberg M, Sheper RJ. Induction of immunological tolerance by oral administration of nickel and chromium. *J Dent Res* 1984;63:124–128.
40. Vreeburg KJJ, van Hoogstraten IMV, von Blomberg BME, de Groot K, Scheper R. Oral induction of immunological tolerance to chromium in the guinea pig. *J Dent Res* 1990;69:1634–1639.
41. Waterman AH, Schrik JJ. Allergy in hip arthroplasty. *Contact Dermatitis* 1985;13:294–301.
42. Wilkinson JD. Nickel allergy and orthopedic prostheses. In: Maibach HI, Menné T, eds. *Nickel and the skin: immunology and toxicology*. Boca Raton, FL: CRC Press, 1989:187–193.
43. Wrangsjö K, Wahlberg JE, Axelsson IGK. IgE-mediated allergy to natural rubber in 30 patients with contact urticaria. *Contact Dermatitis* 1988;19:264–271.

Biological, Material, and Mechanical Considerations of Joint Replacement, edited by B. F. Morrey. Raven Press, Ltd., New York © 1993.

Discussion of Toxicity and Allergy

Barbara D. Boyan

Department of Orthopaedics, University of Texas Health Science Center at San Antonio, San Antonio, Texas 78284-7774

A panel of 18 surgeons and scientists discussed the toxic and allergenic aspects of joint replacement and arrived at the following conclusions.

CONSENSUS

Biomaterials have the potential to cause adverse biologic reactions in patients.

Biomaterials change over time in the body with respect to chemical composition, material properties, and mechanical characteristics.

There is a differential biologic and mechanical response to bulk, particulate, and ionic materials, and this response is material specific.

There is host variability in the response to the biomaterials that includes humoral, cellular, tissue, organ, and whole animal aspects; systemic and local factors are involved.

Orthopedic biomaterials may elicit hypersensitivity reactions in susceptible persons, i.e., persons capable of immunologic reactions directly associated with specific antigens (allergens/haptens).

CONTENTIONS

It is unknown whether allergic reactions can precipitate events leading to implant loosening.

It is unknown whether sensitization or tolerance to orthopedic implant materials exists.

It is unknown at this time whether biomaterials are carcinogenic when used as orthopedic implants. (Active surveillance is occurring to monitor this potential relationship.)

FUTURE NEEDS

Clinical Studies

Development of prospective databases to monitor patients with respect to adverse reactions to biomaterials at the cellular, mechanical, and material levels and correlation of implants with history of disease and incidence of morbidity and mortality.

Need for standardized retrieval data and estimation of risk/benefit ratio by outcome studies based in part on function and on patient-derived satisfaction.

Utilization of appropriate epidemiologic tools and reference groups for determining outcomes.

Basic Research Approaches

The following needs or initiatives are recognized:

Development of standardized and relevant reference materials and animal models.

Development of better tests for assessing individual variability in response to biomaterials.

Use of characterized materials for *in vivo* and *in vitro* testing. Use of these materials to improve understanding of the similarities and differences in animal models and their comparison with comparable events in humans.

Assess bioreactivity of biomaterials in terms of host response appropriate to the application (biocompatibility) and in so doing determine whether the systemic effects of biomaterials are due to particles, ions, cytokines and growth factors, and/ or mechanical forces.

Understand the role of the biomaterial as a reactive surface.

Need for appropriately designed multifactorial experiments and a multidisciplinary approach to biomaterial research.

Understanding the interaction of material properties and the musculoskeletal system with respect to bone remodeling, conditioning and adaptation of the material by cells and fluids, conditioning of the cells by the material, and modulation of both by mechanical factors.

Biological, Material, and Mechanical
Considerations of Joint Replacement,
edited by B. F. Morrey.
Raven Press, Ltd., New York © 1993.

30

New Directions in Manufacturing

Roy D. Crowninshield and Jack E. Parr

Zimmer, Inc., Warsaw, Indiana 46581-0708

New developments in biomaterials and new manufacturing technologies are closely tied. Manufacturability is required to transform successful biomaterials research into a successful medical product. New manufacturing technologies can be successfully applied to orthopaedic implants if the technologies provide functional advantages that are commensurate with their cost and if they can receive regulatory approval. The technologies' functional advantage can be applicable to the manufacturer, patient, or health care provider. The cost effectiveness of technology includes not only the incremental manufacturing cost (or savings) to apply the technology to a product but also includes the investment in technology development. Throughout the world's major orthopaedic markets, the regulatory approval of new technologies requires increasingly exact and time-tested demonstrations of both safety and efficacy. The investment in technology development, to include regulatory approval, needs to be recovered during technology commercialization and is a factor in the products' economic viability.

In the past decade, there have been many new technologies introduced into orthopaedics and many more are currently under development. Many new technologies have already demonstrated functionality, cost effectiveness, and regulatory approvability. Many of these successful technologies, which are built on or are modifications of previously existing technologies, are evolutionary steps in technological progression. Some more revolutionary technologies, while holding promise, are commercially unproven whereas others are surrounded by considerable question as to their ability to achieve functionality, cost effectiveness, and regulatory approval.

The following discussion of orthopaedic manufacturing technologies progresses from successful innovations of evolutionary nature to scientifically intriguing advanced technologies that may, or may not, achieve commercial success.

SURFACE TREATMENT TECHNOLOGIES

Technologies oriented to the treatment of implant surfaces have made important contributions to orthopaedic surgery. Most of the successful surface treatment technologies are improvements in existing implant surfaces by manufacturing processes that introduce no significant questions of product safety. These technologies have affected both the articular surface and the biologic interface surface of implants.

The use of titanium alloys for total joint applications has been very successful due to high levels of biocompatibility, excellent mechanical properties, and clinically sound prosthetic device designs (16). The increased clinical attention to issues of implant wear and particle release has inspired the development of improvements in titanium surface properties that have advanced titanium implant function.

Implant Surface Polishing and Nitriding

The easiest new manufacturing technologies to implement are technologies that in fact are not new but are rather reinvented technologies that find renewed application due to new understandings of implant function. Implant surface polishing and nitriding are both old technologies that have renewed interest.

Prosthetic-debris generation in and around orthopaedic implants and its associated biologic response is a current topic in orthopaedic research. Bone lysis has been shown clinically with cemented, cementless, porous, and smooth implants made of both titanium alloy and cobalt-chrome alloy. This apparent particulate debris-induced response can be affected by reducing particulate generation at the implant interface with the body.

Many metal orthopaedic implants have been traditionally finished utilizing abrasive blasting, typically glass-bead blasting to produce a uniform matte surface. The appearance of glass bead-blasted titanium alloy and cobalt-chrome alloy implant surfaces is shown in Fig. 1. These surfaces contain bits of metal loosely attached to the implant surface as well as blast medium embedded in the implant surface. In contrast, the magnified appearance of a polished and nitrided titanium alloy surface is shown in Fig. 2. This surface is cleaner and smoother without the fragments of metal and blast medium typical of blasted implant surfaces. Although relatively highly polished implant surfaces are not a new technology, they are a technology of renewed interest, particularly when combined with surface-hardening technologies.

The formation of titanium nitride can be thermally induced within a titanium-based implant surface through a furnace-nitriding process. This process traces its origins back to the early 1970s when it was first used to prepare the surface of titanium fracture fixation devices. This process produces a nitrogen-rich region within the prosthesis surface that reacts with the titanium on the surface to form titanium nitride. As a result, the prosthesis surface hardness and abrasion resistance (Fig. 3) are substantially increased while the potential for particulate release is substantially reduced.

Polishing and thermally induced nitriding of titanium implants have manufacturing efficiency and can improve implant function. These renewed applications of earlier developed technologies are currently utilized on several implant systems.

Ion Implantation

The second easiest new manufacturing technologies to be implemented are technologies that, although new to orthopaedics, are borrowed from other industries.

Ion implantation has been demonstrated to increase the hardness, abrasion resistance, and corrosion resistance of titanium-based implants (1,14). The process (Fig. 4) of ion implantation causes elemental ions to be embedded in the surface of a

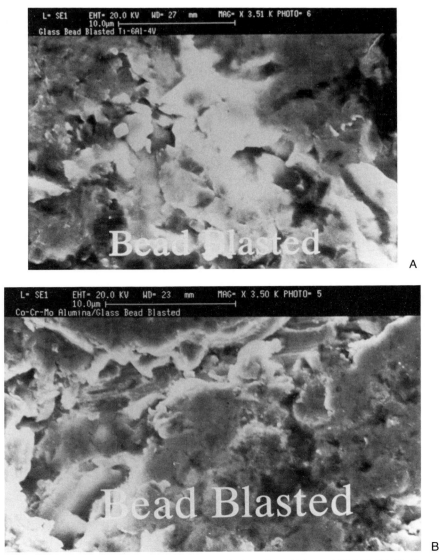

FIG. 1. A: Scanning electron photomicrograph of glass-bead blasted Ti-6Al-4V. **B:** Scanning electron photomicrograph of glass-bead blasted Co-Cr-Mo.

material. Ion implantation is done under vacuum conditions at relatively high (80–100 KeV) electric potentials and low current (0.5–1.0 mA). Nitrogen gas (N_2) is introduced into the system at the ion source where elements from an incandescent tungsten filament collide with the neutral gas to create a wide range of ionic nitrogen. Motivated by the electrical potential, the ionized gas exits from the source, is electronically filtered to yield the desired ionic species, and is accelerated and focused on the surface of the implant. The ballistic interaction of the nitrogen ions and im-

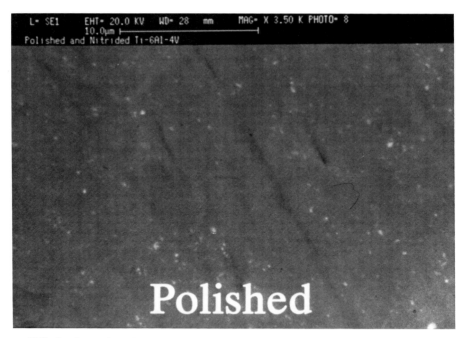

FIG. 2. Scanning electron photomicrograph of polished and nitrided Ti-6Al-4V.

plant surface results in ions entering the implant surface and coming to rest in a gaussian distribution concentration within the near surface. The equipment and processes utilized in ion implantation of orthopaedic implants are sophisticated and specialized. The development cost of this technology was, however, largely borne by other industries from which orthopaedics borrowed the technology.

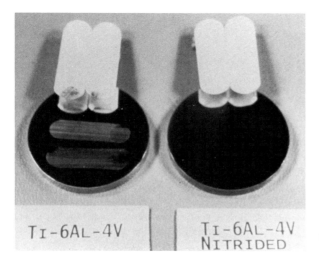

FIG. 3. Pin-on-disk wear results. Ti-6Al-4V (*left*) and nitrogen-hardened (*right*) Ti-6Al-4V.

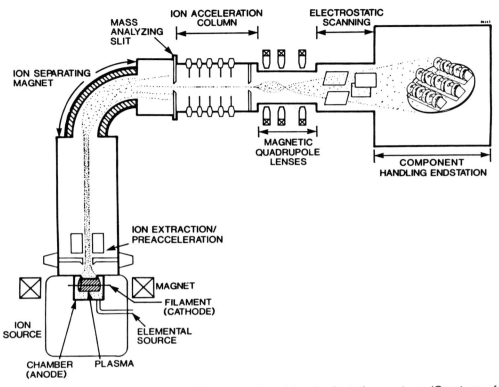

FIG. 4. Schematic representation of mass analyzed ion implantation system. (Courtesy of Spire Corporation, Bedford, MA.)

Since this technology utilizes materials with previously demonstrated biocompatibility (nitrogen and titanium alloys), the demonstration of technology safety was straightforward. Agar overlay techniques have demonstrated no adverse cytotoxicity response, and 30-day rabbit muscle implant studies have demonstrated no adverse histological affects. Ion-implanted titanium-alloy surfaces have demonstrated excellent biocompatibility at a cellular level.

The functionality of ion implantation has been demonstrated in a variety of laboratory protocols employed to investigate the effects of the technology. Basic mechanical and chemical properties of ion-implanted surfaces have been demonstrated by Buchanan et al. (1), Lucas et al. (14), and Sioshansi (17). The improved wear performance in orthopaedic applications has been demonstrated in the hip by McKellop et al. (16) and in the knee by Crowninshield et al. (5). These improvements in mechanical performance of titanium-alloy implant surfaces are due to the increased surface hardness resulting from the ion implantation-induced formation of nitride, oxide, and carbide participates within the near implant surface.

Orthopaedic ion implantation has been developed to a practical level of application and is routinely used in implant manufacture. Ion implantation of titanium-based implants has been demonstrated to improve implant function in a cost-effective manner. The safety of the process has been demonstrated, and the technology has received regulatory approval for use in several manufacturers' implants in many countries.

Plasma Spraying

Plasma spraying is another borrowed manufacturing technology. This process is well established as a means of depositing dense metal coatings on mechanical components. The process was first modified to apply porous metal coatings for orthopaedic applications and more recently to apply orthopaedic ceramic coatings.

Calcium-phosphate ceramics and their ability to enhance fixation have been studied extensively for the past decade (3,9). This research effort has supported the introduction of calcium-phosphate ceramics as coatings on orthopaedic implants. The data to support improved functionality of implants provided with these coatings and the corresponding regulatory approval of the technologies vary greatly across the global orthopaedic practice.

Calcium phosphates are a class of materials that encompass a large number of chemical entities. One of the most common forms is hydroxyapatite (HA). Research has shown that synthetic HA is chemically similar to naturally occurring bone mineral and is biocompatible with bone.

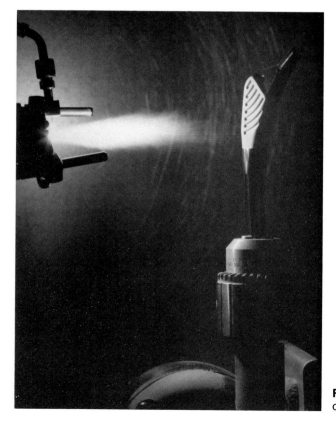

FIG. 5. Plasma spraying of HA coating onto a hip prosthesis.

The manufacturing technology utilized in HA coatings is plasma spraying (Fig. 5). The calcium-phosphate ceramic in a powder form is fed into a gas plasma. The gas plasma is formed when a gas such as argon is passed between electrodes that are at high potential. The plasma can reach temperatures of 3,000° K with velocities around 1,000 km/hr. The powder is partially melted in the plasma while being propelled toward a properly prepared implant surface. A thin adherent layer of calcium-phosphate material can be deposited on the implant surface. Although utilizing rather sophisticated equipment, this manufacturing method is effective and efficient.

In the past decade, the use of high-purity HA coatings has extended from dentistry to orthopaedics. Much of the early orthopaedic evaluation of these coatings occurred in Europe (11,18). Orthopaedic implants coated with HA are widely available throughout much of Europe and Asia. Proponents of this technology cite evidence of enhanced biologic fixation resulting from bone-to-implant attachment induced by the biologic activity of synthetic HA. In contrast, within the United States, recent Food and Drug Administration (FDA) approval of HA-coated devices is based on the determination that HA-coated devices are not functionally better than noncoated press-fit devices. As with many new implant technologies, plasma-sprayed HA coatings have a somewhat controversial scientific and regulatory standing.

Perhaps an ultimately more functional use of calcium phosphates as implant coatings will be found in the treatment of porous orthopaedic implants. Calcium-phosphate coatings, particularly coatings of more biologically active chemistries than high-purity HA, offer the potential to enhance bone-ingrowth fixation of total joint prostheses. Outside the United States, calcium phosphate-coated porous orthopaedic implants are available and are gaining clinical acceptance. Within the United States, demonstrated scientific and clinical safety and efficacy are required to support FDA approval of the technology.

NEW SYNTHETIC IMPLANT MATERIALS

A variety of synthetic materials that do not have a tradition of orthopaedic use are being considered for new implants. Each of these materials has associated with it novel manufacturing technologies. Since many of these materials are without substantial prior medical applications, issues of material safety as well as product efficacy need to be resolved prior to commercialization.

Resorbable Materials

The resorbable materials most commonly considered for orthopaedic application include polylactic and polyglycolic acid. Each of these materials has been utilized as nonorthopaedic implant products, thus safety is less of an issue than demonstrated efficacy or functionality. The resorption of these polymeric materials is initiated by hydrolysis and results in biocompatible compounds that are metabolized by the body. Considerable effort has lead to commercialization of low load applications such as pins and screws (7).

Pins have been developed and are in limited use for finger and ankle fracture fixation. Screws for use in the pelvis and near articular surfaces are under investigation. The development of higher strength bioresorbable devices is a requirement for any widespread penetration into the metal-dominated fixation market.

Intermedullary plugs for cemented femoral stems have been developed using bioresorbable polymers in an effort to minimize debris generation during potential revision surgery.

Because these polymers are highly sensitive to heat, humidity, and radiation, the manufacturing technologies utilizing these materials require careful controls. The resulting orthopaedic product can have a predictable rate of bioresorption and associated mechanical properties that support the use of the material in temporary functioning situations.

Composite Materials

Materials that are composites of polymers and reinforcing fibers have been considered for orthopaedic implants (8). Total hip femoral components and fracture fixation devices are generally considered the most realistic application of composite materials. In comparison to an equivalent metal device, a composite device can have increased structural flexibility. Although the reinforcing fibers strengthen the polymer matrix, the achievement of strength comparable to high strength metallic devices is a substantial challenge for a composite device. From a manufacturing point of view, composite devices may depart radically from conventional orthopaedic manufacturing practices and present many new challenges. Much of the work in composite orthopaedic device fabrication has tended to utilize elements of tradi-

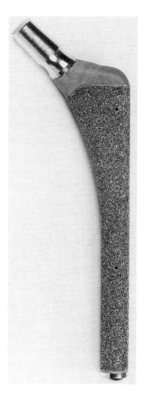

FIG. 6. Macro composite of metal and polymer elements that offer promise for a biocompatible, high-strength, flexible, and extensively ingrown prosthesis.

tional prosthetic device manufacture while not fully utilizing the special features of composite fabrication. Many of the present orthopaedic composite devices obtain their final implant geometry by machining in a manner very similar to that utilized in the manufactured of equivalent metal devices (2,15). In the machined composite approach, the composite manufacturing steps of, for example, lamination and compression molding are utilized only to fabricate a block of composite material from which conventional machining can produce the final composite implant. Other industries have successfully utilized composite fabrication techniques that result directly in the final product geometry.

Despite considerable interest and activity for more than a decade, both within the industry and the research community, fiber-reinforced polymer-composite orthopaedic devices have to date not been successfully developed at a commercial level. This new manufacturing technology has experienced difficulties in achieving cost effectiveness and fulfilling product design requirements. Achieving designed flexibility, strength, fixation, biocompatibility, and manufacturability simultaneously has been difficult.

A total hip femoral component that is a macro composite of metal and polymer elements is illustrated in Fig. 6. This device obtains its strength from a forged metallic core, its flexibility through a polymer encasement, and its fixation through a porous metal surface. The implant shape is achieved through a series of forging and molding steps that efficiently achieve the anatomic requirements. This approach utilizes a blend of proven technologies with innovative technologies.

BIOLOGIC TECHNOLOGIES

Orthopaedic products have been traditionally dominated by metallurgical and organic polymer technologies. There is, however, a growing scientific interest in biologically based orthopaedic products. These potential biologic products represent perhaps the greatest manufacturing challenge to the medical industry. The successful development of biologically based orthopaedic products requires unique demonstrations of biologic activity, immunologic acceptability, reproducible manufacture, and commercial practicality.

Collagen-Based Implants

The simplest biologic products are based on existing tissue structures or elements. Xenografts and tissue transplants have been used in a variety of medical products.

Collagen is a natural polymer fiber that has potential applications in many orthopaedic situations. Current scientific and clinical orthopaedic activity utilizing collagen-based implants has centered on ligament reconstructions and bone-graft substitutes. Both of these applications have utilized xenograft-collagen implants.

Ligament replacement with xenograft implants has been widely used in Europe and has been the subject of controlled clinical trials within the United States. The manufacturing technology used in xenograft ligament replacement was glutaraldehyde cross-linking borrowed from heart valve applications. Although successful in heart valve replacement, the early orthopaedic applications have resulted in disappointing long-term clinical results due to mechanical and biologic limitations of the devices. Harvesting and transplanting of cartilage and ligament structures, both autogenic and allogenic, have shown some promise for restoration of joint function, although with a reduction of capability. Additional work with second-generation approaches to collagen scaffold replacement of ligaments is ongoing (13).

Synthetic bone-graft substitutes have been the subject of extensive research efforts in recent years (6). Highly purified fibrillar collagen, when combined with calcium-phosphate ceramic and autogenous bone marrow, has been demonstrated to be an effective bone-defect filler (10). Randomized controlled clinical trials of this material have demonstrated equivalent function to autogenous bone graft in the treatment of long-bone fractures (4). This material, subject to final FDA approval, will soon be available in the United States.

Xenograft collagen implants are perhaps the most conceptionally simple biologically based orthopaedic products. Other biologic product possibilities are based on far more advanced manufacturing.

Growth Factors

The induction of orthopaedically desirable tissue growth has been, and remains, an intriguing technological possibility. Perhaps the earliest clinical and commercial activities in this area are found in the still somewhat controversial use of electric fields to induce tissue growth. More recently, much scientific and commercial activity has been directed to the isolation, identification, and synthesis of protein-based tissue growth factors (6,12). The tissues of greatest interest include the dermis, bone, and articular cartilage.

Although it has been long identified that tissue growth is regulated by so-called growth factors, the commercial development of products based on these biologic technologies has proven to be a difficult and expensive endeavor. Development of growth factor-based orthopaedic products has been hampered by complexities in biology, patents, protein synthesis, and regulatory requirements. Despite the achievement of scientific advances in this area, commercial developments have been disappointingly slow. It is not clear at present when, how, and if growth factor-based technologies will become commonly utilized orthopaedic products.

CONCLUSIONS

Over the past decade, the orthopaedic industry has contemplated many new implant concepts and associated manufacturing technologies. The greatest successes in the development of new manufacturing methods have been associated with changes to otherwise traditional plastic and metal implants. Many of the "new" manufacturing technologies are in fact old orthopaedic technologies with new applications or are technologies borrowed from other industries and are thus only new to orthopaedics. Many new technologies are popularized on the basis of their scientific interest; however, the successfully commercialized technologies provide valuable implant function, utilize efficient manufacturing methods, and successfully achieve regulatory approval. The future for orthopaedic technologies does remain bright; however, the continuously changing orthopaedic marketplace and regulatory environment require careful consideration of the effort required and the benefit obtained in the pursuit of manufacturing technology development.

REFERENCES

1. Buchanan RA, Rigney ED Jr, Williams JM. Ion implantation of surgical Ti-6Al-4V for improved resistance to wear accelerated corrosion. *J Biomed Mater Res* 1987;21:355–366.
2. Chang F-K, Perez JL, Davidson JA. Stiffness and strength tailoring of a hip prosthesis made of advanced composite materials. *J Biomed Mater Res* 1990;24:873–899.
3. Cook S, Kay JF, Thomas KA, et al. Interface mechanics and histology of titanium and hydroxylapatite coated titanium for dental applications. *Int J Oral Maxillofac Implant* 1987;2:15–22.
4. Cornell CN, Lane JM, Chapman M, et al. Multicenter trial of collagraft as bone graft substitute. *J Orthop Trauma* 1991;5:1–8.
5. Crowninshield R, Lower J, Gilbertson L, et al. Simulating total knee replacement wear in vitro: comparison of Ti-6Al-4V and nitrogen-ion implanted Ti-6Al-4V. *J Bone Joint Surg [Am]* 1990;14:470–471.
6. Damien CJ, Parson JR. Bone graft and bone graft substitutes: a review of current technology and applications. *J Appl Biomater* 1991;2:187–208.
7. Daniels AU, Chang MKO, Andrian KP. Mechanical properties of biodegradable polymers and composites proposed for internal fixation of bone. *J Appl Biomater* 1990;1:57–78.
8. Davidson JA. The challenge and opportunity for composites in structural orthopaedic applications. *J Compos Tech Res* 1987;9:151–161.
9. deLange GL, Donath K. Interface between bone tissue and implants of solid hydroxyapatite or hydroxyapatite-coated titanium implants. *Biomaterials* 1989;10:121–125.
10. Flatley TJ, Lynch KL, Benson M. Tissue response to implants of calcium phosphate ceramic in the rabbit spine. *Clin Orthop* 1983;179:246–252.
11. Geesink RGT. Experimental and clinical experience with hydroxyapatite-coated hip implants. *Orthopedics* 1989;12:1239–1242.
12. Johnson EE, Urist MR, Finerman GAM. Bone morphogenetic protein augmentation grafting of resistant femoral nonunions. *Clin Orthop* 1988;230:257–265.
13. Kato YP, Dunn MG, Zawadsky JP, Tria AJ, Silver FH. Regeneration of Achilles tendon with a collagen tendon prosthesis. *J Bone Joint Surg [Am]* 1991;73:561–574.
14. Lucas DC, Lee JE, Lemons JE, et al. In vitro corrosion investigations of TiN coated and nitrogen implanted Ti-6Al-4V alloy. *Trans 31st Ann Meeting Orthop Res Soc* 1985;10:323.
15. Magee FP, Weinstein AM, Longo JA, Koeneman JB, Yapp RA. A canine composite femoral stem. *Clin Orthop* 1988;235:237–252.
16. McKellop HA, Sarmiento A, Schwinn CP, et al. In vivo wear of titanium-alloy hip prostheses. *J Bone Joint Surg [Am]* 1990;72:512–517.
17. Sioshansi P. Improving the properties of titanium alloys by ion implantation. *J Miner Metal Mater Soc* 1990-(March):30–31.
18. Soballe K, Hansen ES, Brockstedt-Rasmussen H, et al. Hydroxyapatite coating enhances fixation of porous coated implants. *Acta Orthop Scand* 1990;61:299–306.

Biological, Material, and Mechanical Considerations of Joint Replacement, edited by B. F. Morrey. Raven Press, Ltd., New York, 1993.

31

ISO Standard 10993-1: Biological Evaluation of Medical Devices

Part 1: Guidance on Selection of Tests

*James M. Anderson and †David H. Mueller

*Institute of Pathology, Case Western Reserve University, School of Medicine, Cleveland, Ohio 44106-4907; †Medtronic, Inc., Minneapolis, Minnesota 55432

This chapter presents Part 1, Guidance on Selection of Tests, of the ISO Standard 10993-1: Biological Evaluation of Medical Devices. Impetus for the development of this standard has been provided, in part, by the needs of the European Economic Community (EEC) to have a commonly accepted standard for the biological evaluation of medical devices. This part of ISO 10993 is a combination/harmonization of numerous international and national standards and guidelines. It is intended to be the overall guidance document for the selection of tests enabling evaluation of biological responses relevant to material and device safety.

ISO 10993 consists of the following parts, under the general title "Biological Evaluation of Medical Devices":

Part 1: Guidance on selection of tests
Part 2: Animal welfare requirements
Part 3: Tests for genotoxicity, carcinogenicity, and reproductive toxicity
Part 4: Selection of tests for interactions with blood
Part 5: Tests for cytotoxicity: *in vitro* methods
Part 6: Tests for local effects after implantation
Part 7: Ethylene oxide sterilization residuals
Part 8: Clinical investigation
Part 9: Degradation of materials related to biological testing
Part 10: Tests for irritation and sensitization
Part 11: Tests for systemic toxicity
Part 12: Sample preparation and reference materials

The overall Part 1 document contains informative (nonofficial) components: Foreword, Introduction, and Rationale (Annex A), which are included for perspective and components that are the official part of the document and provide a framework in which to plan the biological evaluation. The official components of the Part 1 document include:

1. Scope
2. Normative references
3. Definitions
4. General Principles Applying to Biological Evaluation of Materials and Devices
5. Categorization of Medical Devices
6. Testing
7. Guidance on Selection of Biological Evaluation Tests
8. Assurance of Test Methods

The official component of the document also contains two annexes: (A) rationale and (B) Bibliography of International and National Standards and Regulations.

This introduction summarizes salient points and provides perspective from the Foreword, Introduction, and Rationale components of the document. The official contents of the document are provided in the following sections of this chapter. Finally, the reference list or Bibliography of International and National Standards and Regulations is provided as Annex B.

The following comments are taken from the Foreword, Introduction, and Rationale (Annex A) components of the Standard and are included here to provide perspective and overview. The selection and evaluation of any material or device intended for use in humans require a structured program of assessment. In the design process, an informed decision should be made that weighs the advantages/disadvantages of the various material and test procedure choices. To give assurance that the final product will perform as intended and be safe for human use, the program should include a biological evaluation. The role of this document, Part 1: Guidance on Selection of Tests, is to serve as a framework in which to plan such a biological evaluation that minimizes the number and exposure of animals. The biological evaluation should be planned and carried out by knowledgeable and experienced individuals capable of making informed decisions based on the advantages and disadvantages of the various materials and test procedures available. The protection of humans is the primary goal of ISO 10993. The appropriate selection and interpretation of biological evaluation tests require an understanding of the rationale behind such testing.

This part of ISO 10993 is concerned with the safety-in-use of medical devices and materials. It is intended to assess the biological response of devices and materials as part of the overall evaluation and development of devices and materials. It addresses the determination of the effects of devices and materials on tissue in a general way, rather than for specific individual applications. This part of ISO 10993 thus classifies devices into broad categories and indicates, in matrices, the biological tests that are thought to be relevant for consideration for each device category.

The range of biological hazards with medical devices is wide. The tissue interaction of the material cannot be considered in isolation from the overall device design. The best material with respect to tissue interaction may result in a less functional device, tissue interaction being only one characteristic of a material. Where the material is intended to interact with tissue in order for the device to perform its function, evaluation takes on dimensions not generally addressed in standards and guide-lines to date.

Biological reactions that are adverse for a material in one application may not be adverse for the use of the material in a different application. Biological testing relies on animal models, and a material cannot, therefore, be conclusively shown to have the same tissue reactions in humans. In addition, differences between humans suggest that some patients may have adverse reactions even to well-established materials. Currently, biological testing relies on animal models. However, as scientific knowledge advances our understanding of basic mechanisms, preference should be given to *in vitro* models in situations in which scientific evidence reveals equally relevant information.

For devices and materials the application of a rigid set of test methods and pass/fail criteria may result in either an unnecessary restriction or a false sense of security in their use. Where a particular application warrants, experts in the product or application area involved may choose to establish specific tests and criteria specified in a product-specific vertical standard.

This part of ISO 10993 is not, therefore, intended to be a set of definitive statements to be followed by individuals not qualified by training and experience; it should be applied with interpretation and judgment by the appropriate professionals qualified by training and experience taking into consideration the factors relevant to the device/material, its intended use, and the current knowledge of the device/material provided by scientific literature and previous clinical experience.

The official organization responsible for the development of Part 1 of the ISO 10993 standard is the American Association of Medical Instrumentation, AAMI, 3330 Washington Boulevard, Suite 400, Arlington, VA 22201-4598. Additional information on the respective parts of the ISO 10993 international standard may be obtained from AAMI.

1 SCOPE

This part of ISO 10993 gives guidance on

a. the fundamental principles governing the biological evaluation of medical devices:
b. the definition of categories of devices based on the nature and duration of contact with the body;
c. the selection of appropriate tests.

ISO 10993 does not cover testing of materials and devices that do not come into contact with the patient's body directly or indirectly. Nor does it cover biological hazards arising from any mechanical failure. Other parts of ISO 10993 cover specific tests as indicated in the foreword. (See A.2, clause 1 Scope.)

2 NORMATIVE REFERENCES

The following standards contain provisions which, through reference in this text, constitute provisions of this part of ISO 10993. At the time of publication, the editions indicated were valid. All standards are subject to revision, and parties to agreements based on this part of ISO 10993 are encouraged to investigate the possibility of applying the most recent editions of the standards indicated below. Members of IEC and ISO maintain registers of currently valid International Standards.

ISO 9001:1987, *Quality systems—Model for quality assurance in design/development, production, installation, and servicing.*
ISO 9004:1987, *Quality management and quality system elements—Guidelines.*

3 DEFINITIONS

For the purposes of ISO 10993, the following definitions apply.

3.1   Medical Device: Any instrument, apparatus, appliance, material, or other article, including software, whether used alone or in combination, intended by the manufacturer to be used for human beings solely or principally for the purpose of:

—diagnosis, prevention, monitoring, treatment or alleviation of disease, injury, or handicap;
—investigation, replacement, or modification of the anatomy or of a physiological process;
—control of conception;

and which does not achieve its principal intended action in or on the human body by pharmacological, immunological, or metabolic means, but which may be assisted in its function by such means.

NOTES

1   Devices are different from drugs and their biological evaluation requires a different approach.
2   Use of the term "medical device" includes dental devices.

3.2   Material: Any synthetic or natural polymer, metal, alloy, ceramic, or other nonviable substance, including tissue rendered nonviable, used as a device or any part thereof.

3.3   Final product: Medical device in its "as used" state.

4   GENERAL PRINCIPLES APPLYING TO BIOLOGICAL EVALUATION OF MATERIALS AND DEVICES

4.1   In the selection of materials to be used in device manufacture, the first consideration should be fitness for purpose having regard to the characteristics and properties of the material, which include chemical, toxicological, physical, electrical, morphological, and mechanical properties.

4.2   The following should be considered for their relevance to the overall biological evaluation of the device:

a. the material(s) of manufacture;
b. intended additives, process contaminants and residues;
c. leachable substances;
d. degradation products;
e. other components and their interactions in the final product;
f. the properties and characteristics of the final product.

NOTE 3   If appropriate, identification and quantification of extractable chemical entities of the final product should precede biological evaluation.

4.3   Tests and their interpretation to be used in the biological evaluation should take into account the chemical composition of the materials including the conditions of exposure as well as the nature, degree, frequency, and duration of the device or its constituents to the body. By following these principles devices can be categorized to facilitate the selection of appropriate tests. This guide is concerned with the tests to be carried out on materials and/or the final product.

The range of potential hazards is wide and may include:

a. short-term effects (e.g., acute toxicity, irritation to the skin, eye and mucosal surfaces, sensitization, haemolysis, and thrombogenicity);
b. long-term or specific toxic effects (e.g., subchronic and chronic toxic effects, sensitization, genotoxicity, carcinogenicity (tumorigenicity), and effects on reproduction including teratogenicity).

4.4   All potential biological hazards should be considered for every material and final product but this does not imply that testing for all potential hazards will be necessary or practical (see clause 7).

4.5   Any *in vitro* or *in vivo* tests shall be based on end-use applications and appropriate good laboratory practice followed by evaluation by competent informed persons. Whenever possible, *in vitro* screening should be carried out before *in vivo* tests are commenced. Test data, complete to the extent that an independent analysis conclusion could be made, should be retained.

4.6   The materials or final product shall be considered (see A.2, subclause 4.6) for biological reevaluation if any of the following occurs:

a. any change in the source or in the specification of the materials used in the manufacture of the product;
b. any change in the formulation, processing, primary packaging, or sterilization of the product;
c. any change in the final product during storage;
d. any change in the intended use of the product;
e. any evidence that the product may produce adverse effects when used in humans.

4.7   The biological evaluation performed in accordance with this part of ISO 10993 should be considered in conjunction with the nature and mobility of the ingredients in the materials used to manufacture the device and other information, other non-clinical tests, clinical studies, and post-market experiences for an overall assessment (see A.2, subclause 4.7).

5   CATEGORIZATION OF MEDICAL DEVICES

The testing of any device that does not fall into one of the following categories should follow the general principles contained in this part of ISO 10993. Certain devices may fall into more than one category, in which case testing appropriate to each category should be considered.

5.1   Categorization by Nature of Contact

5.1.1   Non-contact Devices

These are devices that do not contact the patient's body directly or indirectly and are not included in ISO 10993.

5.1.2   Surface-Contacting Devices

These include devices in contact with the following:

a. **Skin:** devices that contact intact skin surfaces only; examples include electrodes, external prostheses, fixation tapes, compression bandages, and monitors of various types;
b. **Mucosal membranes:** devices communicating with intact mucosal membranes; examples include contact lenses, urinary catheters, intravaginal and intraintestinal devices (sigmoidoscopes, colonoscopes, stomach tubes, gastroscopes), endotracheal tubes, bronchoscopes, dental prostheses, orthodontic devices, and IUDs;
c. **Breached or compromised surfaces:** devices that contact breached or otherwise compromised body surfaces; examples include ulcer, burn, and granulation tissue dressings or healing devices and occlusive patches.

5.1.3   External Communicating Devices

These include devices communicating with the following:

a. **Blood path, indirect:** devices that contact the blood path at one point and serve as a conduit for entry into the vascular system; examples include solution administration sets, extension sets, transfer sets, and blood administration sets;
b. **Tissue/bone/dentin communicating:** devices and materials communicating with tissue, bone, and pulp/dentin system; examples include laparoscopes, arthroscopes, draining systems, dental cements, dental filling materials, and skin staples;
c. **Circulating blood:** devices that contact circulating blood; examples include intravascular catheters, temporary pacemaker electrodes, oxygenators, extracorporeal oxygenator tubing and accessories, dialyzers, dialysis tubing and accessories, haemoadsorbents, and immunoadsorbents.

5.1.4 Implant Devices

These include devices in contact with the following:

a. **Tissue/bone:** devices principally contacting bone; examples include orthopaedic pins, plates, replacement joints; bone prostheses, cements, and intraosseous devices. Devices principally contacting tissue and tissue fluid; examples include pacemakers, drug supply devices, neuromuscular sensors and stimulators, replacement tendons, breast implants, artificial larynxes, subperiosteal implants, and ligation clips;

b. **Blood:** devices principally contacting blood; examples include pacemaker electrodes, artificial arteriovenous fistulae, heart valves, vascular grafts, internal drug delivery catheters, and ventricular assist devices.

5.2 Categorization by Duration of Contact

Contact duration may be categorized as follows:

a. **Limited exposure (A):** devices whose single or multiple use or contact is likely to be up to 24 h;

b. **Prolonged exposure (B):** devices whose single, multiple (cumulative), or long-term use or contact is likely to exceed 24 h, but not 30 days;

c. **Permanent contact (C):** devices whose single, multiple (cumulative) or long-term use or contact exceeds 30 days.

If a material or device may be placed in more than one duration category, the more rigorous testing requirements should apply. With multiple exposures, the decision into which category a device is placed should take into account the potential cumulative effect, bearing in mind the period of time over which these exposures occur.

6 TESTING

6.1 General

In addition to the general principles laid down in clause 4, the following should be applied to biological testing of medical devices.

a. Testing should be performed on the final product, or representative samples from the final product or materials.

b. The choice of test procedures shall take into account:
   1. the nature, degree, duration, frequency, and conditions of exposure to or contact of humans to the device in the normal intended use;
   2. the chemical and physical nature of the final product;
   3. the toxicological activity of the chemicals in the formulation of the final product;
   4. that certain tests (e.g., those designed to assess systemic effects) may not be

applicable where the presence of leachable materials has been excluded, or where leachables have a known and acceptable toxicity profile;

5. the relationship of device surface area to recipient body size;
6. the existing information based on the literature, experience, and non-clinical tests;
7. the protection of humans is the primary goal of this document: a secondary goal is to ensure animal welfare to minimize the number and exposure of animals.

c. If extracts of the devices are prepared, the solvents and conditions of extraction used should be appropriate to the nature and use of the final product.
d. Positive and negative controls should be used where appropriate.
e. Test results cannot ensure freedom from potential biological hazard, thus biological investigations should be followed by careful observations for unexpected adverse reactions or events in humans during clinical use of the device.

Annex B provides a Bibliography of International Standards and Guidelines on biological response test methods.

6.2   Initial Evaluation Tests

The initial biological response tests that should be considered are as given in 6.2.1 to 6.2.9.

6.2.1   *Cytotoxicity*

With the use of cell culture techniques, these tests determine the lysis of cells (cell death), the inhibition of cell growth, and other effects on cells caused by devices, materials, and/or their extracts.

6.2.2   *Sensitization*

These tests estimate the potential for contact sensitization of devices, materials, and their extracts, using an appropriate model. These tests are appropriate because exposure or contact to even minute amounts of potential leachables can result in allergic or sensitization reactions.

6.2.3   *Irritation*

These tests estimate the irritation potential of devices, materials and their extracts, using appropriate site or implant tissue such as skin, eye, and mucous membrane in a suitable model. The test(s) performed should be appropriate for the route (skin, eye, mucosa) and duration of exposure or contact to determine irritant effects of devices, materials, and potential leachables.

6.2.4 *Intracutaneous Reactivity*

These tests assess the localized reaction of tissue to device extracts. These tests are applicable where determination of irritation by dermal or mucosal tests are inappropriate (e.g., devices having access to the blood path). These tests may also be useful where extractables are hydrophobic.

6.2.5 *Systemic Toxicity (Acute)*

These tests estimate the potential harmful effects of either single or multiple exposures, during a period of less than 24 h, to devices, materials, and/or their extracts in an animal model. These tests are appropriate where contact allows potential absorption of toxic leachables and degradation products.

Pyrogenicity tests are included to detect material-mediated pyrogenic reactions of extracts of devices or materials. No single test can differentiate pyrogenic reactions that are material-mediated from those due to endotoxin contamination.

6.2.6 *Sub-chronic Toxicity (Sub-acute Toxicity)*

These tests determine the effects of either single or multiple exposures or contact to devices, materials and/or their extracts during a period of not less than 24 h to a period not greater than 10% of the total life-span of the test animal (e.g., up to 90 days in rats). These tests may be waived for materials with chronic toxicity data. The reason for waiving of the tests should be included in the final report. These tests should be appropriate for the route and duration of contact.

6.2.7 *Genotoxicity*

These tests apply mammalian or non-mammalian cell culture or other techniques to determine gene mutations, changes in chromosome structure and number, and other DNA or gene toxicities caused by devices, materials, and/or their extracts.

6.2.8 *Implantation*

These tests assess the local pathological effects on living tissue, at both the gross level and microscopic level, of a sample of a material or final product that is surgically implanted or placed into an implant site or tissue appropriate to the intended application (e.g., special dental usage tests have been described). These tests should be appropriate for the route and duration of contact. For a material, these tests are equivalent to sub-chronic toxicity tests if systemic effects are also investigated.

6.2.9   Haemocompatibility

These tests evaluate effects on blood or blood components by blood-contacting devices, materials or using an appropriate model or system. Specific haemocompatibility tests may also be designed to simulate the geometry, contact conditions, and flow dynamics of the device or material during clinical applications.

Haemolysis tests determine the degree of red blood cell lysis and the release of haemoglobin caused by devices, materials, and/or their extracts *in vitro*.

6.3   Supplementary Evaluation Tests

The supplementary biological evaluation tests that should be considered are as given in 6.3.1 to 6.3.4.

6.3.1   Chronic Toxicity

These tests determine the effects of either single or multiple exposures to devices, materials, and/or their extracts during a period of at least 10% of the life-span of the test animal (e.g., over 90 days in rats). These tests should be appropriate for the route and duration of exposure or contact.

6.3.2   Carcinogenicity

These tests determine the tumorigenic potential of devices, materials, and/or their extracts from either a single or multiple exposures or contacts over a period of the total life-span of the test animal. These tests may be designed in order to examine both chronic toxicity and tumorigenicity in a single experimental study. Carcinogenicity tests should be conducted only if there are suggestive data from other sources. These tests should be appropriate for the route and duration of exposure or contact.

6.3.3   Reproductive and Developmental Toxicity

These tests evaluate the potential effects of devices, materials, and/or their extracts on reproductive function, embryonic development (teratogenicity), and prenatal and early postnatal development. Reproductive/developmental toxicity tests or bioassays should only be conducted when the device has potential impact on the reproductive potential of the subject. The application site of the device should be considered.

6.3.4   Biodegradation

Where the potential for resorption and/or degradation exists, such tests may determine the processes of absorption, distribution, biotransformation, and elimination of leachables and degradation products of devices, materials, and/or their extracts.

TABLE 1. *Guidance for initial evaluation tests*

Device categories			Biological effect							
Body contact (see 5.1)		Contact duration (see 5.2) A-limited ($\leq$ 24 h) B-prolonged (> 24 h to 30 days) C-permanent (> 30 days)	Cytotoxicity	Sensitization	Irritation or intracutaneous reactivity	Systemic toxicity (acute)	Sub-chronic toxicity (sub-acute toxicity)	Genotoxicity	Implantation	Haemocompatibility
Surface devices	Skin	A	X	X	X					
		B	X	X	X					
		C	X	X	X					
	Mucosal membranes	A	X	X	X					
		B	X	X	X					
		C	X	X	X		X	X		
	Breached or compromised surfaces	A	X	X	X					
		B	X	X	X					
		C	X	X	X		X	X		
External communicating devices	Blood path, indirect	A	X	X	X	X				X
		B	X	X	X	X				X
		C	X	X		X	X	X		X
	Tissue/bone/dentin communicating	A	X	X	X					
		B	X	X				X	X	
		C	X	X				X	X	
	Circulating blood	A	X	X	X	X				X
		B	X	X	X	X		X		X
		C	X	X	X	X	X	X		X
Implant devices	Tissue/bone	A	X	X	X					
		B	X	X				X	X	
		C	X	X				X	X	
	Blood	A	X	X	X	X			X	X
		B	X	X	X	X		X	X	X
		C	X	X	X	X	X	X	X	X

Note: Each device shall be considered on its own merits.

TABLE 2. *Guidance for supplementary evaluation tests*

Device categories		Biological test				
Body contact (see 5.1)		Contact duration (see 5.2) A-limited (≤ 24 h) B-prolonged (> 24 h to 30 days) C-permanent (> 30 days)	Chronic toxicity	Carcinogenicity	Reproductive/developmental	Biodegradation
Surface devices	Skin	A				
		B				
		C				
	Mucosal membranes	A				
		B				
		C				
	Breached or compromised surfaces	A				
		B				
		C				
External communicating devices	Blood path, indirect	A				
		B				
		C	X	X		
	Tissue/bone/ dentin communicating	A				
		B				
		C		X		
	Circulating blood	A				
		B				
		C	X	X		
Implant devices	Tissue/bone	A				
		B				
		C	X	X		
	Blood	A				
		B				
		C	X	X		

Note: Each device shall be considered on its own merits.

7 GUIDANCE ON SELECTION OF BIOLOGICAL EVALUATION TESTS

Table 1 identifies the initial evaluation tests that shall be considered for each device and duration category. Table 2 identifies the supplementary evaluation tests that shall be considered for each device and duration category.

Due to the diversity of medical devices, it is recognized that not all tests identified in a category will be necessary or practical for any given device. It is indispensable for testing that each device shall be considered on its own merits: additional tests not indicated in the table may be necessary.

It is strongly recommended that the rationale for selection and/or waiving of tests be recorded.

8 ASSURANCE OF TEST METHODS

8.1 Test Method Assurance

The test methods used in the biological evaluation shall be sensitive, precise, and accurate. The test results should be reproducible (interlaboratory) as well as repeatable (intralaboratory).

8.2 Continued Assurance

The assurance that a material is initially acceptable for its intended use in a product, and its continued acceptability in the long term, is an aspect of a quality system. (See A.2, subclause 8.2.)

ISO 9001:1987, clause 4 specifies the requirements for such quality assurance systems. ISO 9004 provides more detailed guidance for designing and manufacturing products.

ANNEX B
(informative)

Bibliography of International and National Standards and Regulations

NOTE 4 Titles of all standards and regulations in this bibliography are given in English: this should not, however, be taken to imply that the documents are necessarily available in this language.

B.1 International Organization for Standardization (ISO)

[1] ISO/TR 9966:1989, *Implants for surgery—Biocompatibility—Selection of biological test methods for materials and devices.*

[2] ISO/TR 7405:1984, *Biological evaluation of dental materials.*

[3] ISO 9000:1987, *Quality management and quality assurance standards—Guidelines for selection and use.*

[4] ISO 9001:1987, *Quality systems—Model for quality assurance in design/development, production, installation, and servicing.*

[5] ISO 9004:1987, *Quality management and quality system elements—Guidelines.*

B.2　The Joint European Standards Institution (CEN/CENELEC)

[6] EN 29 001:1989, *Quality systems—Model for quality assurance in design, development, production, installation, and servicing.*

[7] EN 46 001:1990, *Specific requirements for the application of* EN 29 001 *for medical devices.*

B.3　Canada

[8] CAN 3 Z 310.6M 84, *Biocompatibility testing.*

B.4　France

[9] AFNOR S 90-700, *Medico-surgical equipment—Choice of tests enabling assessment of biocompatibility of medical materials and devices.*

[10] AFNOR NF 90-701, *Medico-surgical equipment—Biocompatibility of medical materials and devices; Extraction methods.*

[11] AFNOR NF S 90-702, *Medico-surgical equipment—Evaluation* in vitro *of cytotoxicity of medical materials and devices.*

B.5　Germany

[12] DIN V 13 930-09 90, *Dentistry; Biological testing of dental materials.*

B.6　Italy

[13] UNI 9582-1, *Biocompatibility of medical materials and devices—Part 1: Terminology, samples preparation and test choice.*

[14] UNI 9582-2, *Biocompatibility of medical materials and devices—Part 2: Cytotoxicity.*

[15] UNI 9582-3, *Biocompatibility of medical materials and devices—Part 3: Bone implant test.*

[16] UNI 9582-4, *Biocompatibility of medical materials and devices—Part 4: Pyrogen test.*

[17] UNI 9582-5, *Biocompatibility of medical materials and devices—Part 5: Oral mucoses membrane irritation.*

[18] UNI 9582-6, *Biocompatibility of medical materials and devices—Part 6: Mutagenicity (Ames' Assay).*

[19] UNI 9582-7, *Biocompatibility of medical materials and devices—Part 7: Systemic toxicity.*

B.7   Switzerland

[20] SN 119809-1990, *Biological evaluation of dental materials.*

B.8   Tripartite Agreement (United Kingdom, Canada, United States)

[21] *Biocompatibility guidance for medical devices.*

B.9   United Kingdom

[22] BS 5736-1:1989, *Evaluation of medical devices for biological hazards—Part 1: Guide for the selection of biological methods of test.*

[23] BS 5736-2:1990, *Evaluation of medical devices for biological hazards—Part 2: Method of testing by tissue implantation.*

[24] BS 5736-3:1981, *Evaluation of medical devices for biological hazards—Part 3: Method of test for systemic toxicity; assessment of acute toxicity of extracts from medical devices.*

[25] BS 5736-4:1981, *Evaluation of medical devices for biological hazards—Part 4: Method of test for intracutaneous reactivity of extracts from medical devices.*

[26] BS 5736-5:1982, *Evaluation of medical devices for biological hazards—Part 5: Method of test for systemic toxicity; assessment of pyrogenicity in rabbits of extracts from medical devices.*

[27] BS 5736-6:1983, *Evaluation of medical devices for biological hazards—Part 6: Methods of test for sensitization; assessment of the potential of medical devices to produce delayed contact dermatitis.*

[28] BS 5736-7:1983, *Evaluation of medical devices for biological hazards—Part 7: Method of test for skin irritation of extracts from medical devices.*

[29] BS 5736-8:1984, *Evaluation of medical devices for biological hazards—Part 8: Method of test for skin irritation of solid medical devices.*

[30] BS 5736-9:1986, *Evaluation of medical devices for biological hazards—Part 9: Method of test for eye irritation.*

[31] BS 5736-10:1988, *Evaluation of medical devices for biological hazards—Part 10: Method of test for toxicity to cells in culture of extracts from medical devices.*

[32] BS 5736-11:1990, *Evaluation of medical devices for biological hazards—Part 11: Method of test for haemolysis.*

[33] BS 5828:1989, *Methods of biological assessment of dental materials.*

[34] BS 7254-4:1990, *Orthopaedic implants—Part 4: Recommendations for retrieval and examination of implants and associated tissues.*

B.10   United States

[35] ANSI/ADA 41-1979, *Biological evaluation of dental materials.*

[36] ASTM F-748-87, *Practice for selecting generic biological test methods for materials and devices.*

[37] ASTM F-981-87, *Practice for assessment of compatibility of biomaterials (non-porous) for surgical implants with respect to effect of materials on muscle and bone.*

[38] ASTM F-720-81(1986), *Practice for testing guinea pigs for contact allergens: Guinea pig maximization test.*

[39] ASTM F-750-87, *Practice for evaluating material extracts by systemic injection in the mouse.*

[40] ASTM F-813-83(1988), *Practice for direct contact cell culture evaluation of materials for medical devices.*

[41] ASTM F-895-84, *Test method for agar diffusion cell culture screening for cytotoxicity.*

[42] ASTM F-763-87, *Practice for short-term screening of implant materials ASTM E-1262: Standard Guide for Performance of the Chinese Hamster Ovary Cell/ Hypoxanthine Guanine Phosphoribosyl Transferase Gene Mutation Assay.*

[43] ASTM E-1280, *Standard Guide for Performing the Mouse Lymphoma Assay for Mammalian Cell Mutagenicity.*

[44] ASTM F-619, *Standard Practice for Extraction of Medical Plastics.*

[45] ASTM F-719, *Standard Practice for Testing Biomaterials in Rabbits for Primary Skin Irritation.*

[46] ASTM F-749, *Standard Practice for Evaluating Material Extracts by Intracutaneous Injection in the Rabbit.*

[47] ASTM F-756, *Standard Practice for Assessment of the Hemolytic Properties of Materials.*

[48] ASTM F-1027, *Standard Practice for Assessment of Tissue and Cell Compatibility of Orofacial Prosthetic Materials and Devices.*

[49] USP 1987, *Biological Reactivity Tests,* In-Vitro.

[50] USP 1988, *Biological Reactivity Tests,* In-Vivo.

[51] USP, XXII, 1990, *U.S. Pharmacopeia National Formulary.*

B.11   Organization for Economic Co-operation and Development (OECD)

[52] *Guidelines for testing of chemicals—Section 4: Health effects.*

*Biological, Material, and Mechanical
Considerations of Joint Replacement,*
edited by B. F. Morrey.
Raven Press, Ltd., New York, 1993.

32

Federal Support for Research on Joint Replacements

Stephen L. Gordon

*Musculoskeletal Diseases Branch, National Institute of Arthritis and Musculoskeletal
and Skin Diseases, National Institutes of Health, Bethesda, Maryland 20814*

The National Institutes of Health (NIH) and other federal agencies support a large number of basic, applied, and clinical projects that are specifically targeted toward prosthetic joint replacements. In addition there is a broad range of basic science research in related areas that receives substantial federal support. For example, basic bone biology investigations have led to the discovery of many local growth and regulatory factors that control bone remodeling. In some cases these agents are now being considered as a means to enhance the growth of bone into porous implants. Therefore, the total federal support for joint replacement research is only partially reflected by the specific grant activities described below.

NIH RESEARCH SUPPORT

The Musculoskeletal Diseases Branch of the National Institute of Arthritis and Musculoskeletal and Skin Diseases (NIAMS) is the focal point for joint replacement research within the NIH. Grant support utilizes several mechanisms, which include regular research grant, first independent research support and transition (FIRST) awards, career development awards, individual projects within center grants, training grants, and small business grants. The spectrum of projects covers biomaterials, biomechanics, and biology of the device and bone-device interface. Table 1 presents examples of individual research projects supported by NIAMS.

In fiscal year 1991, NIAMS expended over $5 million in projects related to joint replacements. As indicated above, there is a much larger base of support for fundamental projects on bone biology and bone healing that may lead the way for future projects applied to joint replacements.

There is a surprisingly diverse source of research support for projects from other components of the NIH that are directed toward improving the outcome of prosthetic joint surgery. Examples of these other funding sources were identified from the NIH Division of Research Grants computer database. There may be additional related research projects that were not determined from the computer search. Table 2 identifies some specific projects funded by other components of the NIH.

TABLE 1. *Examples of NIAMS supported research areas*

Biological/clinical
  Biochemical and cellular response to biomaterials
  Bacterial colonization of orthopaedic biomaterials
  Bone ingrowth/remodeling in cementless knee replacement
  Patient education in total joint arthroplasty
  Bone mass in hip replacements
  Experimental models for joint replacement
  Robotic surgical assist device
Biomaterials
  In vitro and *in vivo* corrosion of orthopaedic implants
  Degradation of polyethylene joint components
  Calcium phosphate coatings for joint prostheses
  Fabrication of high-performance prostheses
  Mechanisms of ion release from titanium
  Surface failure in ultrahigh molecular weight polyethylene joint components
  Fracture mechanics in design of joint replacements
Biomechanics
  Gait analysis of total knee replacement
  Systemic implications of total joint replacements
  In vivo measure of hip forces
  Bone-cement interface biomechanics

OTHER FEDERAL RESEARCH SUPPORT

The Department of Veterans Affairs (VA) supports a large basic science program in biomaterials and biomechanics research on joint replacements. Projects are supported on a competitive basis through collaborations with investigators from VA Medical Centers. Examples of supported projects include pulsed laser hydroxyapatite coatings, all plastic knee replacement, quantitative stress/strain analysis, wear debris assessment, and high viscosity bone cements.

The National Institute for Disability and Rehabilitation Research (NIDRR) supports research on joint replacements at one of its Rehabilitation Engineering Centers and through individual projects under the Field Investigator Initiative Research Program. Examples of supported projects at NIDRR include assessment of clinical and surgical approaches, surface properties and biological adherence, new device materials, and postsurgical rehabilitation.

The Agency for Health Care Policy and Research has two large projects to determine patient management approaches and outcomes in (i) total knee joint replacements and (ii) total hip joint replacements. These are part of the recently initiated

TABLE 2. *Examples of NIH (excluding NIAMS) supported research areas*

Modular joint replacement device after tumor resection
Predictors of recovery from hip fracture and joint replacement
Thrombosis prevention in surgical joint replacement
Neuropsychological disorders in elderly with joint replacement
Psychological and coping factors affecting total joint replacement recovery
Prophylactic use of Foley catheter in total joint replacement
Knee replacement and transcutaneous electrical nerve stimulation therapy
Patient-controlled analgesia in total joint replacement
Clinical study of joint exercise prior to total joint replacement

Patient Outcome Research Team projects to determine the results of various treatment approaches and their cost effectiveness for several major surgical procedures and disease conditions. The objective is to guide practitioners in the selection of appropriate and effective care and to best utilize health care resources.

IMPACT AND FUTURE DIRECTIONS

Support from federal sources is only a component of the total funding for basic, applied, and clinical studies in joint replacement. Many important journal articles on outcome studies for various procedures or devices are supported through clinical department funds. Industry provides substantial funding both to university-based investigators and to in-house scientists. Finally, there are several foundations (e.g., Whitaker Foundation and Orthopaedic Research and Education Foundation) that support research studies and the development of academic orthopaedic research careers. The composite research portfolio of federal, private, and industrial support has resulted in continual advances and new approaches to joint replacement. In one example of collaborative funding, the NIAMS provided Phase I and II support under the Small Business Innovative Research Award to develop an ion coating for titanium joint replacement surfaces. The development of this improved wear and friction coating was completed with Phase III industrial support. This materials manufacturing process is now used in most titanium joint replacements.

Joint replacements successfully offer patients dramatic relief from pain and disability from diseased and/or injured joints. Although the newer concepts await the test of time in clinical trials and patient outcome studies, there is hope for improved long-term results.

This volume is an outstanding resource for investigators seeking to obtain funding for research. The state of knowledge, gaps in current understanding, and opportunities for future investigations are clearly identified. The NIAMS continues to have a strong programmatic interest in projects related to prosthetic joint replacement. Highly meritorious grant applications will be funded within the total available resources appropriated by Congress. Potential applicants are encouraged to contact the Chief, Musculoskeletal Diseases Branch for specific advice regarding their proposed project.

*Biological, Material, and Mechanical
Considerations of Joint Replacement,*
edited by B. F. Morrey.
Raven Press, Ltd., New York, 1993.

33

Regulation of Biomaterials and Medical Devices

Donald E. Marlowe

*Center for Devices and Radiological Health, U.S. Food and Drug Administration,
Rockville, Maryland 20852*

This topic will be discussed in the context of the U.S. Food and Drug Administration's (FDA) Center for Devices and Radiological Health as a whole and the present and future in terms of regulation of and research in biomaterials. In that context, the Safe Medical Devices Act (SMDA) of 1990 will be reviewed and the FDA's goals and activities in the international arena as they affect our responsibilities in this area will be briefly discussed.

THE PRESENT

On May 28, 1976, President Gerald R. Ford signed into law the Medical Device Amendments to the Federal Food, Drug, and Cosmetic Act (3). The purpose of the Amendments is to ensure that medical devices are safe and effective and properly labeled for their intended use. To accomplish this mandate, the amendments provide the FDA with the authority to regulate devices during most phases of their development, testing, production, distribution, and use. The FDA's approach to this regulation focuses heavily on both the pre- and postmarket phases of a product's lifetime. During the premarket phase, the FDA concentrates on providing a reasonable assurance that new products are adequately evaluated for safety and effectiveness. Implicit in this assessment is the concept of risk to benefit. If the benefits significantly outweigh the risks for the intended application, the product would most likely be approved for marketing in the United States. Since risk/benefit assessments for new technology involve considerable clinical judgment, the FDA consults with expert panels composed of clinicians, engineers, toxicologists, and other experts familiar with the devices to make these assessments. These panels review the data provided by the manufacturer to support the claims for product safety and effectiveness. If the advisory panel believes the data support the manufacturer's claims, an approval for marketing recommendation is made to FDA.

Once a product has been approved for use in the United States, the FDA's role shifts to the postmarket monitoring of product performance and manufacturing practices. This activity ensures that the product design, which was approved during the premarket phase, is in fact the product that is manufactured and sold. To do this, the

FDA periodically inspects the medical device manufacturers to ensure compliance with Good Manufacturing Practices (GMPs) (4). Further, the FDA evaluates failures reported under a variety of systems to determine whether appropriate actions have been taken by the manufacturer to reduce the risk to the users.

Note that the above discussion has focused on medical devices, not biomaterials. The regulation of biomaterials is an often-confused area for developers of new medical devices. Many believe that the FDA regulates all materials used in medical devices, in addition to regulating the device itself. Hence, the FDA is regularly confronted with the following types of questions: (a) How does a biomaterial get approved by the FDA? (b) How does one get a list of the approved materials for use in medical devices?

The answers to these questions depend entirely on the intended application of the materials. The FDA regulates the end product (medical device), not the materials from which it is made. The FDA does not approve biomaterials. Therefore, the FDA does not maintain a list of approved biomaterials nor does it provide guidance on how to get a biomaterial approved for general application. There are, however, instances in which a biomaterial is the end product, e.g., polymethylmethacrylate bone cement, block silicone, injectable collagen. In these cases, the claims made for the material by the manufacturer are for specific applications and the manufacturer has provided adequate *in vitro* and *in vivo* testing to demonstrate the safety and efficacy for those applications.

The FDA does, however, provide premarket evaluation guidance for a wide variety of medical devices (2). Although this guidance does, in some instances, address materials considerations, it is fundamentally directed at demonstrating safety and effectiveness of specific devices.

Since the FDA does not evaluate or approve device materials per se, but does approve devices in regard to their safety and effectiveness, a safe biological response to the material is obviously an important aspect of the review process. In 1986, the FDA, Health and Welfare of Canada, and Department of Health and Social Services of the United Kingdom issued the "Tripartite Biocompatibility Guidance for Medical Devices" (6). This guidance has been used by FDA reviewers (7), as well as manufacturers of medical devices, in evaluating the toxicological effects of the device. Recently the International Standards Organization developed a standard, "Biological Testing of Medical and Dental Materials and Devices—Part 1: Guidance on Selection of Tests" (ISO 10993-1) (1), which uses an approach similar to that of the "Tripartite Biocompatibility Guidance."

THE FUTURE

Reevaluating "Old" Products

One area of immediate concern to the agency is the safety and effectiveness of products that have been on the market for some time. A recent article in the *New York Times* portrayed this program as a "crackdown" on pre-Amendments devices and listed a number of devices as imminent candidates for premarket approval (PMA) submissions. While this is an important program for FDA, the word "crackdown" overstates the reality a bit.

Let us put this into perspective. Yes, we are concerned about the safety and effectiveness of "old" products on the market. By "old" is meant products that were on the market before 1976 and also products that were brought to market soon after the Device Amendments were enacted. The idea is to identify those products that have a weak safety foundation and then use the appropriate mechanisms to reduce or eliminate unacceptable risks to the patient. We expect to focus our efforts on implants, or on devices in which malfunctions could be life-threatening.

Internally, we have been using the acronym RAISE, (Re-Assessment of Information on Safety and Effectiveness) to describe this program, but it is actually just a part of our overall strategy for monitoring and reevaluating products currently on the market. The Safe Medical Devices Act recognizes the need to look back at already-marketed devices and gives us several tools for gaining additional information about them. We will use these new postmarket tools, plus the information tools we had before, such as Mandatory Device Reporting, recalls, inspections for GMPs, and reviews of the scientific literature.

For a long time, we have been using this information to set priorities on which devices should be required to have PMAs, and in which order. In 1983, we published a list of 13 pre-Amendments devices that we planned to require to have PMAs. We have called for PMAs for seven of these and are considering reclassification of two others. In January 1989, we published a similar list of 31 more devices. Silicone gel-filled breast implants were on that list.

As we reevaluate marketed products, we are likely to find that requiring PMAs is not the only solution to the problems we might find. For example, user education, better performance standards, or improved labeling may resolve problems with a device that stem from user error rather than·device materials, design, or manufacturing.

Still, calling for PMAs for grandfathered products will be an integral part of our program. In the coming year or so, we are expecting to call for PMAs for five products. These products are

1. Saline-filled breast implants
2. Testicular implants
3. Penile implants
4. Cardiovascular bypass devices
5. Cranial electrotherapy stimulators.

As an aside, it should be noted that our experience with the PMAs for silicone gel-filled breast implants can serve as an example for the future. Any company making an important device that was "grandfathered" under the 1976 Medical Device Amendments that may pose a significant risk can anticipate that we are going to be calling for PMAs on that product.

If there is anything to be learned from the silicone breast implant situation, perhaps it is this: companies should be collecting the relevant data before the FDA asks for it. This cannot be stressed strongly enough. This is especially true when safety could be an issue and the product has not been adequately tested. The safety of an old device is not established simply because it has been in existence for a long time. The current uncertainty about the safety of silicone breast implants is the result of PMAs that were submitted with inadequate data.

For the companies, the results of submitting inadequate PMAs have been terrible, including tarnished reputations, and, for some firms, eventual closing. For the Center, it has been a difficult and labor-intensive project, one that is still time and energy consuming. Again, it must be emphasized strongly that manufacturers must do their part to prevent such a situation from ever occurring again.

SMDA Provisions for Pre-1976 Class III Devices

Under the 1976 Amendments, the FDA is supposed to call for safety and effectiveness data for each class III device that was on the market before the Amendments were enacted.

This still holds true, but the SMDA sets both a deadline (December 1, 1995) and procedures for reclassifying appropriate devices and setting a schedule for calling for PMAs for the remaining 130 or so types of pre-Amendments class III devices. First, the FDA is to publish a notice for companies to submit a summary of information on their devices including sources of the data and any outstanding reports on device problems. Second, we must develop a proposed regulation for each device, either keeping it in class III or reclassifying it. Third is a final regulation on the status of each pre-Amendments' class III product. Finally, within a year of any regulation keeping a product in class III, the FDA is to issue a schedule for requiring a PMA for that product.

Trust—But Verify

Of course, it is not sufficient to simply obtain data. Their accuracy must be confirmed.

The FDA has had some earlier problems with data fraud, although not in the area of devices. Still, it is an important concern for us. In the future, the Center will be focusing more on the accuracy of the data submitted to us.

We are increasing our attention to bioresearch monitoring, focusing on the truth of the information supporting product approvals—so-called "trust but verify." As part of this effort, we will also be looking more closely at industry's promotion of investigational products.

Risk Assessment

An important focus on the Center's future activities is risk assessment. There is a great need in the device area to weigh a product's risks against its benefits. In some cases the calculation is straightforward. For a heart valve, the morbidity and mortality from the untreated disease with the morbidity and mortality using the valve are compared. For many other devices, the equation is less clear. How do we measure the benefits of a breast implant? How do we measure the risks of a material like silicone gel or oil, when its basic toxicology and pharmacokinetics are still uncertain. Straightforward or not, the process is difficult.

Mention should be made of some concern with the societal messages associated with risk assessment. Unfortunately, many people have been led to believe that no amount of risk from a medical product is acceptable and that our job in government is to guarantee that the products we regulate are absolutely safe. That view is unrealistic, of course, and it greatly hampers our ability to communicate effectively with people about a host of risk-benefit issues.

We must all work together to change this situation. We must educate the public to understand that some risks may be acceptable, whereas others are not, and help them to judge which are which. In this complex world, and particularly in the area of medical devices, "scientific literacy" is essential to gain an understanding of important health issues. If we can help the public to better recognize the risks of daily living and to be able to compare those risks with the risks of certain medical devices, we will have made an important contribution to the scientific literacy of our society. It may be the most important contribution we can make in the months and years to come.

Biomaterials Research and Compendium

Biomaterials is an important issue for the Center and for the device industry. We do not know enough about many of the materials used to make medical devices, their chemical makeup, how the body reacts to them, and how the materials themselves react to the body. Implanted devices are of particular concern. Silicone gel in breast implants is an obvious example, but the problem of latex allergy is a good example of how devices that are not implanted can have unexpected effects too.

We would like to see the Center provide some leadership in the area of biomaterials research. We are already working on certain biomaterials questions, but this is a broad area of research and we must divide our research staff and resources between many device-related issues. Obviously this is a task that requires the cooperative effort of industry, academia, and many government agencies and funding from many sources. We have described the research needs in this area in the *Research Agenda for the 90s*. This document has been circulated widely.

One exciting project on the horizon is a new program that will set up a systematic way to retrieve and study explanted devices on a national level. We plan to work with university medical centers, professional societies, and standards organizations to establish research protocols and a uniform database for collecting, storing, and analyzing information about the fate of implanted devices in the body. This kind of information, if widely disseminated and shared, can be very valuable to both the FDA and the industry. We hope to develop this project further by the end of this fiscal year.

In a second project, we envision an effort in which we all work together and pool our results to develop a compendium of knowledge about the performance and potential risks of specific biomaterials in specific environments, a biomaterials database. Such a compendium could be a resource for both manufacturers and government, particularly to streamline product approval. Conceptually, this compendium could be compared with the drug master file used by drug manufacturers to develop "me-too" pharmaceuticals with a minimum of testing.

For example, if a new product were manufactured from a certain formulation of a material listed in the compendium, we might not require preclinical testing. In essence, it would already be done. It is even possible that, eventually, such a biomaterials compendium could be one element of internationally harmonized procedures for premarket approval.

SMDA—A General Overview

After 14 years of experience with the Federal Food, Drug, and Cosmetic Act, Medical Device Amendments of 1976, a number of limitations in the regulation were identified. Most notable of these with regard to biomaterials is the difficulty in predicting long-term performance of certain devices (implants) from *in vitro,* animal, and limited human studies. To address this, in 1990, Congress modified the Act (5) in ways that will change several aspects of the approval of devices fabricated from new materials. Among the changes are provisions that require the manufacturer to establish systems for tracking certain devices and selected implants, provisions requiring studies of device performance after the device has been approved and distribution has begun, and provisions requiring health care facilities to report all mortality and several types of morbidity associated with device problems to the FDA.

For selected permanent implant devices and life-sustaining devices used in the home, the new tracking provisions require that the device manufacturer establish a system by which the devices can be located at any time, even down to the user level. This tracking system must be able to locate devices in a relatively short time and remain in place for the useful lifetime of the device. The intention of these provisions is to facilitate product recall and patient notification when problems have been identified.

The Postmarket Surveillance Study provisions of the Act are probably the most far reaching and immediate for devices manufactured from new materials. Two types of studies are outlined in the new law: mandatory and discretionary. Manufacturers of permanent implant devices and life-sustaining and life-supporting devices that are brought to market after January 1, 1991 are required by law to conduct postmarket studies of the performance characteristics of their products. In addition, the FDA has the discretion to require the manufacturer of any device to initiate such a study of the device's performance, regardless of when the device was first marketed or classified. Congress' intention for these studies is expansion of the information available on the performance of the device over a larger population and for a longer period of time beyond that gathered during the premarket testing. The FDA will likely define the aspects of the device that are to be studied, e.g., specific populations may be targeted for study as high risk with the use of a new material, the qualifications of the principal investigator, and the characteristics of an acceptable study. The study protocol and qualifications of the principal investigator require FDA approval prior to initiation of the study. When a medical device fails in service and causes death, the health care facility is required to report that information to the FDA and the manufacturer. When the failure results in a serious injury, this information must be reported to the manufacturer. This user reporting provision is an extension of the existing mandatory device reporting regulation that required manufacturers to report death and serious injury information. It is possible to envision an information system linking these three provisions. User reporting provides information of the experience of users with the device in service. Device tracking is able to locate devices having similar problem characteristics. Postmarket surveillance studies would be initiated to explore the long-term behavior of the new materials in the actual service environment.

All the mandatory regulations have been drafted and, if not yet published, are somewhere in the review process from the FDA, at the agency level, through the

Public Health Service, the Department of Health and Human Services, and, finally, the Office of Management and Budget.

What does this new law mean to the industry? In the most basic sense, it shifts the emphasis of our regulatory programs from premarket review to postmarket surveillance. However, this shift is actually a trade-off. An important feature of SMDA is that it codifies our 510(k) procedures into law.

Although industry was comfortable with how we handled the 510(k) program, Congress definitely was not, and the program was vulnerable to court challenge. Whereas Congress grew to accept and institutionalize the Center's 510(k) procedures, it also increased the postmarket surveillance and enforcement side of the law. In the long run, it is a fair trade.

INTERNATIONAL ACTIVITIES

We have heard much recently about international trade issues and the nation's problems with the trade deficit. The medical device industry is one area in which the United States has a trade surplus. The SMDA recognizes the importance of international trade and fostering international relations. We have already been involved in international activities for some time.

We have two basic goals in the international area. First, to harmonize our GMP regulations with those of other nations. As a step in that direction, we will make sure that our revised GMP regulations are consistent with international requirements, as long as the changes do not lessen our product requirements here at home. Specifically, the new regulations will incorporate the provisions of ISO 9001. We have a working agreement on GMPs with the United Kingdom, under which we recognize their GMP inspections of device manufacturers as equal to our own and vice versa. This obviates the need for the FDA to conduct GMP inspections in the United Kingdom or for the United Kingdom to inspect device manufacturers here. We also have preliminary discussions underway for similar agreements with Switzerland, Australia, Malaysia, Japan, and the European Community.

Our second major goal in this area is to harmonize the product evaluation process as much as possible. Progress has also been made here. For example, as noted previously, we have an agreement with the United Kingdom and Canada on test protocols to establish many aspects of device material biosafety. Last fall in Brussels, we cosponsored with the European Community and Canada the first international workshop on the harmonization of nomenclature for health care products.

Finally, on the issue of voluntary standards for medical devices, we have had a long history of commitment and direct involvement in the voluntary standards-setting process. We believe they are a viable alternative to the expense and time required to promulgate mandatory standards, such as those developed under the Radiation Control for Health and Safety Act. We have worked for years helping to set standards both in the United States and internationally, and we plan to continue that commitment. In fact, strong voluntary standards should go a long way toward harmonizing regulations. Perhaps we can expect equal commitments from the device industry and surgeons. We must all work together to establish voluntary standards.

CONCLUSION

Several important aspects in the approval of devices manufactured from new biomaterials have been discussed. We recognize all too well that the medical device industry is an immensely important part of our nation's health care and economy, in many cases at the cutting edge of technology. The Center for Devices and Radiological Health is committed to working with industry and the medical community to ensure that innovative and life-saving devices reach the patient as soon as possible and that all products on the market are both safe and effective.

REFERENCES

1. Biological testing of medical and dental materials and devices, part 1: Guidance on selection of tests. ISO International Standard 10993-1.
2. FDA Guidance Documents. Guidance documents for assessing new medical device safety and effectiveness can be obtained from an FDA operated electronic bulletin board in Rockville, Maryland. The EBBS operates 24 hours per day and can be accessed by modem on (301) 443-7496.
3. Medical Device Amendments of 1976. Federal Food, Drug and Cosmetic Act as amended and related laws. Washington, DC: U.S. Government Printing Office, 1990:0-248–576 QL3.
4. Regulations establishing good manufacturing practices for the manufacture, packing, storage, and installation of medical devices. Federal Register (43 FR 31508) July 21, 1978.
5. Safe Medical Devices Act of 1990. Conference report. 101st Congress, 2nd session. House of Representatives report 101-959 (1990).
6. Toxicology Subgroup Tripartite Subcommittee on Medical Devices. Tripartite Biocompatibility guidance for medical devices. Washington, DC: U.S. Department of Health and Human Services, 1986.
7. West D-L. *Coll Toxicol* 1988;7:499.

Biological, Material, and Mechanical Considerations of Joint Replacement, edited by B. F. Morrey. Raven Press, Ltd., New York, 1993.

34

Regulatory Perspective for Orthopedic Devices

Mark N. Melkerson, Martin A. Yahiro, and Nirmal K. Mishra

Orthopedic Branch, Division of General and Restorative Devices, Office of Device Evaluation, Center for Devices and Radiological Health, U.S. Food and Drug Administration, Rockville, Maryland 20850

Orthopedic surgery, by its very nature, is a device-dependent specialty. As orthopedic surgeons, researchers, manufacturers, and consumers, we often equate advances in technology with medical progress. Over the past 40 years, developments in electronics, polymers, ceramics, composites, metallurgy, and fiberoptics have greatly contributed to a surgeon's ability to diagnose and treat orthopedic conditions. Surgeons and the public now have available to them a wide array of devices that are reliable, safe, and effective. It is only natural that surgeons have come to expect modern science to produce safe and effective devices. In spite of their dependence on these devices, surgeons are unaware of how vulnerable they are to device-related problems.

Although surgeons derive much of their device information from the orthopedic literature and scientific meetings, they may make crucial decisions regarding the choice of implants by relying on information from advertising claims, sales pitches, anecdotal reports, and premature reports of early clinical findings. Most orthopedic surgeons assume that all of this information is correct. Many believe that all commercially available devices have been thoroughly tested by the U.S. Food and Drug Administration (FDA) and have undergone clinical trials to demonstrate their utility and safety. In fact, many assume that all devices that are commercially available are "FDA approved." In reality, the FDA infrequently tests medical devices for market clearance, and there are very few orthopedic devices that have actually completed FDA's Premarket Approval (PMA) process. Despite these misconceptions, it is important for orthopedists to know that they can have confidence in the devices they use and on what this confidence is based. By understanding how the devices come to be marketed, how they are regulated, what nonclinical and clinical testing information is supplied in support of device submissions, and to what degree the information available about them can be relied on, the orthopedist will be better equipped to make important decisions regarding safety and efficacy issues.

This chapter is solely the authors' own perspectives of the U.S. Food and Drug Administration and its role in the regulation of orthopedic medical devices. It does not constitute an official FDA position or opinion for medical devices, is not binding on the FDA, and is not meant to be representative of any legal or regulatory policy and should not be used as such.

BACKGROUND

The FDA is one of the nation's oldest consumer protection agencies. Its approximately 8,900 employees regulate and monitor the manufacture, import, transport, storage, and sale of $570 billion worth of products annually. It does cost the taxpayer approximately $2 per person per year. Enforcing the laws enacted by the U.S. Congress and the regulations promulgated by the Agency to protect the public health and safety is a difficult, sometimes impossible, task, but one that the FDA has been legally mandated to fulfill. To carry out its mission the FDA employs approximately 2,100 scientists and clinicians from a variety of backgrounds, including engineering, material science, toxicology, pathology, statistics, and medicine, as well as 1,100 investigators and inspectors across the country. The Orthopedic Devices Branch and the Restorative Devices Branch of the Office of Device Evaluation are the components of the FDA's Center for Devices and Radiological Health that are responsible for the scientific review of all orthopedic devices submitted for evaluation. These evaluations are required by law for almost all medical devices intended for release into interstate commercial distribution or for clinical investigation.

The laws by which the FDA regulates are the Federal Food, Drug, and Cosmetic (FD&C) Act, Fair Packaging and Labeling Act, Sections of the Public Health Service Act relating to biological products for human use and control of communicable diseases, Radiation Control for Health and Safety Act, Medical Device Amendments of 1976 (MD Amendments), and Safe Medical Devices Act of 1990 (SMDA) (Table 1). The FD&C Act is the basic food and drug law for the United States. With its numerous amendments it is the most extensive law of its kind in the world. These laws are intended to assure the consumer that foods are pure and wholesome, safe to eat, and produced under sanitary conditions; that drugs and devices are safe and effective for their intended uses; that cosmetics are safe and made from appropriate ingredients; and that all labeling and packaging is truthful, informative, and not deceptive.

The MD Amendments charge the FDA with the responsibility of assuring that medical devices are safe, effective, and properly labeled for their intended use. To accomplish this, the MD Amendments, enacted May 28, 1976, provide the FDA the authority to regulate devices during most phases of their development, testing, production, distribution, and use. The MD Amendments provide a broad definition of the term medical device (Table 2). The MD Amendments also give the FDA author-

---

TABLE 1. *History of medical device evaluation*

1906 Pure Food and Drug Act
  Created the early FDA
  No device regulations
1938 Federal Food, Drug, and Cosmetic Act
  Regulated misbranded and adulterated devices only
1976 Medical Device Amendments
  The first legislation providing for comprehensive regulation of devices
1990 Safe Medical Devices Amendments
  Extend definitions and powers
1992 Medical Device Amendments of 1992
  Outline postmarket surveillance, device trading and device reporting requirements and revises
    device repair, replacement, and refund regulations

TABLE 2. *Medical device definition*

Definition: Medical device is defined as "any instrument, apparatus, implement, machine, contrivance, implant, *in vitro* reagent, or other similar or related article, including any component, part, or accessory, which is:
- recognized in the official National Formulary, or the United States Pharmacopeia, or any supplement to them;
- intended for use in the diagnosis of disease or other conditions, or in the cure, mitigation, treatment, or prevention of disease, in man or other animals; or
- intended to affect the structure or any function of the body of man or other animals; and
- does not achieve any of its principal intended purposes through chemical action within or on the body of man or other animals and which is not dependent upon being metabolized for the achievement of any of its principal intended purposes."

From the Medical Device Amendments of 1976.

ity to classify devices and to require PMA of devices, registration and listing, and adherence to Good Manufacturing Practices (GMPs).

The SMDA gives FDA new authority and expands and modifies the requirements of the MD Amendments. The provisions of the SMDA include new enforcement authority for the FDA including the reporting of medical device problems to the FDA by user groups and distributors. Other requirements and provisions of the SMDA affect device classification and reclassification, Premarket Notification (510(k)) and PMA processes, and GMP requirements. Some of the provisions went into effect when signed by President Bush on November 28, 1990, whereas others have future effective dates or require implementing regulations.

GETTING A DEVICE TO MARKET

As described in Table 2, medical devices include several thousand health products, from simple articles such as splints, elastic bandages, and crutches to external fixators, total joint replacements, prosthetic ligaments, and bone substitutes. The term devices also includes components, parts or accessories of devices, diagnostic aids, and test kits for *in vitro* diagnosis of disease and other conditions. Prior to the 1976 passage of the MD Amendments, a manufacturer could market most medical devices without any government approval or notification. Even though the FD&C Act of 1938 specifically addressed medical devices, it did not give the FDA authority to require any premarket testing or approval of medical devices. Consequently, defective, fraudulent, quack, or otherwise unsafe devices could only be taken off the market after the fact. The passage of the MD Amendments remedied this situation. The regulation of the devices depends on whether the device is a pre-Amendments device or a new device. Those devices in commercial distribution before May 28, 1976, are regulated as old, or "pre-Amendments" devices, whereas those introduced to the market after May 28, 1976, are regulated as new devices. In very rare cases, such as in the case of a custom device, a device may be exempt from certain regulations (see below).

Figure 1 illustrates the overall device evaluation process. Essentially, a device is (i) a device in pre-Amendments use; (ii) a new device that is substantially equivalent to a pre-Amendments device; or (iii) an entirely new device or one that was found

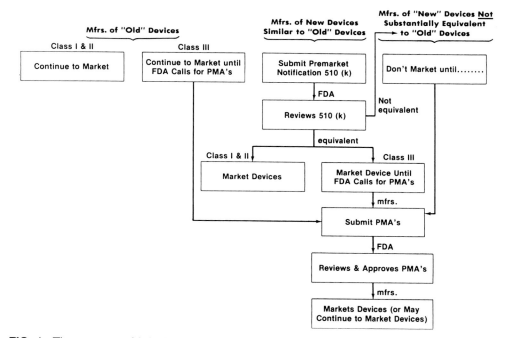

FIG. 1. The process of bringing a device to market follows this logic tree. Pre-Amendments devices may continue to market; Class III devices must be prepared to submit PMA applications when requested. New devices must be cleared through the 510(k) (Premarket Notification) process before marketing. If the device is not cleared, it must obtain PMA.

to be not substantially equivalent to a pre-Amendments device. A device is regulated accordingly in one of three device classifications.

It should be emphasized at this point, no matter which of these three categories a device belongs to, the basic purpose of FDA review remains the same. Any device will be reviewed from the standpoint of safety, efficacy, and clinical utility prior to marketing clearance or approval, although the standard of acceptable proof may be slightly different in each case.

DEVICE CLASSIFICATIONS

The MD Amendments directed the FDA to classify all pre-Amendments devices into one of three regulatory control categories, Class I, II, or III, depending on the degree of regulation necessary to provide reasonable assurance of their safety and effectiveness (Table 3). The class in which a device is placed determines the requirements that must be met before a manufacturer may distribute a device in interstate commerce.

Class I consists of devices for which General Controls are sufficient to assure safety and effectiveness. General Controls (Table 4) include requirements for manufacturer registration and product listing with the FDA, premarket notification, the establishment and maintenance of manufacturing records and filing reports with re-

TABLE 3. *Medical device classification: Medical Device Amendments, May 28, 1976*

Regulatory category	Definition	Examples of orthopedic devices
Class I: General Controls	Least stringent regulatory category, consists of devices for which General Controls are sufficient to assure safety and effectiveness	Manual surgical instruments; noninvasive traction components; elastic bandages, crutches
Class II: Special Controls	General Controls alone are not sufficient to assure safety and effectiveness, but enough information is available to develop special controls to provide adequate assurance	Intramedullary rods; cemented total hip replacements; cerclage wire; bone screws and plates
Class III: Premarket Approvals	Most stringent category; adequate data are not available to assure safety and effectivenss	Total shoulder and ankle replacements; prosthetic ligaments; bone substitutes

spect to device marketing experience, and adherence to GMPs. Some typical Class I orthopedic devices are manual surgical instruments not unique to the implantation of another orthopedic device, cast materials, crutches, and wheelchairs. Class II consists of those devices for which General Controls are insufficient to assure safety and effectiveness. However, there exists sufficient information to establish special controls that may include performance standards to provide such assurance. Intramedullary nails, bone screws, and plates when used for long bone fractures, cemented hip replacements, and cerclage wire are Class II devices. Class III, the most stringent category, is reserved for entirely new devices or device found not substantially equivalent for which there is insufficient information to assure their safety and effectiveness. The majority of ligament replacements and bone substitutes are Class III. Currently classified orthopedic devices are identified in the Code of Federal Regulations (21 CFR 888 Subpart D).

Manufacturers of Class I and II pre-Amendments devices are allowed to continue marketing their products, providing that the GMP regulations and special controls are observed (Fig. 1). Manufacturers of Class III pre-Amendments devices may also continue to market but must be prepared to submit PMA applications demonstrating

TABLE 4. *General controls*

Consist of the basic requirements of the Amendments that apply to all medical devices:
  Adulteration
  Misbranding
  Banned devices
  Notification, repair, replacement, refunds
  Records and reports
  Restricted devices
Also require device manufacturers to perform the following activities:
  Establishment registration and device listing
  Premarket Notification 510(k)
  Adherence to GMPs

the device's safety, effectiveness, and clinical utility when requested by the FDA (see below).

POST-AMENDMENTS DEVICES

For any device that is being introduced into the market after May 28, 1976, a manufacturer must submit to the FDA a Premarket Notification (the so-called 510(k)) or a PMA application. Section 510(k) of the MD Amendments contains the 510(k) requirements. The purpose of the 510(k) is to permit the FDA to determine whether the device is substantially equivalent in terms of design, materials, and intended use to a legally marketed predicate device, that is, a device already on the market in the United States prior to the May 28, 1976 (the enactment date of the Amendments) or a device marketed after that date that has already been determined to be SE. Premarket notification is required whenever a device is being introduced into the market for the first time, when a new device is being introduced that may already be marketed by another manufacturer, when a device currently in commercial distribution is about to be significantly changed or modified, or there is a change in the intended use of the device.

The determination of substantial equivalence (SE) is made by the scientific staff of the FDA. With the signing of the SMDA, SE means that a device has the same intended use and the same technological characteristics as the legally marketed predicate device, or it has the same intended use and different technological characteristics but it can be demonstrated that the device is as safe and effective as the legally marketed predicate device and does not raise different questions of safety and efficacy than the predicate device. Nonclinical laboratory testing and/or clinical testing may be used to demonstrate SE of a device with the same intended use but with new technological characteristics. It is incumbent on the manufacturer to supply any information that the FDA requires to make a determination. The amount and type of information required to determine equivalence vary with the complexity of the device. For the most part, the FDA performs no device testing on its own. All information required for the determination of SE is submitted by the manufacturer. Based on the information contained in a device submission, the FDA determines whether the device is substantially equivalent to a device that was or is being marketed (Fig. 2). If the device is determined to be substantially equivalent to a pre-Amendments device, it is placed in the same regulatory class as the device to which it is found equivalent and it can be then be legally marketed. If the FDA determines that the device is not substantially equivalent (NSE) to a predicate device, it is automatically in Class III and therefore must obtain FDA approval of a PMA before it can be legally marketed.

It must be emphasized that devices are only cleared for marketing for a specific intended use. Any promotion or labeling for an intended use other than that which was the basis of substantial equivalence would constitute misbranding. For example, most porous-coated knee prostheses were cleared for marketing under a 510(k) for cemented use only when they were found substantially equivalent to the cemented predicate devices. If a manufacturer promoted the device for uncemented use, biological fixation, or bone ingrowth, this would be a new intended use and would therefore constitute misbranding under the Act.

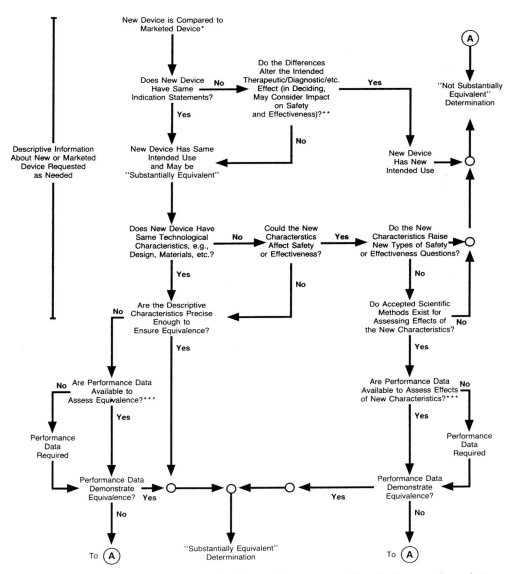

FIG. 2. 510(k) Premarket Notification decision-making process. The device must be substantially equivalent to legally marketed predicate devices in terms of intended use and technological characteristics to be cleared for marketing under the 510(k) process. If the device has a new intended use, the device's new technological characteristics raise new types of safety or effectiveness questions, or there are no accepted methods to assess the effects of the new characteristics, the device should be found Not Substantially Equivalent. On the other hand, if the device has the same intended use and the technological characteristics are the same or do not affect the safety or effectiveness of the device, it should be found Substantially Equivalent. *510(k) submissions compare new devices to marketed devices. The FDA requests additional information if the relationship between marketed and "predicate" (pre-Amendments or reclassified post-Amendments) devices is unclear. **This decision is normally based on descriptive information alone, but limited testing information is sometimes required. ***Data may be in the 510(k)s, other 510(k)s, the Center's classification files, or the literature.

The 510(k) process provides a high degree of public protection by allowing the FDA to identify devices that present significant unanswered questions of safety and effectiveness. The 510(k) process also allows manufacturers to achieve marketing equity by allowing manufacturers of new devices that are substantially equivalent to pre-Amendments devices to go to market without facing greater regulatory burdens than those faced by manufacturers of the pre-Amendments devices.

It is important to note that the FDA does not actually "approve" devices in response to 510(k) submissions; rather it determines whether the proposed device is substantially equivalent to a type of device that was on the market before May 28, 1976. This equivalence determination by the FDA clears the device for marketing, because it is considered to be as safe and effective as other legally marketed devices, but does not approve it.

PREMARKET APPROVAL

Manufacturers of new Class III devices, including those determined to be not substantially equivalent to marketed devices, must obtain PMA from the FDA before their devices may be marketed. The PMA process is a rigorous scientific analysis of the device's safety, effectiveness, and clinical utility (Fig. 3). A granted PMA is, in effect, a private license granted to the applicant for marketing a particular medical device.

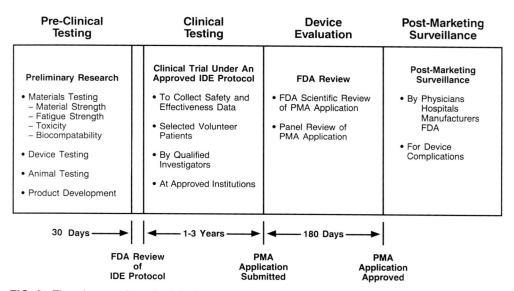

FIG. 3. The phases of medical device development. Preliminary research is performed to provide reasonable assurance that the use of the device in humans will be safe. The manufacturer submits to the FDA an IDE protocol for a well-controlled clinical trial. After FDA approval, the manufacturer may conduct the clinical investigation. When adequate preclinical and clinical data are available, the manufacturer may submit a PMA application. After a thorough scientific review by the FDA staff and the panel, the PMA application may be approved. Postmarket surveillance allows continued assessment of the devices safety.

The review procedure of a PMA is a multistep process that initially consists of an in-depth scientific review of valid scientific evidence submitted by the manufacturer. A PMA generally will include data from nonclinical laboratory tests, a well-controlled clinical trial, and statistical analyses of the data from a comparison of the device to controls. In contrast, anecdotal information often given in case-report form in the literature is not considered valid scientific evidence. The supporting nonclinical, clinical, and statistical information provided may then be reviewed by an FDA advisory committee (the "panel") for their comments and recommendations. The FDA then considers the recommendations of the panel and makes a final decision of whether to approve the device. Whether or not a PMA for a device is granted, the FDA prepares and publishes a summary of the safety and effectiveness data to support its determination.

The panel is a group of experts from outside the government who provide advice and recommendations to the FDA on PMA device applications, as well as in other matters. The Orthopedic and Rehabilitation Devices Panel is one of 16 operating medical device advisory committees appointed by the FDA. Each panel is composed of nine members, seven voting and two nonvoting, appointed to 3-year terms. Voting members are appointed from relevant scientific disciplines, such as orthopedics or engineering. The current panel consists of many distinguished members of the scientific community (Table 5). The FDA has the flexibility to alter the makeup of the panel in order to utilize other consultants with particular areas of expertise, or to eliminate the possibility of a conflict of interest, by temporarily removing a member or swearing in another panel member. One nonvoting member represents the medical devices industry and another represents consumer interests.

TABLE 5. *Orthopedics and Rehabilitation Advisory Panel Members (as of February 1992)*

Michael B. Mayor, M.D.	M. Clinton Miller III, Ph.D.
(Panel Chairman)	Professor and Chairman
Associate Professor	Department of Biometry
Dartmouth-Hitchcock Medical Center	Medical University of South Carolina
Lebanon, NH	Charleston, SC
Daniel R. Benson, M.D.	Donald E. Sweet, M.D.
Professor	Chairman and Registrar
Department of Orthopedic Surgery	Orthopedic Pathology
University of California, Davis	Armed Forces Institute of Pathology
Sacramento, CA	Washington, DC
Thomas L. Craig[a]	Bernard F. Morrey, M.D.
Industry Representative	Professor and Chairman
Director, Regulatory Affairs	Department of Orthopedic Surgery
Smith & Nephew Richards	Mayo Clinic
Memphis, TN	Rochester, MN
A. Seth Greenwald, D.Phil. (Oxon)	Peter A. Torzilli, Ph.D.
Director	Associate Professor
Orthopaedic Research Laboratories	Department of Biomechanics
Mt. Sinai Medical Center	The Hospital for Special Surgery
Cleveland, OH	New York, NY
	Vacant
	Consumer Representative[a]

[a]Nonvoting member.

Only after the PMA has been granted can the manufacturer proceed to market the device. Manufacturers may only label and promote the device for the indications specifically approved by the FDA under the PMA. Any promotion or labeling of the device not specifically included in the approval would constitute misbranding under the Act. For example, several porous-coated hip replacements were granted PMA for uncemented use. However, during the PMA process, the manufacturers were unable to conclusively demonstrate actual bony ingrowth as the means of fixation. The devices were found to function similarly to the "press-fit" hip prostheses and were approved for labeling as such. Therefore, any labeling or promotion of these devices for bony ingrowth would constitute misbranding under the Act. A post-Amendments Class III device that fails to obtain PMA cannot be marketed.

INVESTIGATIONAL DEVICE EXEMPTION

To encourage the discovery and development of useful medical devices, the MD Amendments provided exemptions for investigational devices from many of the controls of the Act, such as 510(k) and PMA. An Investigational Device Exemption (IDE) permits a device to be shipped in interstate commerce for clinical investigation to demonstrate that it is as safe and effective as a legally marketed predicate device for the purposes of a 510(k), to determine its safety and effectiveness for the purposes of a PMA, or to allow for the collection of safety and effectiveness data. Although the IDE regulation exempts the device from certain requirements of the Act, it still requires safeguards for humans who are subjects of investigations, maintenance of sound ethical standards, and procedures to assure the development of reliable scientific data.

All clinical investigations of devices conducted in the United States must have an approved IDE or be exempt from the IDE regulation. The IDE regulation distinguishes between significant and nonsignificant risk device studies. The determination of whether a device study presents a significant risk is initially made by the sponsor. A significant risk device is defined as an implant, one used in supporting or sustaining human life, or one that is important in diagnosing or treating disease. For example, nearly all orthopedic implants are considered significant risk devices by the FDA. A proposed study is then submitted to an Institutional Review Board (IRB) for review. If the IRB agrees with the sponsor that the device study presents a nonsignificant risk, no IDE submission is required. However, the FDA maintains the final authority on decisions regarding significant risk. A sponsor of a significant risk device investigation is required to obtain both IRB and FDA approval of the IDE before beginning the study in the United States.

An IDE application must include a complete report of prior nonclinical and clinical investigations, published and unpublished information on device problems, and a summary of all other unpublished information that is relevant to an evaluation of the safety and effectiveness of the device. For instance, data from materials testing for composition, physical characteristics and biocompatibility, conformance to voluntary testing standards, sterilization methods, device design considerations, device testing, and proposed uses are all required for evaluation relative to safety or risk. For the clinical study itself, an investigational plan, including a statistical basis of evaluation and sample size with all calculations, a description of the evaluation methods, inclusion and exclusion criteria, success and failure criteria, valid control group, informed consent, and methods of data analysis must be supplied.

Once the IDE application is approved, the sponsor may begin the investigation on a specified number of cases at a specified number of sites, strictly adhering to the investigational protocol. In order to further safeguard the human subjects in the investigation, the sponsors are required to immediately notify the FDA of any unanticipated adverse reactions and conduct an evaluation of any unanticipated adverse device effects. If the adverse device effect presents an unreasonable risk to subjects, the sponsor must terminate the investigation.

CUSTOM DEVICES

Clinical investigations of a significant risk device may be exempted if it is a custom device. Custom medical devices defined by regulation to be those devices meeting all five criteria specified in the IDE regulations. They are devices that: necessarily deviate from devices generally available; are not generally available to, or used by, other physicians; are not generally available in their finished form for purchase or for dispensing upon prescription; are not offered for commercial distribution through labeling or advertising; and are intended for use by an individual patient named in an order of a physician and are to be made in a specific form for that patient. Except for 510(k), such devices must comply with all general control requirements relating to GMPs, investigational use of devices, banning, restriction, adulteration, and misbranding. There are very few bona fide orthopedic devices that fulfill the custom device definitions. For instance, even so-called "made-to-order" or "patient-matching" joint prostheses are not considered to be custom devices in the regulatory sense. They must conform to all materials, design, and intended use restrictions under which they are cleared. By restricting the dimensions, geometry, and materials of these prostheses to certain defined and tested limits, the safety and effectiveness can still be assured for the purposes of a 510(k) or PMA.

EVALUATION OF ORTHOPEDIC DEVICES

General Submission Elements

No matter what form an orthopedic device submission takes, 510(k), IDE, or PMA, there is general information needed that is common to all. Each requires identification of a device name, including the trade or proprietary name and the common or usual name. All submissions require labels, labeling including package inserts and/or surgical technique manuals, and advertisements sufficient to describe the intended use and directions for use. Device descriptions, including photographs or drawings of the assembled device, materials used in the manufacture, surface treatments, or processing, and engineering drawings with dimensions and tolerances of each component are also necessary. In addition, each submission must address how the device or its intended use is similar to and/or different from other products in commercial distribution and must accompany these statements with nonclinical and clinical data to support them.

Evaluations of substantial equivalence of 510(k), relative safety or risk of IDEs, and safety, efficacy, and clinical utility of PMAs are based on descriptions of the intended use and directions for use, device descriptions, and the nonclinical and clinical information for a device supplied to support a manufacturer's statements or claims. Furthermore, the FDA may make a judgment on the "implicit claim" even when it is not cited as a claim by the sponsor. This is, however, rare and based on the actual history of the device and FDA's knowledge of the marketplace. Most review delays involve incomplete information being supplied for one or any combination of the above areas of evaluation. Identification of the intended use for a device, the most pivotal point of evaluation, should be specific, not broad or general unless supported by data or allowed for other legally marketed predicate devices.

Adequate device descriptions allow for the determination of whether there are new characteristics that could affect safety or effectiveness. Drawings or photographs of the assembled device provide an overall perspective of the device's interaction with the body and other components. Engineering drawings provide needed details of these interactions, such as anatomic and physical limitations. Identification of manufacturing materials and voluntary standards to which these materials conform indicate to the FDA whether additional biocompatibility and toxicologic information is necessary. Nonclinical and clinical data may support specified intended uses, differences in design and manufacture or other technological characteristics, or claims, such as enhanced clinical performance, reduced wear, improved stability or strength, increased fatigue resistance. Although not a requirement, much of the nonclinical and clinical information provided in a submission is in the form of test reports with the remainder supplied in the form of published references.

Nonclinical Records and Reports

Although Good Laboratory Practice (GLP) regulation for nonclinical laboratory studies is not applicable to all nonclinical testing, it does describe sections whose intent should be applied to any nonclinical test provided as part of a submission. The section pertaining to the characterization and handling requirements for test and control articles is a particularly important one. This section requires that the identity, strength, purity, and composition, and other characteristics that will appropriately define the test or control article shall be determined and documented for each batch. Determining and reporting the stability of each test or control article are other requirements. The identification of each storage container for each article by name, code number, lot number, expiration date, and storage conditions is necessary to maintain its identity, strength, purity, and composition. An additional requirement is the retention of test or control articles.

The section relating to the preparation of a written protocol and conduct of a study in accordance with that protocol is another pertinent section for device submissions. A written protocol that identifies the objectives of the study; describes the experimental design including methods for the control of bias; notes the type and frequency of tests, analyses, and measurements to be made; and states the proposed statistical methods to be used should be provided for each nonclinical study. If changes become necessary while conducting a study, all revisions of the protocol should be identified and the reasons for these changes should be documented in device submissions.

Probably the most germane section of the GLP regulations for any nonclinical study is the section on records and reports. It identifies the need for a complete final report and its intent may be extended to interim reports. Any report should identify the name and address of the facility performing the study and contain the names and signatures of the individuals conducting the studies. The introduction should have a brief purpose and procedures section taken from the written protocol for the study including any variations from original protocol. If variations from the original protocol did occur, then the purpose and procedure section of a report should describe why these changes were necessary. Identification of the statistical methods employed in analyzing the data should also be included in any technical report. A description of the composition, purity, strength, and other appropriate characteristics of test and control articles identified by name or code number should be furnished. An explanation of the experimental set-up, sufficient to allow for reconstructing the test, is essential in the evaluation of a nonclinical testing report.

The body of the nonclinical testing report should have four main areas. It should contain the raw data including failure data, if any; provide a description of the transformations, calculations, or operations performed on the data; include a summary and analysis of the raw data, and failure data, if any; and should include the conclusions drawn from the analysis of the data.

Clinical Study Design Considerations

Evaluation of clinical study design is one of the prime elements considered during the evaluation of IDE to ascertain that the proposed study has a reasonable chance to produce scientifically valid data when executed properly.

From a scientific point of view, a clinical study, like most other scientific investigations, can only hope to yield the information for which it was designed. Therefore, it is extremely important that prior to the development of each protocol, careful consideration be given to the basic scientific tenets of clinical trial and associated biostatistics. In general, a hierarchical order of preference for trial design has long been recognized. A prospective randomized concurrent (placebo-controlled, double-blind or alternative treatment-controlled and evaluator-blind) clinical trial design has the best chance to yield bias-free data. Where feasible, such a design should be relied on for safety and efficacy evaluation of orthopedic devices. In several defined situations, patient randomization can be performed prior to selection of the operating surgeon who performs only one of the two alternative procedures. On the other end of the scale, an uncontrolled study or a prospective trial design utilizing retrospective cohort controls (including historical controls from literature) often provide misleading or erroneous conclusions in spite of valiant statistical manipulation of data. The crossover trial is another useful design concept but is often impractical for most orthopedic devices for obvious reasons. Therefore, in spite of various objections cited against randomized controlled trials (e.g., unsubstantiated ethical reasons, difficulty in patient accrual, competitive pressure and economics), no real life valid alternatives exist in trial design that can substitute a prospective bias controlled study for obtaining unambiguous scientific evidence of the safety and efficacy of a new orthopedic device. Every clinical trial of a new device carries some degree of unknown or unanticipated risk to the patient, which, by definition, cannot be totally eliminated. In addition to the probability of benefiting the patient, the study, therefore, must also yield the maximum possible information for societal benefit in the form of new and reliable public health knowledge. This can only be accomplished through a properly controlled study. This concept is consistent with and has been aptly articulated in the Declaration of Helsinki (Article 4. Basic Principle).

Several other aspects or components of clinical trial design that are equally important and merit proper consideration are precise trial objective statement (null hypothesis), appropriate sample size (based on preset error and power levels), unbiased multicenter patient distribution, uniform predefined exclusion and inclusion criteria, objective (quantifiable) clinical and radiographic outcome measurements and observations, surrogate end-point measurements, predefined success/failure criteria based on sound follow-up time, and methods for tracking the entire cohort (including loss to follow-up). Each of these elements affects the future validity of data analysis and therefore should be considered carefully before initiation of the study.

Finally, no trial design is complete until thoughtful consideration is given to how the collected data can be properly analyzed using a proper test of significance. Therefore a comprehensive discussion of statistical evaluation methods (means and ways) should be undertaken in an IDE submission.

A number of guidelines on specific devices such as artificial ligaments and bone-growth stimulators are available from the FDA that may be of assistance to the sponsors of other devices for conceptual purposes.

Clinical Records and Reports

Although the IDE regulation and proposed International Standards Organization of (ISO) draft standard for clinical studies (TC194/WG4) are not applicable to all clinical studies, they do describe a section pertaining to records and reports that should be applied to any report of a clinical study provided as part of a device submission. An interim or final clinical report should include a complete accounting of the devices shipped, implanted, inventoried, returned, and disposed. For each investigational site a report should identify the names and addresses of the investigator and IRB chairperson and the dates of IRB approval, first shipment of devices, and first implantation of the device. A complete written and approved protocol should accompany any final report of a clinical investigation of an orthopedic device and should identify the purpose of the study, supply the statistical basis for the evaluation and sample size, identify the types of controls, and describe the evaluation methods, inclusion and exclusion criteria, success and failure criteria, and methods of data analysis.

Each group or subgroup, based on a device configuration or prognostically distinct indication, involved in a clinical study should be reported on separately before any attempts to pool these groups or subgroups are made. For each group and subgroup involved in a clinical study, complete patient demographics should be supplied in any interim or final submission report. Adequate patient accounting in the form of a time course distribution also should be supplied for each stratification of subjects. Both interim and final clinical study reports should include a time course of the distributions of the number of subjects having each clinical and radiographic evaluation parameter required by the approved protocol; reporting complications, device related or not, stratified into systemic and operative site; experiencing revisions stratified by the component; and requiring additional operations at the operative site but not revision of the device. For each subject of a group or subgroup reporting device-related complications, experiencing device revisions, or involving a protocol violation, a patient summary should be supplied that documents the patient's current status and dates of onset and correction of that occurrence.

The remainder of an interim or final report should discuss relevant observations, including anticipated or unanticipated adverse device effects as they pertain to safety, effectiveness, corrective actions, and future plans.

MATERIALS AND DEVICE TESTING

Due to increasingly sophisticated materials used in manufacturing medical devices, requests for testing, validation of biocompatibility and integrity testing, and characterization of device designs and materials have been more prevalent for most types of orthopedic device submissions (see Chapter 33).

Biocompatibility

Historically, biocompatibility testing has not been an issue for most orthopedic device submissions if the manufacturing materials conform to voluntary standards for medical-grade implant materials with known or documented biocompatibility. Within the past few years there has been an increasing move to new polymer, composite, ceramic, and metallic alloy materials with unknown or undocumented biocompatibility. The Office of Device Evaluation (ODE) of FDA's Center for Devices and Radiological Health has developed and supplied general guidance in the evaluation and review of new biomaterials in the form of a general program memorandum based on the Tripartite Biocompatibility Guidance for Medical Devices as early as 1987. The ODE continues its efforts to provide and develop general guidance in the evaluation and review of new biomaterials through its efforts to develop voluntary standards through organizations such as the Association for the Advancement of Medical Instrumentation (AAMI), American National Standards Institute (ANSI), American Society of Testing and Materials (ASTM), and the ISO. Although these efforts continue, the ODE still bases its evaluation of new biomaterials on the Tripartite Biocompatibility Guidance, which outlines the fundamental principles of toxicity evaluation for medical devices and provides a rational framework for their application.

The scope and application of the Tripartite guidance, specifically designed for polymers, can be extrapolated to all new materials if the general intent of the suggested testing is followed. The application of these principles requires the assignment of a given medical device to a category defined by the nature of contact of the device with the body, the time of contact, and the materials of manufacture interaction with the body for the intended use. The Tripartite guidance contains a table of suggested tests related to the nature and duration of contact for the safety evaluation of medical devices. The FDA expects a device submission to contain data addressing each type of suggested test or to present a sound argument why the information is not needed for the evaluation with supporting documentation. It should also be underscored that the Tripartite guidance is an outline for sets of toxicologic parameters to be considered in the evaluation process. Under special situations, various other toxicologic tests may also be needed for risk evaluation and/or management.

Device Design Integrity

The possible combinations of materials, design features, and manufacturing methods have made evaluation of orthopedic devices much more of a challenge than in the past. No longer can a reviewer be expected to look at a picture or engineering drawing and determine that an orthopedic device is as safe and effective as another legally marketed device for the purposes of a 510(k), is relatively safe for the purposes of clinical investigation under an IDE, or is safe and effective for the purposes of a PMA without testing or analyses of the proposed device.

The acceptable methods of addressing new design features and new manufacturing methods include complete engineering analyses with validation of the models used, nondestructive evaluation using documented methods, and mechanical characterization through static and fatigue testing. Voluntary standard test methods developed by organizations such as the AAMI, ANSI, ASTM, and ISO should be used whenever possible and identified as such in a submission. If the test methods used are not in conformance with draft or final voluntary standards in a device submission, identification of variations and justification for these variations should be provided. If no draft or final voluntary standard exists, the information regarding nonclinical testing described above should be followed. No matter which method is used, a comparison to legally marketed controls should be conducted and submitted as part of any device submission.

At the present time manufacturers of orthopedic devices incorporating new materials, especially nonmetals, will have a difficult task justifying equivalence with anything other than mechanical characterization through static and fatigue testing. Testing methods should follow the same suggestions outlined for design and manufacturing changes.

Manufacturing and design methods used in orthopedic devices such as made-to-order or patient-matching, inappropriately called "custom" by many manufacturers, are subject to the Reviewer Guidance for Computer-Controlled Medical Devices. Devices incorporating software in the design and manufacturing are of major concern because failures or latent design flaws could result in serious injury. Devices with a major level of concern require the submission and review of functional requirements and system specifications, software design and development techniques, verification and validation protocol or other quality assurance testing performed, test results and analysis of the data verification and validation testing, certification of adherence to good quality control procedures, and that the test results demonstrate the system specifications and functional requirements were met.

CONCLUSION

For more than 75 years, the FDA has adapted to rapidly improving and increasingly sophisticated medical devices. Regulatory controls for these devices have been developed to encourage the expeditious but responsible marketing clearance of the majority of medical devices, while at the same time upholding the public safety. The tiered regulatory framework for devices, with different degrees of safety concerns, allows for both rapid screening of devices through the 510(k) process and deliberate and intense scrutiny of new devices for safety and efficacy issues through the PMA process. Gradual stepwise advances in technology are allowed to be incorporated into devices through the 510(k) process as slight technological improvements are found substantially equivalent to recently cleared devices. Greater technological advances usually involve important unanswered questions of safety and effectiveness. These require greater scrutiny and are appropriately subjected to the more rigorous evaluation through the PMA process. In this way, the practitioner and the patient have prompt access to up-to-date, yet proven, medical devices, while unproven devices are kept off the market until their safety and effectiveness are adequately demonstrated. Although it has been the FDA's responsibility to regulate the medical device market, it is only through mutual cooperation between the FDA, manufacturers, physicians, and patients that safe and effective medical devices will continue to be available to the public.

ACKNOWLEDGMENTS

The authors acknowledge the invaluable assistance of Julie Gantenberg, M. Kendrick McDermott, Samie Niver, Stephen Rhodes, Hollace Saas, and Theodore Stevens of the Orthopedic Branch of the Office of Device Evaluation, Center for Devices and Radiological Health, U.S. Food and Drug Administration.

GLOSSARY OF TERMS

510(k)	The Section of the 1976 Medical Device Amendments to the Federal Food, Drug, and Cosmetic Act that contains the Premarket Notification requirement.
Adulteration	Defined under Section 501 as products that are defective, unsafe, filthy, or manufactured under unsanitary conditions.
Amendments	Medical Device Amendments to the Food, Drug, and Cosmetic Act, enacted May 28, 1976.
CFR	Code of Federal Regulations. The CFR is the general and permanent rules published in the Federal Register by the executive departments and agencies of the federal government.
General Controls	Basic requirements of the Amendments that apply to all medical devices.
GMP	Good Manufacturing Practices.
FDA	Food and Drug Administration. Under the Department of Health and Human Services (HHS), Public Health Service.
IDE	Investigational Device Exemption.
MDR	Medical Device Reporting regulation, 21 CFR Part 803, which requires manufacturers to report to the FDA any device-related injuries.
Misbranding	Defined under Section 502 as mislabeling.
NSE	Not substantially equivalent to a predicate device.
ODE	Office of Device Evaluation.
PMA	Premarket approval.
Pre-Amendments devices	Devices in commercial distribution on or before May 28, 1976.
Predicate	A legally marketed device that is used for comparison.
SE	Substantially equivalent to a predicate device.

BIBLIOGRAPHY

Code of Federal Regulations, Food and Drugs, Title 21, Office of the Federal Register National Archives and Records Administration, U.S. Government Printing Office, revised as of April 1, 1991.

Everything you always wanted to know about the medical device amendments . . . and weren't afraid to ask, HEW/FDA publication #77-5006, U.S. Department of Health, Education, and Welfare, Public Health Service, Food and Drug Administration, Bureau of Medical Devices, October 1977.

The Food and Drug Administration: An Overview. *FDA Backgrounder* February 1991.

Frisch E. An economic evaluation of premarket regulatory requirements. Medical Device & Diagnostic Industry, October 1980.

Highlights of the Safe Medical Devices Act of 1990 (Public Law 101–629), HHS/FDA publication #91-4243, U.S. Department of Health and Human Services, Public Health Service, Food and Drug Administration, Office of Training and Assistance, Division of Small Manufacturers Assistance, August 1991.

Premarket Notification: 510(k), HHS Publication FDA 90-4158, U.S. Department of Health and Human Services, Public Health Service, Food and Drug Administration, Center for Devices and Radiological Health.

Regulatory Requirements for Medical Devices, 4th ed., HHS publication FDA 89-4165, U.S. Department of Health and Human Services, Public Health Service, Food and Drug Administration, Center for Devices and Radiological Health.

Requirements of laws and regulations enforced by the U.S. Food and Drug Administration, HHS/FDA publication #81-1115, U.S. Department of Health and Human Services, Public Health Service, Food and Drug Administration, 1985.

Reviewer guidance for computer-controlled medical devices, U.S. Department of Health and Human Services, Public Health Service, Food and Drug Administration, Center for Devices and Radiological Health, Office of Device Evaluation, August 29, 1991.

Tripartite biocompatibility guidance, U.S. Department of Health and Human Services, Public Health Service, Food and Drug Administration, Center for Devices and Radiological Health, Office of Device Evaluation, General Program Memorandum #87-1, April 24, 1987.

Biological, Material, and Mechanical
Considerations of Joint Replacement,
edited by B. F. Morrey.
Raven Press, Ltd., New York © 1993.

Discussion of Regulatory Issues

Michael B. Mayor

Dartmouth Biomedical Engineering Center, Dartmouth College,
Hanover, New Hampshire 03755

Seven experts convened to discuss the context in which clinical research and regulatory affairs are conducted; the environment in which we are working is clearly extending to a global scale of effort. Issues of safety and efficacy of devices and procedures challenge the existing methodology.

CONSENSUS

Mechanisms must be developed to enhance the dialogue among clinicians and their professional organizations, industry, and government. Coordination of the process of developing the scientific foundation on which requirements are based must be achieved. Rational frameworks would then exist to support the development of effective clinical research projects. Mechanisms to convey this foundation to regulatory agencies must be developed to satisfy their need for information to demonstrate safety and efficacy.

The process of producing and evaluating clinical data to guide decisions both within and outside the regulatory framework is undergoing profound changes. These changes create the impression of a moving target, when in fact they are an unavoidable property of a field in which science is advancing rapidly.

Common goals exist among clinicians, producers, and regulators. Perspectives differ within each of the groups. Cost, for instance, may be considered critical to the producer, important to the clinician, and inconsequential by the regulators. In this context it was observed that user fees are a highly probable element that will emerge in our legislative and regulatory future in the United States.

Good science remains a universal sine qua non for all three. As the state of the art advances through the efforts of all three entities, safety, efficacy, and utility remain basic and critical criteria. Clinical utility requires a clear demonstration of impact on the disease entities targeted by the treatment modality under study.

The universality of standards is a highly desirable goal, one that is difficult to achieve because of provincial interests that create concerns on the part of individuals participating in the process of standards writing. A model for monitoring and evaluating the work we do does emerge, if slowly and painfully, from the process of producing such standards. Standards writing work, as done by the American Society of Testing and Materials, emerges as an ideal arena to conjoin the efforts of clinicians, producers, and regulators. Standards guidance documents and regulations themselves are resting on the same foundation. The foundation is built of bricks whose substance depends on good science. Specific standards are included in this text.

FUTURE WORK

The Safe Medical Devices Act creates the requirement for substantial scientific support for assertions of safety and efficacy. This requirement has recently been extended to relate to the process of a 510(k) (substantially equivalent) application. Investigational devices (ID), ID approvals, 510(k) applications, and premarket approvals (PMAs) all require good science, and that good science is context sensitive, both in terms of the development of the science itself and in terms of the specific device or treatment modality being researched.

Additionally, the continuing development of our fund of knowledge creates the impression of a moving target for those designing clinical studies. A forum in which dialogues can be initiated and continued is a highly desirable, even necessary, element as we look to the near and more distant future. It is the responsibility of the clinical organization, industrial associations, and regulatory agencies to search diligently and effectively for forums in which these common goals and concerns can be shared constructively.

All three entities with their representatives at the breakout session expressed commitment to pursuing the effort to develop participation in such forums to satisfy those common interests and enhance the mechanisms to produce the identified results. In this context, the American Academy of Orthopaedic Surgeons has established a task force to pursue integrating these interests with objective and consistent standards governing both the development of a device and its surveillance following approval for the marketplace.

Biological, Material, and Mechanical
Considerations of Joint Replacement,
edited by B. F. Morrey.
Raven Press, Ltd., New York © 1993.

35

The Local Cellular Response to Components of Total Hip Arthroplasty Experiencing Massive Osteolysis

Halina Witkiewicz, Russell T. Turner, Michael G. Rock, Bernard F. Morrey, and Mark E. Bolander

Department of Orthopaedics, Mayo Clinic, Rochester, Minnesota 55905

Total hip arthroplasty (THA) is in most cases a successful procedure, yet, in some patients, bone resorption around the implant is so extensive that the prosthesis becomes loose and revisions are necessary. At revision the zone of resorbed bone is filled not with a liquid exudate but with a membrane having the structural features of an organized tissue. This unique tissue between implant and bone may be directly and/or indirectly involved in the bone resorption. Cases of massive periprosthetic osteolysis suggest that very aggressive cellular mechanisms are active locally; however, there is no direct evidence of the specific cell types involved. This chapter will discuss the biological nature of the periprosthetic membrane, its heterogeneity, and possible interactions among the cell subpopulations of the membrane and bone cells that control normal bone remodeling. Identifying cellular mechanisms responsible for bone resorption in this unique clinical situation is the first step toward evaluating the feasibility of inhibiting the process after it has been initiated.

CURRENT CONCEPTS ON MECHANISMS OF THE ASEPTIC LOOSENING OF HIP IMPLANTS

Factors Inducing Bone Resorption

Prosthetic Wear Debris

Studies of the aseptic loosening of hip implants have focused on wear debris that is generated by the implants and found in periprosthetic soft tissue retrieved during THA revisions. These investigations suggest that mechanical wear of the implants and the response of the tissue to the particles is the primary etiology of loosening (7,19). Characterization of the biological response in these cases fails to show typical features of immunological rejection, i.e., accumulation of high numbers of activated B and T lymphocytes (32,36). However, all components of the prostheses (Ti, Ti-Al-V, high-density polyethylene, polymethylmethacrylate) induce accumulation of macrophages and giant cells when abraded into particles even though they are biocompatible in block form (38). There seems to be agreement in the literature that the formation of periprosthetic tissue represents a foreign-body response phenomenon; it has some elements of immunological reaction but not all of them. Cells responsible for removing debris (multinucleate giant cells and monocyte macrophages) are present in abundance, but activated lymphocytes (antigen-presenting T cells and antibody-producing B cells) are not common.

Macrophages may mediate bone resorption through various mechanisms. *In vitro* experiments demonstrating that isolated mouse macrophages stimulate bone resorption when they phagocytose particles provide indirect support for the concept that macrophage-secreted prostaglandin E2 (PGE2) initiates bone resorption (30). Wear particles of metal and polymer have been identified intracellularly, within the macrophages and giant cells in the tissue surrounding loose implants (18). PGE2, considered to be a potent stimulator of osteoclastic bone resorption, was detected in cell and organ cultures of the membrane surrounding loose prostheses, whereas membranes around nonloose prostheses produced negligible amounts of PGE2 (13,14). More recently, however, elevated levels of PGE2 were reported in membranes from both loose and fixed hips, suggesting that the role of PGE2 in bone resorption remains undefined (8). In addition to the indirect, PGE2-mediated bone resorption, macrophages and foreign-body giant cells of the periprosthetic membrane may also be capable of resorbing bone directly, as cells derived from the joint capsule after arthroplasty were shown to produce small resorption pits and some superficial resorption of the bone surface when cultured on cortical bone slices *in vitro* (3).

Factors Other than Particulate Debris

Elevated levels of locally bound metal ions found in synovial fluids of loose and fixed, cemented and cementless hips (8), together with the capability of $CoCl_2$ to stimulate production of the neutral proteinases (collagenase, gelatinase, and caseinase) by human synoviocytes cultured *in vitro* (12), suggest that soluble metal ions may induce proteinases and initiate bone resorption even when no particulate debris is found in the membrane by microscopy.

Altered mechanical loading or stress shielding are factors that also may contribute to periprosthetic bone resorption. Even though the molecular basis for mechanically induced bone remodeling is poorly understood, there are situations suggesting a causative relationship between mechanical factors and bone resorption. Increased air pressure, for example, induces localized bone resorption in a rodent model of osteoclastic bone resorption (6). Also, mechanical deformation of murine calvarial ostoeblasts *in vitro* significantly increases release of bone resorbing factors by these cells (33). Consequently, a role of osteoblasts as receptors that detect changes in mechanical force and initiate bone remodeling activity has been suggested (22).

THA as a Biological Phenomenon

A clear-cut difference has been noticed histologically between the common lesion accompanying prosthetic loosening and the massive osteolysis described as aggressive granulomatous lesions, namely, the relative lack of activated fibroblasts in granulomatosis. The reason for this imbalance between the monocyte-macrophage response and the fibroblast response has not been understood. Therefore, in spite of suspecting that aggressive granulomatosis and aseptic loosening might be part of a spectrum of a single condition, the authors suggested considering them as distinct conditions (35). From a different perspective, the single condition (of which the aggressive granulomatous lesions seen in massive osteolysis and the ligament-like tissue found in successful cases of THA are two opposite extremes) may be seen as a wound-healing process.

The body responds to injury or wounding by initiating a repair process. The response to THA can be categorized as a wound-healing process with three classic phases, inflammation, cell proliferation, and tissue remodeling. The *inflammatory* phase includes (i) initial tissue breakdown resulting in release of growth factors such as basic fibroblast growth factor and transforming growth factor β (TGF β) that are present in extracellular matrix; (ii) blood coagulation with degranulation of platelets and release of platelet-derived growth factor and TGF β; (iii) cellular release of growth factors and cytokines by stimulated cells present at the site of injury and by incoming macrophages, neutrophils, and lymphocytes. The *proliferative* phase includes divisions of mesenchymal cells attracted into the wound by the growth factors and cytokines during the inflammatory phase. Current concepts suggest that cell differentiation of these pluripotential cells is determined by the local, tissue-specific, matrix-bound growth factors. The *remodeling* phase results in production of new extracellular matrix by the differentiated cells and the reconstruction of this matrix into the specific tissue that will repair the wound and stabilize the prosthesis.

Tissues that suffer injury during THA include bone and bone marrow. However, insertion of the implant changes the tissue environment of the wound at the time of healing. Removing the bone marrow from the medullary canal of the femur in rodents results in formation of bone. The central portion of the bone is subsequently replaced with new bone marrow (26). Based on this observation and on the fact that during THA the periosteum remains intact, one would not expect callus but rather intramedullary bone formation at the site of the THA surgery. Indeed, bony ingrowth into the porous coating of a prosthesis is seen in many cases. Regeneration of the bone marrow does not occur, however, as the medullary space is filled with the prosthesis.

Yet, soft tissue rather than bone is frequently found adjacent to the implant. This tissue, commonly referred to as the periprosthetic membrane, has been said to have a synovium-like appearance. It has been suggested that the development of a membrane with a synovial lining might be an appropriate biological response to the mechanical microenvironment generated when bone and implant, each with a different elastic modulus, are subjected to weight bearing (13). Extrapolating from the observation that embryological synovial tissue fails to develop in the absence of motion, motion of the interface was implicated as the biological signal that stimulates differentiation of mesenchymal cells into synovial tissue (17). Another composite anatomic structure of the body, attachment of the tooth to the jaw, is an alternative analogy to the implant in the medullary canal of femur. The periodontal ligament connection between the tooth and jaw stabilizes the tooth but allows for limited micromotion. Significantly, the presence of a thin, ligament-like, membrane around hip implants is not usually accompanied by clinically detectable loosening of the prosthesis (14).

The membrane between the implant and bone may vary greatly in thickness and morphology; both well-organized and poorly organized tissues are observed. Histologically, its appearance ranges from that of a ligament-like tissue to granulation tissue. Signs of mineralization have been noticed in the extracellular matrix of the fibrous tissue, suggesting its potential to further adjust structurally to functional requirements (Fig. 1). This variability in the histological characteristics of the membrane is seen between patients, but also along a single femur or acetabulum. Presumably, when the prosthesis becomes loose, changes in the tissue reflect the degree to which it is irritated by the secondary injury, related to mechanical problems with the implant. If the amount of debris exceeds the phagocytic capacity of macrophages, this late, secondary injury to the periprosthetic tissue becomes chronic and leads to local degenerative changes of the ligament-like tissue simultaneously with the massive lysis of the bone.

The tissue recovered at revisions of failed THA may vary in its nature. In cases of morphologically well-organized fibrous connective tissue, there are two possible origins. First, the wound-healing process could, potentially, be arrested at the proliferative phase, continuing to produce undifferentiated fibroblasts that are prevented from further differentiation by the persistent chronic injury. Thus, the membrane would represent scar tissue, not fully differentiated and remodeled, therefore structurally unsuited to support the prosthesis. Alternatively, the membrane may represent well-differentiated ligament-like tissue that can accommodate the micromovement between the bone and implant. In the latter case prosthesis loosening would occur as a result of secondary injury to both the ligamentous lining and underlying bone. Poorly organized tissue recovered at the revision can be categorized histologically as granulation tissue. One can speculate that a granuloma forms when resorption of the tissues capable of maintaining stability of the implant occurs very quickly.

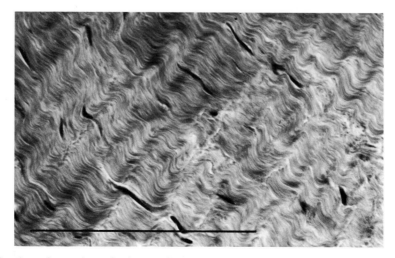

FIG. 1. Section of a periprosthetic membrane stained according to Goldner's method. Elongated, spindle-like cells are separated from each other with substantial fibrillar extracellular matrix, which appears birefringent in polarized light. The histologic appearance resembles ligamocytes embedded in collagen-rich matrix. In the original color slide, large patches of the matrix appear green indicating local mineralization. Bar = 100 μm.

This situation might correspond to an arrest of the wound-healing process initiated by the chronic injury at the inflammatory phase.

CELLS INVOLVED IN BONE RESORPTION

Physiological Bone Remodeling

Studies of bone resorption and remodeling in various systems have provided a basic understanding of these processes. It is clear that ascribing bone-destructive activity to osteoclasts and bone-forming activity to osteoblasts would be an oversimplification of the actual cellular relationships. Osteoblasts not only synthesize significantly more collagenase, predisposing bone surfaces to osteoclastic resorption (5), but also produce factors that induce osteoclasts to resorb the mineral component. Cellular receptors for bone-resorptive hormones are located on osteo*blasts* as well as osteo*clasts* (1,9,21). Additionally, resorption pit formation by osteoclasts is influenced by the viability of osteo*cytes* (39,40). Thus, one should not exclude any of these cell subpopulations from consideration of the molecular mechanisms controlling localized bone resorption.

In Vitro Studies Related to Periprosthetic Bone Resorption

The spectrum of bone resorption around implants ranges from little or no to massive osteolysis described as an aggressive granulomatous lesion (10,34,35). The latter suggests very active local mechanism(s) of bone resorption. The finding that the membrane deposited in place of resorbed bone has a capacity to produce collagenase (8,13) suggests direct involvement of this membrane in the degradation of bone matrix (29). However, another possibility is that the physiological mechanisms of bone remodeling may be influenced by extracellular factors secreted by injured cells of the benign, periprosthetic membrane, similar to the factors secreted by bone tumors.

The role of periprosthetic macrophages and foreign-body giant cells in local resorption of bone is to some extent controversial. Analysis of diffusible factors secreted by tissue and organ cultures of the periprosthetic membrane *in vitro* provides indirect evidence of their potential to stimulate bone resorption *in vivo*. The questionable value of extrapolating the data from one system to another can be exemplified by PGE2, considered to be a potent stimulator of bone resorption. In the context of THA, the presence of PGE2 in the periprosthetic membrane tissue and organ cultures has been interpreted as the potential of the membrane to stimulate bone resorption *in vivo*. In contrast, recent reports demonstrate in rats a positive effect of PGE2 on preventing disuse-induced bone loss by stimulating more bone formation than resorption (2,24).

Contradictory results have been reported on the capacity of macrophages and giant cells to resorb bone directly, utilizing *in vitro* bone resorption assays. Inflammatory cells derived from the joint capsule of hip arthroplasties have been reported to be capable of low-grade bone resorption, possibly of pathogenic significance in the loosening of prosthetic implants (3). In another study, macrophages and giant cells from failed total hip replacements did not form resorption pits on the bone substrates *in vitro,* implying that bone resorption around implants is mediated by bone cells (31). The usefulness of morphologic characteristics, including the resorption pits formed on bone substrate *in vitro,* in evaluating bone resorption suggested that bone fragments recovered at revisions might prove informative about *in vivo* bone-resorbing activities of morphologically distinct cells.

In Situ Analysis of Massive Periprosthetic Osteolysis

Microscopy is the preferred method for identifying cells involved in massive resorption of human bone around loose hip implants. This experimental approach has some features of the *in vitro* bone-resorption assay and the advantage of dealing with the tissue of interest instead of its animal model. Pieces of bone are commonly found in periprosthetic tissue recovered at revisions, making assessment of bone resorption *in situ* feasible without necessitating bone biopsies. Periprosthetic tissues from 23 patients undergoing hip arthroplasty revision of uncemented prostheses due to massive osteolysis of the femur apparent on x-ray were analyzed. Based on morphology of bone pieces found in the sections, some of them were identified as having bone

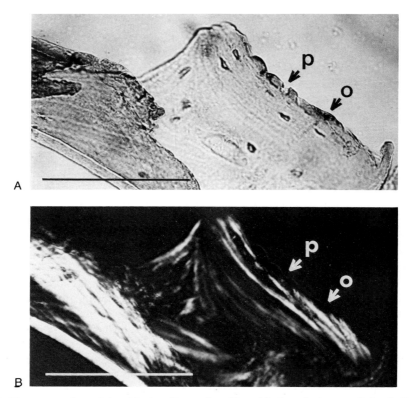

FIG. 2. Frozen section stained to localize cells with acid phosphatase activity. In the original photograph positive cells have their cytoplasm stained red and all cell nuclei appear green. **A:** Resorption pit (p) shown is empty but next to the pit there is a red multinucleate osteoclast (o) still attached to the bone surface. **B:** Same field as in A, photographed in polarized light to visualize collagen fibers with signs of their degradation in vicinity of the pit and osteoclast. Bar = 100 μm.

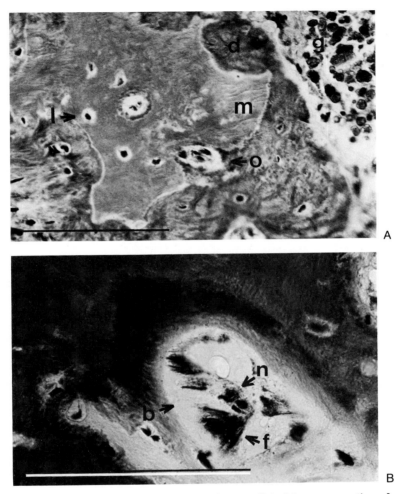

FIG. 3. Osteocytic osteolysis coupled with osteoclast-mediated bone resorption. **A:** Section of the membrane containing fragments of bone, stained according to Goldner's protocol to differentiate between mineralized (m), and demineralized matrix (d). White regions around the osteocyte lacunae (1) indicate lack of both mineral and organic components of the matrix. **B:** Higher magnification of an osteoclast from the same section. Cytoplasm adjacent to ruffled border (b) and the clear zone is devoid of organelles and contains bundles of actin-like filaments (f). Two nuclei (n) are seen in this section plane. Bar = 100 μm.

formation, others had clear signs of bone resorption; the latter were of particular interest. Structural features of the resorbing bone indicated three different cell types participating in the bone destruction: osteoclasts, osteocytes, and cells of the periprosthetic tissue (monocyte macrophages).

Osteoclasts were identified by their size, morphology, and location within characteristic Howship lacunae, i.e., in direct contact with eroded bone surface. In addition, special histological staining methods were applied to visualize acid phosphatase typically present in osteoclasts in contrast to alkaline phosphatase produced by osteoblasts (Fig. 2) and to differentiate between regions of bone that did and did not contain mineral (Fig. 3). The resorbing activity of osteoclasts was evidenced by the scalloped shape of the mineralized part of the bone that was surrounded by nonmineralized matrix, as well as the presence of the osteoclasts. The nonmineralized matrix was highly birefringent in polarized light, but in contrast to osteoid, it was not covered by osteoblasts, indicating demineralization of preexisting bone rather than depositing a new osteoid seam. Apparently, the demineralization occurred faster than degradation of the organic bone matrix. Regions of nonmineralized bone around a centrally located mineralized part without indications of osteoclastic activity were also seen (Fig. 4). Continuity of collagen fibers across the border line and the breakdown of the fibers into shorter fragments at the demineralized bone surface suggested progressive bone resorption in the absence of cells other than histiocytes

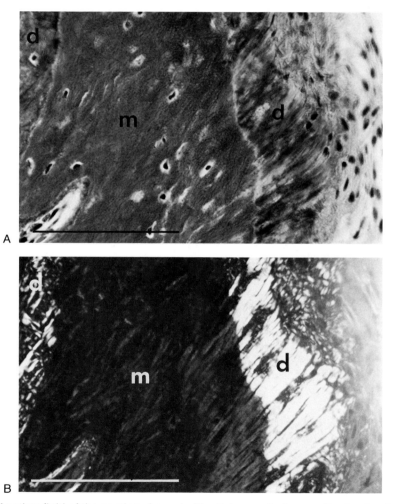

FIG. 4. Another field of the section shown in Fig. 3 demonstrating continuity of collagen fibers across the border between mineralized (m) and demineralized (d) extracellular matrix, indicating bone resorption rather than bone formation. **A**, bright field illumination; **B**, polarized light. Bar = 100 μm.

in direct contact with the bone. In addition, osteocytes were surrounded by colorless zones, implying resorption of both mineral and collagenous matrix beyond the limit of the perilacunar bone (Fig. 3A). The observed histological pattern resembles the one described earlier as osteocytic osteolysis (20). Significantly, the coupling of osteoclastic and osteocytic osteolysis was previously reported in other systems (4).

Larger fragments of bone found in the soft tissue at the time of specimen procurement were analyzed by scanning electron microscopy (SEM). The surface of the resorption pit housing an osteoclast, shown in Fig. 5A, is somewhat less course than the surface of pits formed by isolated osteoclasts on devitalized bone *in vitro* (16). One can interpret this difference as a result of more efficient degradation of matrix

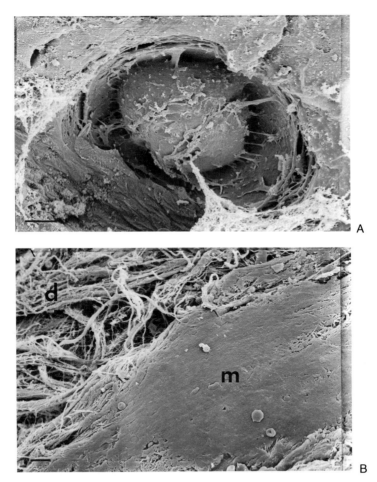

FIG. 5. SEM of bone. **A:** An osteoclast with many peripheral cytoplasmic processes, captured inside a Howship lacuna with a coarse fibrillar surface that was cut open when the bone fractured at surgery. The lacuna was located in close proximity to a blood vessel (not shown); this location is consistent with the hematopoietic origin of the osteoclast precursors. **B:** Surface of a trabecula with a mineralized (m) region surrounded by demineralized (d) bone showing exposed collagen fibers. In contrast to the Howship lacuna, a transition between the two regions is gradual, revealing continuity of the collagen fibers. Bar = 10 μm.

components by the osteoclast captured in the Howship lacuna *in vivo,* i.e., in its native tissue environment. A variation of the *in vitro* bone-resorption assay employing viable instead of nonviable bone as a substrate for osteoclastic activity demonstrated a contribution of osteocytes to the osteoclast-mediated bone resorption; pits formed in viable bone were larger in comparison to those formed in nonviable bone (39,40). The dimensions of the pit, its location in close proximity of the blood vessel, and absence of other cells in the cavity occupied by the osteoclast suggest that all components of the matrix removed to form the cavity were degraded by enzymes secreted or activated by this single cell. This conclusion is consistent with reported proteolytic activities (cysteine proteinases and neutral metalloproteinases) that osteoclasts are capable of expressing in addition to matrix-demineralizing activities (11). Similar to the bone shown in Fig. 4, the trabecular bone in Fig. 5B is not covered with osteoclasts or lining cells, and its smooth surface is gradually converted into rough bundles of fibers. In contrast to the Howship lacuna, this region of exposed (collagen) fibers lacks a well-defined margin and is widespread around the mineralized center, indicating bone-demineralizing activity of cells other than osteoclasts, most likely the surrounding granulomatous tissue. Interpretation of these histological and SEM observations as signs of bone resorption is consistent with massive bone loss seen on radiographs.

APPLICABILITY OF BISPHOSPHONATES IN THA

Our findings suggest that osteoclastic/osteocytic resorption is important in mediating implant loosening. If this conclusion is verified by additional studies, then it may be possible to intervene when evidence of osteolysis is obtained by administering an inhibitor of bone resorption. Bisphosphonates appear to be promising for this purpose. Bisphosphonates are chemotherapeutic compounds that inhibit bone resorption at a cellular level. Chemically they represent a group of pyrophosphate analogues characterized by a central carbon atom linking two phosphate groups and two side chains of variable structure. These side chains affect the spectrum of activity and potency of the bisphosphonates. In a rat model of immobilization osteoporosis, a bisphosphonate was shown to reduce the number of the osteo*cytes* that were actively resorbing bone (28); however, cells that have been most explored experimentally as those affected by bisphosphonates are cells of the osteo*clast* lineage (including monocytes and macrophages [15,41]). The drugs are capable of inhibiting both the resorptive activity of mature osteoclasts and the recruitment of immature cells (27,37). In tissue culture, they reverse the stimulatory effect of a variety of factors known to stimulate bone resorption (parathyroid hormone, calcitriol, prostaglandins, cytokines). This wide spectrum of inhibitory activity suggests that the bisphosphonates act as a distal step in the cellular events that affect bone resorption and for this reason are suitable agents for the management of accelerated osteoclast activity, irrespective of the cause (23). The molecular mechanism by which this action occurs is unknown, but they have been successfully used for treatment of Paget's disease, hypercalcemia due to malignancy, and osteoporosis of various etiologies. Analogous to treatment of metastatic bone resorption with bisphosphonates, one may expect treatment with a drug of this group to extend the durability of artificial hip joints.

Similar to pyrophosphate, biphosphonates are absorbed onto bone mineral, but unlike pyrophosphate, they are resistant to enzymatic hydrolysis. For this reason one could speculate that bisphosphonates would inhibit demineralization regardless of type of cells that produce the hydrolyzing enzymes, i.e., they might inhibit histiocyte-mediated demineralization as well, but this speculation needs to be verified experimentally.

CONCLUDING REMARKS

Histologic analysis of the tissue recovered at revisions of THA has revealed its morphologic heterogeneity and suggests involvement of several cell types in periprosthetic bone resorption. Identifying osteoclasts as one type actively involved allows for immediate benefit from experiments in other systems that resulted in finding pharmacologic inhibitors of osteoclast-mediated bone demineralization. The problem of particulate debris occurs in all types of hip prostheses used so far, implying that optimal material and design of the prostheses remain to be elaborated. Eliminating prosthetic wear debris by improving material quality and design of implants will be beneficial for future recipients of artificial joints, whereas the bisphosphonate treatment may also extend durability of the prostheses that have already been implanted.

The second aspect of the extracellular matrix degradation, i.e., degradation of its organic components in addition to bone demineralization, represents another potential target of therapeutic intervention. We hypothesize that, despite the possibly multiple initiating factors of bone resorption (which may encompass transduction of the mechanical signal into enzymatic processes), degradation of the organic extracellular matrix can be inhibited by inhibiting the final step of the cascade, the activity of proteolytic, matrix-degrading enzymes. The chemical composition of bone matrix suggests which enzymes may be required for its degradation. The observed heterogeneity of the membrane implies the necessity of an *in situ* approach to localize specific molecules to certain cell types and thus provide a functional analysis of the cells. The interaction between the periprosthetic tissue and the underlying bone provides a unique opportunity to study resorption of human bone directly *in situ*. Studies of this tissue may result in a better general understanding of mechanisms that control bone resorption.

REFERENCES

1. Agarwala N, Gay CV. Specific binding of parathyroid hormone to living osteoclasts. *J Bone Miner Res* 1992;7:531.
2. Akamine T, Jee WSS, Ke HZ, Li XJ, Lin BY. Prostaglandin E2 prevents bone loss and adds extra bone to immobilized femoral metaphysics in female rats. *Bone* 1992;13:11.
3. Athanasou NA, Quinn J, Bulstrode CJ. Resorption of bone by inflammatory cells derived from the joint capsule of hip arthroplasties. *J Bone Joint Surg* [*Br*] 1992;74:57.
4. Chambers TJ. The cellular basis of bone resorption. *Clin Orthop* 1980;151:283.
5. Chambers TJ, Darby JA, Fuller K. Mammalian collagenase predisposes bone surfaces to osteoclastic resorption. *Cell Tissue Res* 1985;241:671.
6. Chole RA, Chan DE. Rapid induction of localized bone resorption in the auditory bulla of the mongolian gerbil, *Meriones unguiculatus*, by increased air pressure. *Calcif Tissue Int* 1989;45:318.
7. DiCarlo EF, Bullough PG. The biologic responses to orthopedic implants and their wear debris. *Clin Mater* 1992;9:235.

8. Dorr LD, Bloebaum R, Emmanual J, Meldrum R. Histologic, biochemical, and ion analysis of tissue and fluids retrieved during total hip arthroplasty. *Clin Orthop* 1990;82.
9. Eeckhout Y, Delaisse JM. The role of collagenase in bone resorption. An overview. *Pathol Biol (Paris)* 1988;36:1139.
10. Eskola A, Santavirta S, Konttinen YT, Hoikka V, Tallroth K, Lindholm TS. Cementless revision of aggressive granulomatous lesions in hip replacements. *J Bone Jone Surg [Am]* 1990;72:212.
11. Everts V, Delaisse JM, Korper W, Niehof A, Vaes G, Beertsen W. Degradation of collagen in the bone-resorbing compartment underlying the osteoclast involves both cysteine-proteinases and matrix metalloproteinases. *J Cell Physiol* 1992;150:221.
12. Ferguson GM, Watanabe S, Georgescu HI, Evans CH. The synovial production of collagenase and chondrocyte activating factors in response to cobalt. *J Orthop Res* 1988;6:525.
13. Goldring SR, Schiller AL, Roelke M, ONeil DA, Harris WH. The synovial-like membrane at the bone-cement interface in loose total hip replacements and its proposed role in bone lysis. *J Bone Joint Surg [Am]* 1983;65:575.
14. Goodman SB, Chin RC, Chiou SS, Schurman DJ, Woolson ST, Masada MP. A clinical-pathologic-biochemical study of the membrane surrounding loosened and nonloosened total hip arthroplasties. *Clin Orthop* 1989;182.
15. Holak HM, Szymaniec S, Skriabin A. Effect of dichloromethylene diphosphonate (Cl2-MDP) on bone resorption induced by PHA-stimulated human mononuclear cells in organ culture. *Arch Immunol Ther Exp (Warsz)* 1984;32:77.
16. Holtrop ME. Light and electronmicroscopic structure of osteoclasts. In: Hall BK, ed. *Bone, volume 2: the osteoclast*. Boca Raton, FL: CRC Press, 1992.
17. Huiskes R, Weinans H, Dalstra M. Adaptive bone remodeling and biomechanical design considerations for noncemented total hip arthroplasty. *Orthopedics* 1989;12:1255.
18. Huo MH, Salvati EA, Buly RL. Wear debris in cemented total hip arthroplasty. *Orthopedics* 1991;14:335.
19. Jacobs JJ, Galante JO, Sumner DR. Local response to biomaterials: bone loss in cementless femoral stems. *Am Acad Orthop Surg* 1992 (instruction course Lecture 41):119.
20. Jande SS, Belanger LF. The life cycle of the osteocyte. *Clin Orthop* 1973;94:281.
21. Jo Ousler M, Osdoby P, Pyfferoen J, Riggs BL. Avian osteoclasts as estrogen target cells. *Proc Natl Acad Sci USA* 1991;88:6613.
22. Kahn AJ, Partridge NC. Bone resorption in vivo. In: Hall BK, ed. *Bone, volume 2: the osteoclast*. Boca Raton, FL: CRC Press, 1991:119.
23. Kanis JA, McCloskey EV, Taube T, ORourke N. Rationale for the use of bisphosphonates in bone metastases. *Bone* 1991;12(suppl 1):513.
24. Ke HZ, Jee WSS, Mori S, Li XJ, Kimmel DB. Effects of long-term daily administration of prostaglandin-E2 on maintaining elevated proximal tibial metaphyseal cancellous bone mass in male rats. *Calcif Tissue Int* 1992;50:245.
25. Liang CT, Barnes J, Seedor JG, et al. Impaired bone activity in aged rats: alterations at the cellular and molecular levels. *Bone* 1992.
26. Lowik CW, van der Pluijm G, van der Wee Pals LJ, van Treslong De Groot HB, Bijvoet OL. Migration and phenotypic transformation of osteoclast precursors into mature osteoclasts: the effect of a bisphosphonate. *J Bone Miner Res* 1988;3:185.
27. Martino LJ, Seideman B. The effect of dichloromethylene diphosphonate (Cl2MDP) on osteocyte activity during immobilization osteoporosis in rats. *Metab Bone Dis Relat Res* 1980;2:261.
28. Mundy GR, Eilon G, Altman AJ, Dominguez JH. Non-bone cell mediated bone resorption. In: Horton JE, et al. eds. 1977:229–237.
29. Murray DW, Rushton N. Macrophages stimulate bone resorption when they phagocytose particles. *J Bone Joint Surg [Br]* 1990;72:988.
30. Pazzaglia UE, Pringle JA. Bone resorption in vitro: macrophages and giant cells from failed total hip replacement versus osteoclasts. *Biomaterials* 1989;10:286.
31. Peters KM, Loer F, Hofstadter F, Casser HR. [Immune competence of human tissue lymphocytes in contact with loosened hip joint prostheses. On the topic of cellular or humoral rejection reaction as the mechanism of loosening]. *Chirurgie* 1991;62:414.
32. Sandy JR, Meghji S, Scutt AM, Harvey W, Harris M, Meikle MC. Murine osteoblasts release bone-resorbing factors of high and low molecular weights: stimulation by mechanical deformation. *Bone Miner* 1989;5:155.
33. Santavirta S, Hoikka V, Eskola A, Konttinen YT, Paavilainen T, Tallroth K. Aggressive granulomatous lesions in cementless total hip arthroplasty. *J Bone Joint Surg [Br]* 1990;72:980.
34. Santavirta S, Konttinen YT, Bergroth V, Eskola A, Tallroth K, Lindholm TS. Aggressive granulomatous lesions associated with hip arthroplasty. Immunopathological studies. *J Bone Joint Surg [Am]* 1990;72:252.
35. Santavirta S, Konttinen YT, Hoikka V, Eskola A. Immunopathological response to loose cementless acetabular components. *J Bone Joint Surg [Br]* 1991;73:38.

36. Sato M, Grasser W, Endo N, et al. Bisphosphonate action. Alendronate localization in rat bone and effects on osteoclast ultrastructure. *J Clin Invest* 1991;88:2095.
37. Scales JT. Black staining around titanium alloy prostheses—an orthopaedic enigma. *J Bone Joint Surg [Br]* 1991;73:534.
38. Shimizu H. Different resorption modes on living and devitalized bones by isolated osteoclasts in vitro. The effects of TIMP, E-64, and TGF-alpha. *Dent Jpn* 1990;27:81.
39. Shimizu H., Sakamoto M, Sakamoto S. Bone resorption by isolated osteoclasts in living versus devitalized bone: differences in mode and extent and the effects of human recombinant tissue inhibitor of metalloproteinases. *J Bone Miner Res* 1990;5:411.
40. Stevenson PH, Stevenson JR. Cytotoxic and migration inhibitory effects of bisphosphonates on macrophages. *Calcif Tissue Int* 1986;38:227.

Biological, Material, and Mechanical
Considerations of Joint Replacement,
edited by B. F. Morrey.
Raven Press, Ltd., New York © 1993.

36

Outcomes Research, Shared Decision Making, and the Care of Degenerative Joint Disease

John E. Wennberg

Center for Evaluative Clinical Sciences, Dartmouth Medical School,
Hanover, New Hampshire 03755

In contrast to the well-established basic science of prosthetic replacement discussed elsewhere in the volume, the rationale and relevance of emerging clinically based research seem particularly relevant.

Outcomes research and the shared-decision model provide the profession with a powerful set of tools for dealing with two challenges to professionalism. One is the growing determination among policy makers, employers, and the public at large to do something about rising medical costs, even at the expense of professional autonomy and the doctor-patient relationship. The evidence is obvious to any physician who reads the newspaper or experiences the intrusions of managed care. The other is the growing awareness that the scientific and ethical status of clinical medicine is much weaker than most have assumed. It is increasingly apparent that the large investment in biomedical research and technology has not resulted in a consensus among physicians on the correct way to practice medicine nor resulted in an orderly assessment of treatment theory. To the contrary, biomedical science and related applications of bioengineering and materials sciences, by virtue of their prodigious success, increase uncertainty and confusion by offering an ever-increasing supply of new technology and biomedical ideas. For many reasons, not the least of which is an inadequate national science policy for the evaluative sciences, the necessary studies to evaluate these ideas—to identify the outcomes that matter to patients and to obtain adequate information to estimate their likelihood—have simply not been done.

The weaknesses in the scientific basis of clinical medicine are evident in the practice variation phenomenon. Keller et al. (2) has shown remarkable variations in rates of lumbar disk surgery and other orthopedic procedures among neighboring communities in Maine. Practice variations are as common among communities where most care is received in academic institutions as they are in rural hospital service areas in Maine (3). The residents of Boston have a 75% greater chance of undergoing knee or hip replacement than do the citizens of New Haven (5). This variation almost certainly does not mean that residents of New Haven are going untreated, but rather that they are being treated differently: the clinicians of New Haven more often prefer medical management than do their colleagues in Boston.

But poor science is only one of the reasons for practice variations. They also arise because in most situations, despite the increasing awareness of the requirement for informed consent, patients do not yet make the choice of care. The preferences of clinicians for treatments tend to dominate. This is inevitable under a model for decision making that leaves the choice up to the physician. Thus a policy that seeks to reduce unwanted variations by improving the scientific as well as the ethical basis of clinical medicine must pay attention to learning what patients want as well as how treatments work. It must pay attention to shared decision making, to involving the patient in the choice of treatment as well as outcomes research.

OUTCOMES AND SHARED DECISION MAKING

Outcomes research is clinical research with a new twist. It borrows heavily from the social sciences, statistics, epidemiology, and other disciplines that have typically been applied in health services research projects (7). It focuses on all of the outcomes that matter to patients. It is a global strategy in that it focuses on identifying and evaluating all treatment theories relevant to a particular condition. Certain research strategies or tasks characterize the typical outcomes study, including:

Patient focus groups to learn directly from patients what their points of view are—what matters to them, what outcomes they value, what problems they want resolved, their concerns and expectations, how they differ individually in their concern about their condition, their attitudes toward risks and benefits of different treatments;

Physician focus groups to learn the points of view of the physician, their hypotheses about treatments and outcomes, their explanations for practice style differences and practice variations;

Structured review of the literature to assess the strengths and weakness of published evidence for or against specific treatment hypotheses and to obtain the best possible estimates for the probabilities for outcomes that matter to patients, according to patient subgroup and treatment used;

Large databases to obtain estimates for outcome probabilities based on large samples;

Patient outcome measures and instruments that capture the full dimension of the decision problem from the point of view of the patient, including relevant symptoms, expectations, preferences, and attitudes as well as functional status;

Decision models that capture the complexity of the problem of choice, that can be used to evaluate treatment theories and test for the importance of patient preference in the choice of treatment.

The study designs used in outcomes research are eclectic. Randomized clinical trials (RCTs) are sometimes required, and in a fully developed outcomes research strategy they are necessary if new technology is to be efficiently evaluated, a point that will be discussed below. Retrospective studies are very useful in raising or sharpening hypotheses and they sometimes settle issues. In an outcomes study of the treatment for benign prostatic hyperplasia (BPH), focus groups among physicians revealed that one cause of practice variation was differences in opinion on the value of surgery in extending the life expectancy of patients with early symptoms of BPH. Some physicians believed that early surgery was warranted because most men went on to a progressive course that would ultimately require surgery to relieve life-threatening urinary obstruction. Since patients would at that time be older and sicker and more likely to die from surgery, life expectancy was actually extended by operating early in the course of disease.

A structured literature review, the use of the Medicare claims data, and a decision model were sufficient to demonstrate no indicative evidence for improved life expectancy and the issue could be settled (6). But, as many physicians claimed, did the operation reduce symptoms and improve the quality of life? The question could not be easily answered. Ironically, even though many physicians practiced under the belief that the main reason for surgery was to improve the quality of life, no data were available in the literature. Focus groups were held and outcome measures were developed, followed by a prospective case series study of patients undergoing prostatectomy (1). The results showed a marked improvement in symptoms for most men, much better than the improvement for watchful waiting. It is of interest that this conclusion was reached without a RCT (4).

The global strategy of outcomes research needs to be emphasized. By bringing all treatment theories under evaluation and assessing all of the outcomes that matter to patients, the product of outcomes research is a proper representation of the complexity of the decision problem. It clarifies that there are multiple outcomes that matter to patients and shows how these differ according to treatment. It also shows that individual patients value outcomes and treatments differently, depending on their preferences. Outcomes research thus leads to the shared-decision model. It demonstrates that it is impossible to know what treatment the patient wants on the basis of objective clinical information. In the case of BPH, no element in the clinical history, physical examination, laboratory tests including urine flow, or even symptom state was a reliable surrogate for patient preference. To learn what patients want, they must be asked.

We have been experimenting with ways to develop shared decision making. Using interactive videodisk technology, we developed a uniform way of presenting treatment options to patients. The representation of the decision problem included detailed information about the outcomes that mattered to them—their nature, as described and sometimes illustrated through video and their probabilities, as determined by our studies to be the best estimate for the patient's state of health. The disk was then used by a number of urologists to help them counsel patients who had come to them for advice about their BPH. More than 700 patients have seen the videodisk and we have learned a good deal about the circumstances of choice. When offered a choice among watchful waiting and prostatectomy, many, indeed in our series most, prefer watchful waiting, at least in the short run. This is so even among the most severely symptomatic patients. We are learning that clinical decision making can be structured so the preferences of patients become dominant in the choice of treatment. In marked contrast to our base-line study in Maine where many men undergoing surgery were not bothered very much by their symptoms, shared decision making resulted in decisions that made much more sense: those who chose surgery were those who were bothered most by their symptoms and/or who had little fear of impotence.

Shared decision making and outcomes research are related in a way that has changed my ideas about RCTs. Several years ago, before I became more deeply involved in these issues, I shared the orthodox view that the double-blind, placebo-controlled randomized clinical trial is the optimal strategy for establishing the probabilities for outcomes of alternative treatments. I no longer believe this is always the case. I am not talking about the recognized difficulties of RCTs such as the issue of placebo controls and patient blinding when surgery is involved or the problems of cost, logistics, and changing technology that come into play when the relevant end point requires years of follow-up.

Problem with Randomization

The emphasis that outcomes research places on the multiplicity of relevant outcomes and importance of patient preferences for rational choice raises questions about the role of randomization itself.

First, there are ethical and legal issues. Shared decision making requires the sharing of uncertainty, the full disclosure of what is known and not known. When the outcomes of alternative treatments are asymmetric in some significant way, e.g., known differences in immediate risk of death or incontinence and impotence following watchful waiting versus surgery, patient preferences with regard to what is known about these risks may make it difficult to recruit patients into RCTs. Few activated patients who want to share responsibility for decision making under uncertainty may be indifferent enough about their choice to accept randomization. In this case, the most efficient way to obtain the missing probabilities and characterize patient subgroups may well be a preference trial: the systematic follow-up of patient cohorts where treatment assignments are according to informed patient choice rather than randomization.

But the main point may not be the unwillingness of the informed patient to accept randomization. The preference approach may well provide the information that is most important in clinical practice. It is not intuitively obvious that the probabilities for outcomes estimated using the double-blind trial would be the same as those obtained in preference trial. Patients who agree to randomization after a fair representation of the treatment problem are very likely different from those who want to choose their own treatment. Moreover, I suspect the outcomes associated with freely chosen treatments will be more positive: if patients choose a treatment believing it will help them, the treatment is more likely to have a positive effect. Studies of the effect of patient compliance in double-blinded RCTs show the likely importance of the preference effect.

I have dealt with these issues in more detail elsewhere (3), recommending the need to undertake studies to examine the effect of study design on these issues. (I proposed a randomized trial of the RCT versus preference design to study their differences and biases.) This is an important project because the preference design can be used in every-day practice. Our experience shows that it is acceptable to practicing physicians and their patients will like it. Preference designs make it possible for every-day practice to serve as the basis for patient recruitment into large-scale, cooperative trials for evaluating outcomes. I believe that substantially more patients will elect experimental treatments under the preference design than under randomized designs. If we can become more confident about the limitations and advantages of the preference trial so we can use it effectively, we should be able to greatly speed up and reduce the costs of technology assessment, providing new strategies for phase IV surveillance studies that are much more systematic. Preference trials are inclusive: they offer the opportunity to obtain information relevant to all patient subgroups who, in the real world, are offered treatments.

OUTCOMES RESEARCH AND PROFESSIONAL RESPONSIBILITY

The strategy for organizing outcomes research is nonregulatory. It depends on mobilizing the profession. The strategy for organizing the academic community and assuring that priorities are set and met has relied on the patient outcomes research teams (PORTs) for undertaking the steps listed above for a number of priority conditions. The prospects, however, are utterly dependent on the response of the profession and on the willingness of the professional leadership to accept the ethic of evaluation. In my capacity as Principal Investigator of the Prostate PORT, I have had the extraordinary good fortune of working with the American Urologic Association (AUA). The AUA has provided this type of leadership. It has taken responsibility for organizing a network of some 20 medical centers around the country to undertake a program of assessment of new as well as existing technologies for the treatment of BPH. The idea is not a single trial, but a series of trials that sequentially test new ideas as they become available and undertake systematic evaluation early rather than late in the course of their development. The technologies and theories being brought under evaluation extend across the full spectrum of treatments—new surgical techniques, new devices, and recent U.S. Food and Drug Administration approved drugs as well as drugs approved for other purposes, such as alpha-blockers, which seem to help patients with BPH.

The benefits of a professional leadership model for technology assessment are potentially great. Through its commitment to evaluation, the leadership signals the field that responsible professionalism requires an organized approach for learning from experience and that physicians must be responsible for their own science. It erects a professional barrier to the uncritical acceptance of novelty, protecting patients from exposure to care of unknown value and society against the unnecessary cost.

OUTCOMES RESEARCH, SHARED DECISION MAKING, AND DEGENERATIVE HIP DISEASE

In the context of this volume, outcomes research and shared decision making are highly relevant for degenerative disease of the hip. There are several ways of accomplishing hip replacement; as this book amply demonstrates, new technologies and approaches are continually being invented to redress defects that become apparent in the older ones. Continuous assessments are needed and in a fashion that provides, in as complete a way as possible, a portfolio of probabilities for all relevant outcomes for all relevant treatments and for patients of all relevant subgroups.

One special advantage of the Medicare claims data should be noted that would be helpful in planning outcome studies for joint replacement. Many of the outcomes relevant to evaluating prosthesis failure occur several years after implant. Most hip replacements occur in Medicare patients over 65 years of age. The Medicare database provides a registry of the medical events that makes it possible to find individuals who have had hip replacements in any year since the program began (although improvement in the database has made the task much easier for patients treated since 1983). The charts, operative notes, and, possibly, the records maintained by industry can be retrieved to learn details about operative techniques and prosthetic technologies. Subsequent hospitalizations can be identified by reasons for admission, surgery performed, hospital, data and record number, and charts reviewed for outcome details. If the patient died, this can be ascertained; if patients are alive, they can be located and interviewed for symptoms and functional status. It is thus possible to learn about failure rates from patient records or from direct interview about the longer range outcome from hip replacement.

The registry features of the claims data are extremely useful in prospective designs. At the time of surgery, critical baseline clinical and functional status information can be systematically collected and linked to the claims. Subsequent medical experience can be discovered in the claims data and the patient located for follow-up assessment of functional status. Used systematically, the claims data make the long-term surveillance of large cohorts of hip replacement patients feasible, both technically and economically.

The shared-decision model is particularly relevant. Joint replacement is the prototype of the medical intervention designed to improve the quality of life. For many people it appears to work well. But there are risks and other options and people with the same objective clinical condition, particularly in the earlier stages of the disease, will choose differently, some wanting immediate hip replacement, others wanting to live with their condition and reconsider surgery if they become worse. The large differences in probabilities for treatment between communities such as Boston and New Haven suggest that when decisions are left to physicians, these differences in patient values and utilities are not decisive in the choice of treatment.

One proposed remedy for geographic variations is the control of utilization through detailed guidelines administered by insurance companies or other third parties that specify who should and who should not get a particular treatment. The problem with this strategy is that it ignores the preferences of the patient. Preferences cannot be ascertained by physical examination, laboratory studies, or even objective measures of functional status. To know what patients want, they must be asked.

RELEVANCE OF OUTCOMES STUDIES TO HIP AND KNEE PROBLEMS

The structure of the decision problem for patients with degenerative disease of the hip or knee is ideally suited for shared decision making. Shared decision making, undertaken within the context of the interactive videodisk technology previously discussed, provides an explicit standard for care in which the patient, not the physician or the third-party payer, determines the use of care. When done with care, it converts the medical marketplace from one in which suppliers dominate demand to one in which demand comes from patients. Moreover, when used in the context of the preference trial, it becomes a strategy for organizing outcomes studies and collecting the important clinical information (including functional status) at baseline at the time of treatment choice. It is thus an explicit and ethical way to determine demand and the level of resources required to meet the needs and wants of patients and for organizing networks among the profession's leaders to learn what works.

REFERENCES

1. Barry MJ, Mulley AG, Fowler FJ, Wennberg JE. Watchful waiting vs immediate transurethral resection for symptomatic prostatism. *JAMA* 1988;259:3010–3017.
2. Keller RB, Soule DN, Wennberg JE, Hanley DF. Dealing with geographic variations in the use of hospitals. *J Bone Joint Surg [AM]* 1990;72:1286–1293.
3. Wennberg JE, Freeman JL, Culp WJ. Are hospital services rationed in New Haven or over-utilized in Boston? *Lancet* 1987;1:1185–1188.
4. Wennberg JE, Mulley AG, Hanley D, et al. An assessment of prostatectomy for benign urinary tract obstruction. *JAMA* 1988;259:3027–3030.
5. Wennberg JE, Freeman JL, Culp WJ. Are hospital services rationed in New Haven or over-utilized in Boston? *Lancet* 1987;1:1185–1188.
6. Wennberg JE, Roos N, Sola L, Schori A, Jaffe R. Use of claims date systems to evaluate health care outcomes: mortality and reoperation following prostatectomy. *JAMA* 1987;257:933–936.
7. Wennberg JE. What is outcomes research? In: Gelijns AC, ed. *Medical innovations at the crossroads, volume 1, modern methods of clinical investigation.* Committee on Technological Innovation in Medicine, Institute of Medicine, 1990.

Biological, Material, and Mechanical Considerations of Joint Replacement, edited by B. F. Morrey. Raven Press, Ltd., New York © 1993.

37

Materials

Concluding Observations and Future Directions

*Jack E. Lemons and †Jonathan Black

Laboratory Research, Division of Orthopaedic Surgery, Departments of Surgery and Biomaterials, University of Alabama at Birmingham, Birmingham, Alabama 35294-3295; †Department of Bioengineering, Clemson University, Clemson, South Carolina 29634-0905

CONSENSUS

The general consensus from each group was that the current biomaterials will continue to be utilized for total joint replacement (TJR) over the next years, but there are needs for improvement or development of new materials or designs for articulating surfaces and their attachments to tissue. In this regard, emphasis should be placed on basic characterizations of material properties, standards for evaluation of the materials and devices, and correlations between biomaterial, biomechanical, and clinical factors. The most pressing issues are device resistance(s) to wear phenomena, the debris generated, and the biological consequences of the various products independently and when combined. Model systems for laboratory, laboratory animal, and human clinical trials are very much needed.

DISAGREEMENT

Areas of contention related to a lack of agreement on (i) the basic mechanisms of wear-debris generation and the role(s) of quality control and assessment in minimizing these types of products; (ii) the capabilities of lutes, porosities, or coatings for stabilizing the device to tissue interfaces; and (iii) the synergisms among biomaterial, biomechanical, and clinical factors.

THE FUTURE

General Considerations

The material groups strongly supported the need for (i) improved quality control of existing biomaterials and devices within the industry at large; (ii) multidisciplinary interactions to more fully understand and resolve the critical issues associated with device loss (especially osteolytic phenomena); (iii) relevant model systems within all disciplines; (iv) more research into mechanisms and cause-effect relationships; and (v) improved and/or new biomaterials, designs, and TJR treatment modalities.

Specific Considerations

The discussions focused explicitly on new directions in materials development and application for partial and TJR of the knee and hip. The conclusions from the discussion are divided into six categories: metals, polymers, ceramics, composites, surface coatings/treatments, and others. In each case a consensus effort was made to present each concept as what is known and what is needed for future development.

Metals

Alloy corrosion, with or without concomitant fretting, is regarded as a pressing problem, and it is definitely expected that lower intrinsic corrosion rate alloys will come into use. It is also probable that higher fatigue strength alloys and lower elastic modulus alloys (initially beta titanium-base) will come into clinical use. Finally, it is possible that older alloys no longer in use may be revisited since improved processing and/or coating/surface treatment technologies may render them useful for present and future designs.

Polymers

The failure of ultrahigh molecular weight polyethylene (UHMWPE) to meet the needs as an articulating surface in many current designs will certainly result in the near term in modifications primarily directed toward decreasing surface damage. It is probable that new structural polymers, for use in both bearing and support areas, as well as a new class of elastometric bearing surfaces will be developed. Another probable development is the alteration of materials properties and fabrication approaches to permit alterations of tribological properties of joint articulations to reduce both friction resistance and wear. There are recognized possibilities for new "bone cements" as competitors of polymethylmethacrylate (PMMA) and for resorbable polymeric materials and components as adjuncts to implantation of permanent joint replacement components.

Ceramics

Ceramic components bearing against UHMWPE are a definite emerging feature of modified and new hip and knee designs. In the future it is considered probable that all ceramic articulations will be available for use in the United States, as is already the case in Europe and Asia. Finally, it is probable that additional structural ceramics (other than Al_2O_3 and ZrO_2) will be developed for use as bearing surfaces.

Composites

Although it is possible that composites may come into use for both structural and bearing applications, there is considerable scepticism about the viability of this approach. The development of the technology over the past two decades is considered meager. Yet composite structures, with a single component having different physical properties in different portions, is still desirable. Perhaps this may address problems of modularity. A more likely application for composites, however, is in the development of a ceramic-based composite material to serve as bone graft in augmentation/replacement in cases of massive bone loss.

Surface Coatings/Treatments

This is an area in which near-term developments are considered eminent. Areas of focus will include bearing-surface modification to reduce wear, especially in terms of particulate release, reduction of corrosion, on both bearing and nonbearing surfaces, and the introduction of new surface compositions/textures as alternatives to the current choices for fixation to hard tissue.

Other

There is considerable concern about device modularity. The consensus is that modular designs will increase in the short term but will probably decrease in the longer term. Additional developments are anticipated as the possible use of biological adjuncts (products released from or in the vicinity of implant components) to influence local tissue repair and remodeling as well as acting to suppress osteolysis as a response to debris release.

*Biological, Material, and Mechanical
Considerations of Joint Replacement,*
edited by B. F. Morrey.
Raven Press, Ltd., New York © 1993.

38

Techniques and Models

*Barbara D. Boyan and †Mark E. Bolander

*Department of Orthopaedics, University of Texas Health Science Center at San
Antonio, San Antonio, Texas 78284-7774; †Department of Orthopaedics, Mayo Clinic,
Rochester, Minnesota 55905

CONSENSUS

There have been major advances in our understanding of the local and systemic
factors that regulate bone formation, resorption, and remodeling. Advances in materials science and our understanding of biomechanics have resulted in the development of new devices for use in orthopaedic therapy. However, the interrelationships of biology, biomaterials, and mechanical factors are still not understood. New
methodologies such as molecular technology, growth factor and cytokine research,
and cell culture, as well as imaging techniques such as atomic force electron microscopy, confocal microscopy, magnetic resonance imaging, computer tomography
(CT), and dual x-ray analysis make it possible to better address these critical issues,
especially at the material-biology interface.

FUTURE NEEDS AND DIRECTIONS

1. Development of relevant animal models.
2. Development of appropriate *in vitro* assays and cell culture models.
3. Better understanding of the musculoskeletal system at the molecular, biochemical, cellular, tissue, organ, and immunologic levels.
4. Multidisciplinary and multifactorial studies interrelating biology, materials science, and biomechanics.
5. Development of standardized reference materials and the use of characterized
   materials for *in vivo* and *in vitro* studies.
6. Improved outcome studies based on patient satisfaction.
7. Development of the use of biologic factors to improve biology-material interaction.
8. Studies to understand the effects of cells and biologic fluids on materials, and
   of materials on cells locally and systemically and the role of mechanical forces
   in these events.

9. Better understanding of the basic mechanisms regulating bone remodeling.
10. Improved and standardized use of retrieval and autopsy specimens.

For many questions, the best model is the patient who has had a joint replacement. Recognizing the high value and limited availability of human tissues, the discussion group recommended that steps be taken to maximize the number of samples that are collected at autopsy and revision surgery. Additionally, the discussion group recommended that protocols be established to maximize the potential for analysis of these samples. Several examples of documents that address portions of these protocols or that may serve as models for these protocols include the Hip Society recommendations for retrieving autopsy specimens and the National Institutes of Health/IB recommendation for blood products. The discussion group recommended that protocols be developed that are broad based and expanded from current documents. These protocols should include the collection of basic data on the patient's clinical status, initial disease, radiographs, and serum studies. We recommend that protocols be included for archival storage of tissue and implants. The discussion group emphasized the importance of adhering to guidelines for the protection of health care workers from exposure to blood-borne pathogens.

Autopsy material also represents a potential source of specimens for *in vitro* organ and cell culture studies. The discussion group believed that this material is underutilized at present and that studies of cultured autopsy material could yield clinically significant information.

The discussion group believed that experimental studies in animals would yield information that would add to our understanding of mechanisms that are important in bone resorption. The discussion group emphasized the need to make optimal use of material from animal studies and suggested an emphasis on multidisciplinary analysis of animal material. An additional source of clinically relevant information is the study of veterinary implants. Further studies of this material may be informative.

The controlled conditions afforded by cell culture and organ culture *in vitro* experiments are seen as having an important role in testing and evaluating information gained from animal experiments and evaluation of retrieved human material.

Consistent with these recommendations, the discussion group recommended the formation of a committee to formulate the guidelines.

Subject Index